Pregnancy and Birth
SOURCEBOOK

FOURTH EDITION

Pregnancy and Birth
SOURCEBOOK

FOURTH EDITION

Basic Consumer Health Information about Pregnancy and Fetal Development, Including Facts about Fertility and Conception, Physical and Emotional Changes during Pregnancy, Prenatal Care and Diagnostic Tests, High-Risk Pregnancies and Complications, Labor, Delivery, and the Postpartum Period

Along with Tips on Maintaining Health and Wellness during Pregnancy and Caring for Newborn Infants, a Glossary of Related Terms, and a Directory of Resources for Additional Help and Information

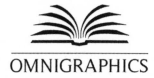

OMNIGRAPHICS

615 Griswold, Ste. 520, Detroit, MI 48226

Bibliographic Note
Because this page cannot legibly accommodate all the copyright notices, the Bibliographic
Note portion of the Preface constitutes an extension of the copyright notice.

* * *

OMNIGRAPHICS
Angela L. Williams, *Managing Editor*
* * *

Copyright © 2019 Omnigraphics

ISBN 978-0-7808-1693-0
E-ISBN 978-0-7808-1694-7

Library of Congress Cataloging-in-Publication Data

Names: Omnigraphics, Inc., issuing body.

Title: Pregnancy and birth sourcebook : health tips about pregnancy and birth.

Description: Fourth edition. | Detroit, MI : Omnigraphics, [2019] | Series: Health
reference series | "Basic Consumer Information about the Reproductive Process;
From Preconception through the Postpartum Period; Fertility, Infertility, and
Pregnancy Prevention, Staying Emotionally and Physically Healthy, and High-Risk
Pregnancies, and Answers Common Questions about Labor and Delivery, Postpartum
Recovery, Newborn Screening, and Infant Care. A Glossary of Related Terms,
Directory of Resources, and Additional Sources for Help and Information are Also
Provided." | Includes index.

Identifiers: LCCN 2018061604 | ISBN 9780780816930 (hard cover : alk. paper) |
ISBN 9780780816947 (ebook)

Subjects: LCSH: Pregnancy--Popular works. | Childbirth--Popular works. |
Pregnancy--Complications--Popular works.

Classification: LCC RG525.P675 2019 | DDC 618.2--dc23

LC record available at https://lccn.loc.gov/2018061604

Table of Contents

Part II: Understanding Pregnancy-Related Changes and Fetal Development

Part III: Staying Healthy during Pregnancy

Part V: Pregnancy Complications

Part VI: Labor and Delivery

Part VII: Postpartum and Newborn Care

Part VIII: Additional Help and Information

Preface

About This Book

Although the months of anticipation before a woman becomes a parent can be joyous and fulfilling, they can also mark a time filled with uncertainty and worry over potential birth defects, pregnancy complications, and chronic health conditions. These worries are not unfounded. Statistics show an increase in preterm deliveries and a decrease in the fertility rate among U.S. women. Fortunately, maternal and fetal monitoring, prenatal care, and healthy habits can reduce the risk of complications and make labor, delivery, and the postpartum period less stressful.

Pregnancy and Birth Sourcebook, Fourth Edition provides health information about the reproductive process—from preconception through the postpartum period. It provides information about fertility, infertility, and pregnancy prevention. The book's chapters explain the physical and emotional changes that occur during pregnancy, and discuss topics related to staying healthy during pregnancy, including eating nutritiously, exercising regularly, obtaining prenatal care, and avoiding harmful substances. Facts about high-risk pregnancies—such as those in women with chronic medical conditions, advanced maternal age, or weight concerns—are included. Finally, the book answers common questions about labor and delivery, postpartum recovery, newborn screening, and infant care. A glossary of terms and a directory of resources for information and support are also provided.

How to Use This Book

This book is divided into parts and chapters. Parts focus on broad areas of interest. Chapters are devoted to single topics within a part.

Part I: Preconception Health: Preparing for Pregnancy provides information about health habits, screenings, and interventions women may need prior to conception. This part also addresses factors that influence fertility, details common causes of infertility, and identifies methods of preventing unintended pregnancies.

Part II: Understanding Pregnancy-Related Changes and Fetal Development provides trimester-by-trimester details about physical changes in the fetus. The part also identifies early signs of pregnancy, suggests strategies for determining conception and due dates, and discusses emotional concerns and physical changes that may occur during pregnancy, including depression, back pain, pelvic floor and bladder problems, and vision and oral changes.

Part III: Staying Healthy during Pregnancy highlights strategies women can undertake to help promote a healthy pregnancy. These include getting prenatal care and related medical tests, using medication safely, eating nutritiously, exercising, preventing excessive weight gain, and avoiding toxic substances and other harmful exposures. This part also offers advice on how pregnant women can stay safe at work or during travel.

Part IV: High-Risk Pregnancies discusses pregnancies at high risk due to maternal age, multiple fetuses, or chronic health conditions, including allergies, asthma, cancer, diabetes, epilepsy, lupus, sickle cell disease, thyroid disease, eating disorders, and obesity.

Part V: Pregnancy Complications describes diseases and disorders that may influence a pregnancy's outcome, such as amniotic fluid abnormalities, birth defects, bleeding, blood clots, gestational diabetes, hypertension, severe nausea and vomiting, placental complications, Rh incompatibility, umbilical cord abnormalities, sexually transmitted diseases, and other infections. This part also offers information about preterm labor and pregnancy loss, including ectopic pregnancy, miscarriage, and stillbirth.

Part VI: Labor and Delivery includes information about planning for labor and delivery by choosing a birthing center or hospital, selecting a birth partner or doula, and preparing a birth plan. This part also provides details on the pain relief during labor, vaginal and cesarean births, and emergency situations that may occur during childbirth.

Part VII: Postpartum and Newborn Care discusses common post-partum concerns, including recovery expectations for new mothers, newborn care and screening tests, breastfeeding and formula-feeding tips, strategies for bonding with a new baby, and considerations for working after a child's birth.

Part VIII: Additional Help and Information includes a glossary of important terms and a directory of organizations that provide help, information, and assistance to low-income pregnant women and their partners.

Bibliographic Note

This volume contains documents and excerpts from publications issued by the following U.S. government agencies: Centers for Disease Control and Prevention (CDC); *Eunice Kennedy Shriver* National Institute of Child Health and Human Development (NICHD); Genetic and Rare Diseases Information Center (GARD); Genetics Home Reference (GHR); National Cancer Institute (NCI); National Heart, Lung, and Blood Institute (NHLBI); National Institute of Diabetes and Digestive and Kidney Diseases (NIDDK); National Institute of Environmental Health Sciences (NIEHS); National Institute of Neurological Disorders and Stroke (NINDS); National Institute on Drug Abuse (NIDA); National Institutes of Health (NIH); National Responsible Fatherhood Clearinghouse (NRFC); NIH Osteoporosis and Related Bone Diseases—National Resource Center (NIH ORBD—NRC); Office of Disease Prevention and Health Promotion (ODPHP); Office on Women's Health (OWH); U.S. Department of Education (ED); U.S. Department of Health and Human Services (HHS); U.S. Department of Labor (DOL); U.S. Environmental Protection Agency (EPA); U.S. Equal Employment Opportunity Commission (EEOC); U.S. Food U.S. National Library of Medicine (NLM) and Youth.gov.

It may also contain original material produced by Omnigraphics and reviewed by medical consultants.

About the Health Reference Series

The *Health Reference Series* is designed to provide basic medical information for patients, families, caregivers, and the general public. Each volume takes a particular topic and provides comprehensive coverage. This is especially important for people who may be dealing with a newly diagnosed disease or a chronic disorder in themselves or in a family member. People looking for preventive guidance, information about disease warning signs, medical statistics, and risk factors for health problems will also find answers to their questions in the *Health Reference Series*. The *Series*, however, is not intended to serve as a tool for diagnosing illness, in prescribing treatments, or as a substitute for the physician/patient relationship. All people concerned about medical symptoms or the possibility of disease are encouraged to seek professional care from an appropriate healthcare provider.

A Note about Spelling and Style

Health Reference Series editors use *Stedman's Medical Dictionary* as an authority for questions related to the spelling of medical terms and the *Chicago Manual of Style* for questions related to grammatical structures, punctuation, and other editorial concerns. Consistent adherence is not always possible, however, because the individual volumes within the *Series* include many documents from a wide variety of different producers, and the editor's primary goal is to present material from each source as accurately as is possible. This sometimes means that information in different chapters or sections may follow other guidelines and alternate spelling authorities. For example, occasionally a copyright holder may require that eponymous terms be shown in possessive forms (Crohn's disease vs. Crohn disease) or that British spelling norms be retained (leukaemia vs. leukemia).

Medical Review

Omnigraphics contracts with a team of qualified, senior medical professionals who serve as medical consultants for the *Health Reference Series*. As necessary, medical consultants review reprinted and originally written material for currency and accuracy. Citations including the phrase "Reviewed (month, year)" indicate material reviewed by this team. Medical consultation services are provided to the *Health Reference Series* editors by:

Dr. Vijayalakshmi, MBBS, DGO, MD
Dr. Senthil Selvan, MBBS, DCH, MD
Dr. K. Sivanandham, MBBS, DCH, MS (Research), PhD

Our Advisory Board

We would like to thank the following board members for providing initial guidance on the development of this series:

- Dr. Lynda Baker, Associate Professor of Library and Information Science, Wayne State University, Detroit, MI

- Nancy Bulgarelli, William Beaumont Hospital Library, Royal Oak, MI

- Karen Imarisio, Bloomfield Township Public Library, Bloomfield Township, MI

- Karen Morgan, Mardigian Library, University of Michigan-Dearborn, Dearborn, MI

- Rosemary Orlando, St. Clair Shores Public Library, St. Clair Shores, MI

Health Reference Series *Update Policy*

The inaugural book in the *Health Reference Series* was the first edition of *Cancer Sourcebook* published in 1989. Since then, the *Series* has been enthusiastically received by librarians and in the medical community. In order to maintain the standard of providing high-quality health information for the layperson the editorial staff at Omnigraphics felt it was necessary to implement a policy of updating volumes when warranted.

Medical researchers have been making tremendous strides, and it is the purpose of the *Health Reference Series* to stay current with the most recent advances. Each decision to update a volume is made on an individual basis. Some of the considerations include how much new information is available and the feedback we receive from people who use the books. If there is a topic you would like to see added to the update list, or an area of medical concern you feel has not been adequately addressed, please write to:

Managing Editor
Health Reference Series
Omnigraphics
615 Griswold, Ste. 520
Detroit, MI 48226

Part One

Preconception Health: Preparing for Pregnancy

Chapter 1

Overview of Reproductive Health

What Is the Reproductive System?

The reproductive system includes the organs involved in producing offspring. In women, this system includes the ovaries, the fallopian tubes, the uterus, the cervix, and the vagina. In men, it includes the prostate, the testes, and the penis.

What Is Reproductive Health?

Reproductive health refers to the diseases, disorders, and conditions that affect the functioning of the male and female reproductive systems during all stages of life. Disorders of reproduction include birth defects, developmental disorders, low birth weight, preterm birth, reduced

This chapter contains text excerpted from the following sources: Text under the heading "What Is the Reproductive System?" is excerpted from "NCI Dictionary of Cancer Terms," National Cancer Institute (NCI), January 23, 2019; Text under the heading "What Is Reproductive Health?" is excerpted from "Reproductive Health," National Institute of Environmental Health Sciences (NIEHS), December 18, 2018; Text under the heading "How the Female Reproductive System Works" is excerpted from "How the Female Reproductive System Works," girlshealth. gov, Office on Women's Health (OWH), April 15, 2014. Reviewed February 2019; Text beginning with the heading "What Are Reproductive Hazards?" is excerpted from "Reproductive Hazards," MedlinePlus, National Institutes of Health (NIH), December 28, 2016.

fertility, impotence, and menstrual disorders. Research has shown that exposure to environmental pollutants may pose the greatest threat to reproductive health. Exposure to lead is associated with reduced fertility in both men and women, while mercury exposure has been linked to birth defects and neurological disorders. A growing body of evidence suggests that exposure to endocrine disruptors, chemicals that appear to disrupt hormonal activity in humans and animals, may contribute to problems with fertility, pregnancy, and other aspects of reproduction.

How the Female Reproductive System Works

The female reproductive system is comprised of all the parts of your body that help you reproduce, or have babies, and most women are born with hundreds of thousands of eggs already in their body.

What's inside the Female Reproductive System?

The ovaries are two small organs in a woman's lower abdomen that are generally stagnant until puberty. During puberty, they "wake up" and start making more estrogen and other hormones. This causes body changes. One important body change is that these hormones trigger your body to begin menstruating.

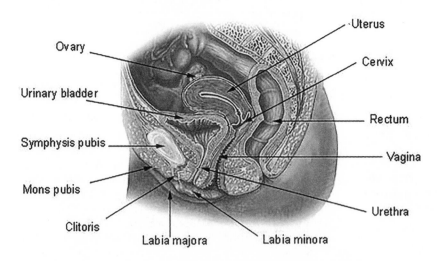

Figure 1.1. *Organs of the Female Reproductive System* (Source: "Female Reproductive System," Surveillance, Epidemiology and End Results Program (SEER), National Cancer Institute (NCI).)

Once a month, the ovaries release one egg (ovum). This is called "ovulation."

The fallopian tubes connect the ovaries to the uterus. During menses, an ovary releases an egg that moves along a fallopian tube.

The uterus—or womb—is where a fetus grows. It takes several days for the egg to get to the uterus.

As the egg travels, estrogen makes the lining of the uterus (called the "endometrium") thick with blood and fluid, which creates an ideal environment in which a fetus can grow. You can get pregnant if you have sex with a male without birth control and his sperm joins the egg (called "fertilization") on its way to your uterus.

If the egg is not fertilized, it will be shed along with the lining of your uterus during your next period.

The blood and fluid that leave your body during your period pass through your cervix and vagina.

The cervix is the narrow entryway between the vagina and uterus. The cervix is flexible so it can expand during childbirth.

The vagina also widens during birth.

The hymen covers the opening of the vagina. It is a thin piece of tissue that has one or more holes in it. The hymen may be stretched or torn when you use a tampon or during your first sexual experience. If it does tear, it may bleed a little bit.

What's outside the Vagina?

The vulva covers the entrance to the vagina. The vulva has five parts: mons pubis, labia, clitoris, urinary opening, and vaginal opening.

The mons pubis is the mound of tissue and skin above your legs, in the middle. This area becomes covered with hair during puberty.

The labia are the two sets of skin folds (often called "lips") on either side of the opening of the vagina.

The labia majora are the outer lips, and the labia minora are the inner lips. It is normal for the labia to look different from each other.

The clitoris is a small, sensitive bump at the bottom of the mons pubis that is covered by the labia minora.

The urinary opening, below the clitoris, is where your urine (pee) leaves the body.

The vaginal opening is the entry to the vagina and is found below the urinary opening.

Those are the basics of a woman's body.

What Are Reproductive Hazards?

Reproductive hazards are substances that affect the reproductive health of women or men. They also include substances that affect the ability of couples to have healthy children. These substances may be chemical, physical, or biological. Some common types include:

- Alcohol
- Chemicals, such as pesticides
- Smoking
- Legal and illegal drugs
- Metals, such as lead and mercury
- Radiation
- Some viruses

You may be exposed to and absorb reproductive hazards through with your skin, by breathing them in, or by swallowing them. This can happen anywhere, but it is more common in the workplace or at home.

What Are the Health Effects of Reproductive Hazards?

The possible health effects of reproductive hazards include infertility, miscarriage, birth defects, and developmental disabilities in children. What type of health effects they cause and how serious they are depends on many factors, including:

- What the substance is
- How much of it you are exposed to
- How it enters your body
- How long or how often you are exposed
- How you react to the substance

How Can Reproductive Hazards Affect Men?

A reproductive hazard can affect a man's sperm and may cause a problem with the number of sperm, their shape, or the way that they swim. It could also damage the sperm's deoxyribonucleic acid (DNA).

Then the sperm may not be able to fertilize an egg. Or it could cause problems with the development of the fetus.

How Can Reproductive Hazards Affect Women?

A reproductive hazard can disrupt a woman's menstrual cycle. It can cause hormone imbalance, which can raise the risk of diseases such as osteoporosis, heart disease, and certain cancers. It can affect a woman's ability to get pregnant.

Exposure to a reproductive hazard during pregnancy can have different effects, depending on when the woman was exposed. During the first three months of pregnancy, it might cause a birth defect or a miscarriage. During the last six months of pregnancy, it could slow the growth of the fetus, affect the development of its brain, or cause preterm labor.

How Can Reproductive Hazards Be Avoided?

To try to avoid reproductive hazards:

- Avoid alcohol and illegal drugs during pregnancy.

- If you smoke, try to quit. And if you are not a smoker, don't start.

- Take precautions if you are using household chemicals or pesticides.

- Practice good hygiene, including handwashing.

- If there are reproductive hazards at your job, make sure to follow safe work practices and procedures.

Chapter 2

Preconception and Prenatal Care

Chapter Contents

Section 2.1

What Is Preconception Health?

This section contains text excerpted from the following sources: Text beginning with the heading "Preconception Health" is excerpted from "Before Pregnancy—Overview," Centers for Disease Control and Prevention (CDC), January 23, 2018; Text beginning with the heading "Why Preconception Health Matters" is excerpted from "Preconception Health," Office on Women's Health (OWH), U.S. Department of Health and Human Services (HHS), June 6, 2018.

Preconception Health

"Preconception health" refers to the health of women and men during their reproductive years. It focuses on taking steps now to protect the health of children you may have sometime in the future.

All women and men can benefit from preconception health, whether or not they plan to have children one day. This is because part of preconception health is staying healthy throughout their lives. Maintaining your health is also important because approximately half of all pregnancies in the United States are unplanned.

Preconception Healthcare

Preconception healthcare is the medical care a patient receives from the doctor or other health professionals that focuses on the particular aspects of health that have been shown to increase the chances of having healthy children.

Preconception healthcare is customized to address each patient's unique needs. Based on those needs, the doctor or other healthcare professional will suggest a course of treatment or follow-up care. If your healthcare provider has not talked with you about this type of care, ask about it.

Healthy Women

Preconception health is important for every woman—not just those planning pregnancy. It means taking control of your own health and well-being by choosing healthy habits. It means living well, being healthy, and feeling good about your life. Preconception health is about making a plan for the future and taking the steps to get there.

Healthy Men

Preconception health is important for men too. It means choosing to be as healthy as possible—and helping others to do the same. As a partner, it means encouraging and supporting the health of your partner. As a father, it means protecting your children. Preconception health is about providing yourself and your loved ones with a bright and healthy future.

Healthy Children

Preconception health considers the possibility that you may bear children and takes steps to increase the likelihood that these children will be healthy. This medical approach means that your children are less likely to be born early (preterm) or have a low birth weight and are more likely to be born without birth defects or other disabling conditions. Preconception health offers children the best chance for a healthy start in life.

Healthy Families

The health of a family depends on the health of all the people in the family. Taking care of your health now will help to ensure a better quality of life (QOL) for yourself and your family in the coming years.

Why Preconception Health Matters

Every woman should be thinking about her health, whether or not she is planning pregnancy. One reason is that about half of all pregnancies are not planned. Unplanned pregnancies are at greater risk of preterm birth and low-birth-weight babies. Another reason is that, despite important advances in medicine and prenatal care, about one in eight babies is born too early. Researchers are trying to find out why and how to prevent preterm birth. But experts agree that women need to be healthier before becoming pregnant. By taking action on health issues and risks before pregnancy, you can prevent problems that might affect you or your child later.

The Five Most Important Things You Can Do to Boost Your Preconception Health

Women and men should prepare for pregnancy before becoming sexually active—or at least three months before getting pregnant.

11

Some actions, such as quitting smoking, reaching a healthy weight, or adjusting medicines should start even earlier. The five most important things you can do for preconception health are:

1. Take 400 to 800 micrograms (400 to 800 mcg or 0.4 to 0.8 mg) of folic acid every day if you are planning or capable of pregnancy to lower your risk of some birth defects of the brain and spine, including spina bifida. All women need folic acid every day. Talk to your doctor about your folic acid needs. Some doctors prescribe prenatal vitamins that contain higher amounts of folic acid.

2. Stop smoking and drinking alcohol.

3. If you have a medical condition, be sure it is under control. Some conditions that can affect pregnancy or be affected by it include asthma, diabetes, oral health, obesity, or epilepsy.

4. Talk to your doctor about any over-the-counter (OTC) and prescription medicines you are using. These include dietary or herbal supplements. Be sure your vaccinations are up to date.

5. Avoid contact with toxic substances or materials that could cause infection. Stay away from chemicals and cat or rodent feces.

Talk to Your Doctor before You Become Pregnant

Preconception care can improve your chances of getting pregnant, having a healthy pregnancy, and having healthy children. If you are sexually active, talk to your doctor about your preconception health now. Preconception care should begin at least three months before you get pregnant. But some women need more time to get their bodies ready for pregnancy. Be sure to discuss your partner's health too. Ask your doctor about:

• Family planning and birth control

• Taking folic acid

• Vaccines and screenings you may need, such as a Papanicolaou (Pap) test and screenings for sexually transmitted infections (STIs), including human immunodeficiency virus (HIV)

• Managing health problems, such as diabetes, high blood pressure, thyroid disease, obesity, depression, eating disorders, and asthma. Find out how pregnancy may affect, or be affected by, the health problems you have.

- Medicines you use, including over-the-counter (OTC), herbal, and prescription drugs and supplements

- Ways to improve your overall health, such as reaching a healthy weight, making healthy food choices, being physically active, caring for your teeth and gums, reducing stress, quitting smoking, and avoiding alcohol

- How to avoid illness

- Hazards in your workplace or home that could harm you or your children

- Health problems that run in your or your partner's family

- Problems you have had with prior pregnancies, including preterm birth

- Family concerns that could affect your health, such as domestic violence or lack of support

Your Partner's Role in Preparing for Pregnancy

Your partner can do a lot to support and encourage you in every aspect of preparing for pregnancy. Here are some ways:

- Make the decision about pregnancy together. When both partners hope for pregnancy, a woman is more likely to get early prenatal care and avoid risky behaviors, such as smoking and drinking alcohol.

- Screening for and treating STIs can help ensure that infections are not passed to female partners.

- Male partners can improve their own reproductive health and overall health by limiting alcohol, quitting smoking or illegal drug use, making healthy food choices, and reducing stress. Studies show that men who drink a lot, smoke, or use drugs can have problems with their sperm. These might cause you to have problems getting pregnant. If your partner won't quit smoking, ask that he not smoke around you in order to avoid harmful effects of secondhand smoke.

- Your partner should also talk to his doctor about his own health, his family health history, and any medicines he uses.

- People who work with chemicals or other should be careful not to expose women in their childbearing years to them. For example, people who work with fertilizers or pesticides should change out of dirty clothes before coming near women. They should handle and wash soiled clothes separately.

Section 2.2

Understanding Genetic Counseling and Evaluation: Is It Right for You?

This section contains text excerpted from the following sources: Text beginning with the heading "What Is Genetic Counseling?" is excerpted from "Genetic Counseling," Centers for Disease Control and Prevention (CDC), October 4, 2018; Text under the heading "Genetic Counselling in Prenatal Period" is excerpted from "Preconception Health," Office on Women's Health (OWH), U.S. Department of Health and Human Services (HHS), June 6, 2018.

What Is Genetic Counseling?

Genetic counseling gives you information about how genetic conditions might affect you or your family. The genetic counselor or other healthcare professional will collect your personal and family health history. They can use this information to determine how likely it is that you or your family member has a genetic condition. Based on this information, the genetic counselor can help you decide whether a genetic test might be right for you or your relative.

Reasons for Genetic Counseling

Your doctor can refer you for genetic counseling based on your personal and family-health history. Your doctor can refer you for genetic counseling. There are different stages in your life when you might be referred for genetic counseling:

- **Planning for pregnancy:** Genetic counseling before you become pregnant can address concerns about factors that might affect your children during infancy or childhood or your ability to become pregnant, including:

14

- Genetic conditions that run in your family or your partner's family
- History of infertility, multiple miscarriages, or stillbirth
- Previous pregnancy or child affected by a birth defect or genetic condition
- Assisted Reproductive Technology (ART) options

- **During pregnancy:** Genetic counseling while you are pregnant can address certain tests that may be done during your pregnancy, any detected problems, or conditions that might affect your children during infancy or childhood, including:

  - History of infertility, multiple miscarriages, or stillbirth
  - Previous pregnancy or child affected by a birth defect or genetic condition
  - Abnormal test results, such as a blood test, ultrasound, chorionic villus sampling (CVS), or amniocentesis
  - Maternal infections, such as cytomegalovirus (CMV), and other exposures such as medications, drugs, chemicals, and X-rays
  - Genetic screening that is recommended for all pregnant women, which includes cystic fibrosis, sickle cell disease (SCD), and any conditions that run in your family or your partner's family

- **Caring for children:** Genetic counseling can address concerns if your child is showing signs and symptoms of a disorder that might be genetic, including:

  - Abnormal newborn screening results
  - Birth defects
  - Intellectual disability or developmental disabilities
  - Autism spectrum disorders (ASD)
  - Vision or hearing problems

- **Managing your health:** Genetic counseling for adults includes specialty areas such as cardiovascular, psychiatric, and cancer. Genetic counseling can be helpful if you have symptoms of a condition or have a family history of a condition that makes you more likely to be affected with that condition, including:

15

- Hereditary breast and ovarian cancer (HBOC) syndrome

- Lynch syndrome (hereditary colorectal and other cancers)

- Familial hypercholesterolemia

- Muscular dystrophy and other muscle diseases

- Inherited movement disorders such as Huntington disease

- Inherited blood disorders, such as sickle cell disease

Following your genetic-counseling session, you might decide to have genetic testing. Genetic counseling after testing can help you better understand your test results and treatment options, help you deal with emotional concerns, and refer you to other healthcare providers and advocacy and support groups.

Genetic Counseling in Prenatal Period

The genes your baby is born with can affect your baby's health in these ways:

- Single gene disorders are caused by a problem in a single gene. Genes contain the information your body's cells need to function. Single gene disorders run in families. Examples of single-gene disorders are cystic fibrosis and sickle cell anemia.

- Chromosome disorders occur when all or part of a chromosome is missing or extra, or if the structure of one or more chromosomes is not normal. Chromosomes are structures where genes are located. Most chromosome disorders that involve whole chromosomes do not run in families.

Talk to your doctor about your and your partner's family-health histories before becoming pregnant. This information can help your doctor find out any genetic risks you might have.

Depending on your genetic risk factors, your doctor might suggest you meet with a genetic professional. Some reasons a person or couple might seek genetic counseling are:

- A family history of a genetic condition, birth defect, chromosomal disorder, or cancer

- Two or more pregnancy losses, a stillbirth, or a baby who died

- A child with a known inherited disorder, birth defect, or intellectual disability

- A woman who is pregnant or plans to become pregnant at 35 years of age or older

- Test results that suggest a genetic condition is present

- Increased risk of getting or passing on a genetic disorder because of one's ethnic background

- People related by blood who want to have children together

During a consultation, the genetics professional meets with a person or couple to discuss genetic risks or to diagnose, confirm, or rule out a genetic condition. Sometimes, a couple chooses to have genetic testing. Some tests can help couples know the chances that a person will get or pass on a genetic disorder. The genetics professional can help couples decide if genetic testing is the right choice for them.

Section 2.3

Genetic Testing

This section contains text excerpted from the following sources:
Text in this section begins with excerpts from "Genetic Testing,"
MedlinePlus, National Institutes of Health (NIH), February 7, 2019;
Text under the heading "What Are the Types of Genetic Tests?" is
excerpted from "What Are the Types of Genetic Tests?" Genetics
Home Reference (GHR), National Institutes of Health (NIH),
February 12, 2019; Text under the heading "What Is Noninvasive
Prenatal Testing and What Disorders Can It Screen For?" is
excerpted from "What Is Noninvasive Prenatal Testing (NIPT)
and What Disorders Can It Screen For?" Genetics Home Reference
(GHR), National Institutes of Health (NIH), February 12, 2019.

Genetic tests are tests on blood and other tissue to find genetic disorders. Over 2,000 tests are available. Doctors use genetic tests for several reasons. These include:

- Finding genetic diseases in unborn babies

- Finding out if people carry a gene for a disease and might pass it on to their children

- Screening embryos for disease

- Testing for genetic diseases in adults before they cause symptoms

- Making a diagnosis in a person who has disease symptoms

- Figuring out the type or dose of a medicine that is best for a certain person

What Are the Types of Genetic Tests?

Genetic testing can provide information about a person's genes and chromosomes. Available types of testing include:

- **Newborn screening:** Newborn screening is used just after birth to identify genetic disorders that can be treated early in life. Millions of babies are tested each year in the United States. All states currently test infants for phenylketonuria (a genetic disorder that causes intellectual disability if left untreated) and congenital hypothyroidism (a disorder of the thyroid gland). Most states also test for other genetic disorders.

- **Diagnostic testing:** Diagnostic testing is used to identify or rule out a specific genetic or chromosomal condition. In many cases, genetic testing is used to confirm a diagnosis when a particular condition is suspected based on physical signs and symptoms. Diagnostic testing can be performed before birth or at any time during a person's life, but is not available for all genes or all genetic conditions. The results of a diagnostic test can influence a person's choices about healthcare and the management of the disorder.

- **Carrier testing:** Carrier testing is used to identify people who carry one copy of a gene mutation that, when present in two copies, causes a genetic disorder. This type of testing is offered to individuals who have a family history of a genetic disorder and to people in certain ethnic groups with an increased risk of specific genetic conditions. If both parents are tested, the test can provide information about a couple's risk of having a child with a genetic condition.

- **Prenatal testing:** Prenatal testing is used to detect changes in a fetus's genes or chromosomes before birth. This type of testing is offered during pregnancy if there is an increased risk that the baby will have a genetic or chromosomal disorder. In some cases, prenatal testing can lessen a couple's uncertainty or help them make decisions about a pregnancy. It cannot identify all possible inherited disorders and birth defects, however.

- **Preimplantation testing:** Preimplantation testing, also called "preimplantation genetic diagnosis" (PGD), is a specialized technique that can reduce the risk of having a child with a particular genetic or chromosomal disorder. It is used to detect genetic changes in embryos that were created using assisted reproductive techniques such as in-vitro fertilization (IVF). In-vitro fertilization involves removing egg cells from a woman's ovaries and fertilizing them with sperm cells outside the body. To perform preimplantation testing, a small number of cells are taken from these embryos and tested for certain genetic changes. Only embryos without these changes are implanted in the uterus to initiate a pregnancy.

- **Predictive and presymptomatic testing:** Predictive and presymptomatic types of testing are used to detect gene mutations associated with disorders that appear after birth, often later in life. These tests can be helpful to people who have a family member with a genetic disorder, but who have no features of the disorder themselves at the time of testing. Predictive testing can identify mutations that increase a person's risk of developing disorders with a genetic basis, such as certain types of cancer. Presymptomatic testing can determine whether a person will develop a genetic disorder, such as hereditary hemochromatosis (an iron-overload disorder) before any signs or symptoms appear. The results of predictive and presymptomatic testing can provide information about a person's risk of developing a specific disorder and help with making decisions about medical care.

- **Forensic testing:** Forensic testing uses deoxyribonucleic acid (DNA) sequences to identify an individual for legal purposes. Unlike the tests described above, forensic testing is not used to detect gene mutations associated with disease. This type of testing can identify crime or catastrophe victims, rule out or implicate a crime suspect, or establish biological relationships between people (for example, paternity).

What Is Noninvasive Prenatal Testing and What Disorders Can It Screen For?

Noninvasive prenatal testing (NIPT), sometimes called "noninvasive prenatal screening" (NIPS), is a method of determining the risk that the fetus will be born with certain genetic abnormalities. This testing analyzes small fragments of DNA that are circulating in a pregnant woman's blood. Unlike most DNA, which is found inside a cell's nucleus, these fragments are free-floating and not within cells, and are, therefore, called "cell-free DNA" (cfDNA). These small fragments usually contain fewer than 200 DNA building blocks (base pairs) and arise when cells die off and get broken down and their contents, including DNA, are released into the bloodstream.

During pregnancy, the mother's bloodstream contains a mix of cfDNA that comes from her cells and cells from the placenta. The placenta is tissue in the uterus that links the fetus and the mother's blood supply. These cells are shed into the mother's bloodstream throughout pregnancy. The DNA in placental cells is usually identical to the DNA of the fetus. Analyzing cfDNA from the placenta provides an opportunity for early detection of certain genetic abnormalities without harming the fetus.

NIPT is most often used to look for chromosomal disorders that are caused by the presence of an extra or missing copy (aneuploidy) of a chromosome. NIPT primarily looks for Down syndrome (trisomy 21, caused by an extra chromosome 21), trisomy 18 (caused by an extra chromosome 18), trisomy 13 (caused by an extra chromosome 13), and extra or missing copies of the X chromosome and Y chromosome (the sex chromosomes). The accuracy of the test varies by disorder.

NIPT may include screening for additional chromosomal disorders that are caused by missing (deleted) or copied (duplicated) sections of a chromosome. NIPT is beginning to be used to test for genetic disorders that are caused by changes (variants) in single genes. As technology improves and the cost of genetic testing decreases, researchers expect that NIPT will become available for many more genetic conditions.

NIPT is considered noninvasive because it requires drawing blood only from the pregnant woman and does not pose any risk to the fetus. NIPT is a screening test, which means that it will not give a definitive answer about whether or not a fetus has a genetic condition. The test can only estimate whether the risk of having certain conditions is increased or decreased. In some cases, NIPT results indicate an increased risk for a genetic abnormality when the fetus is actually unaffected (false positive), or the results indicate a decreased risk for a genetic abnormality when the fetus is actually affected (false negative). Because NIPT analyzes both fetal and maternal cfDNA, the test may detect a genetic condition in the mother.

There must be enough fetal cfDNA in the mother's bloodstream to be able to identify fetal chromosome abnormalities. The proportion of cfDNA in maternal blood that comes from the placenta is known as the "fetal fraction." Generally, the fetal fraction must be above four percent, which typically occurs around the tenth week of pregnancy. Low fetal fractions can lead to an inability to perform the test or a false negative result. Reasons for low fetal fractions include testing too early in the pregnancy, sampling errors, maternal obesity, and fetal abnormality.

There are multiple NIPT methods to analyze fetal cfDNA. To determine chromosomal aneuploidy, the most common method is to count all cfDNA fragments (both fetal and maternal). If the percentage of cfDNA fragments from each chromosome is as expected, then the fetus has a decreased risk of having a chromosomal condition (negative test result). If the percentage of cfDNA fragments from a particular chromosome is more than expected, then the fetus has an increased likelihood of having a trisomy condition (positive test result). A positive screening result indicates that further testing (called "diagnostic testing" because it is used to diagnose a disease) should be performed to confirm the result.

Chapter 3

Promote a Healthy Pregnancy

Can You Promote a Healthy Pregnancy before Getting Pregnant?

For women who are thinking about getting pregnant, following a healthcare provider's advice can reduce the risk of problems during pregnancy and after birth. A healthcare provider can recommend ways to get the proper nutrition and avoid habits that can have lasting harmful effects on a fetus.

For example, taking a supplement containing at least 400 micrograms of folic acid before getting pregnant can reduce the risk of complications such as neural tube defects (NTDs)—abnormalities that can occur in the brain, spine, or spinal column of a developing fetus and are present at birth.

A preconception-care visit with your healthcare provider can improve the chances of a healthy pregnancy. A healthcare provider will likely recommend that you do the following:

This chapter contains text excerpted from the following sources: Text under the heading ""Can You Promote a Healthy Pregnancy before Getting Pregnant?" is excerpted from "Can You Promote a Healthy Pregnancy before Getting Pregnant?" *Eunice Kennedy Shriver* National Institute of Child Health and Human Development (NICHD), January 31, 2017; Text under the heading "Steps to Have the Healthiest Pregnancy Possible" is excerpted from "Healthy Pregnancy," Centers for Disease Control and Prevention (CDC), January 14, 2019.

- Develop a plan for your reproductive life

- Adopt a healthy diet and lifestyle

You can reduce the chance that you will be diagnosed with gestational diabetes (high blood sugar diagnosed during pregnancy) by taking steps to improve your diet and lifestyle before you get pregnant. Gestational diabetes can increase the risk to your health as well as your infant's. In addition, prepregnancy exercise is also associated with lower risk for gestational diabetes, and the benefit increases with more vigorous levels of exercise.

Here are some specific dietary suggestions for women who are planning for a pregnancy:

- Increase your intake of fiber. Eating 10 more grams of fiber in the form of cereals, fruits, and vegetables is associated with 26 percent lower risk of gestational diabetes.

- Reduce consumption of sugar-sweetened cola. Women who drank five or more such beverages per week before they got pregnant were at greater risk of gestational diabetes.

- Eat less red meat, processed meats, and limit intake of animal fats and cholesterol. Eating less of these foods before pregnancy can decrease your chances of developing diabetes when you are pregnant.

- Replace animal protein with protein from nuts to lower your risk of gestational diabetes. Studies have shown that substituting vegetable protein for animal protein before pregnancy can decrease risk of gestational diabetes by about half.

Steps to Have the Healthiest Pregnancy Possible

- Be sure to take 400 micrograms (mcg) of folic acid every day.

  - Folic acid is important because it can help prevent some major birth defects of the fetus's brain and spine. These birth defects develop very early during pregnancy when the neural tube—which forms the early brain and spinal cord—does not close properly. Start taking folic acid at least one month before becoming pregnant and continue taking during pregnancy.

- Book a visit with your healthcare provider before stopping or starting any medicine.

- Many women need to take medicine to treat a health condition during pregnancy. If you are planning to become pregnant, discuss your current medicines with a healthcare provider, such as a doctor or pharmacist. Creating a treatment plan for your health condition before you are pregnant can help keep you and the fetus healthy.

- Become up-to-date with all vaccinations, including the flu shot.

  - Vaccines help protect you and the fetus against serious diseases. Get a flu shot and whooping cough vaccination (called "Tdap") during each pregnancy to help protect yourself and the fetus.

    - Flu: You can get the flu shot before or during each pregnancy.

    - Whooping Cough: You can get the whooping cough vaccine in the last three months of each pregnancy.

- Before you get pregnant, try to reach a healthy weight.

  - An unhealthy weight increases the risk for several serious birth defects and other pregnancy complications. If you are underweight, overweight, or obese, talk with your healthcare provider about ways to reach and maintain a healthy weight before you get pregnant. Focus on a lifestyle that includes healthy eating and regular physical activity.

- Boost your health by avoiding harmful substances during pregnancy, such as alcohol, tobacco, and other drugs.

  - Alcohol: There is no known safe amount of alcohol use during pregnancy or when trying to get pregnant. There is also no safe time during pregnancy to drink. All types of alcohol are equally harmful, including all wines and beer. Alcohol can cause problems for a fetus throughout pregnancy, so it's important to stop drinking alcohol when you start trying to get pregnant.

  - Tobacco: Smoking causes cancer, heart disease, and other major health problems. Smoking during pregnancy can also harm the fetus and can cause certain birth defects. It's best to quit smoking before you get pregnant. But if you are already pregnant, quitting can still help protect you and the fetus from health problems. Quitting smoking will help you feel better and provide a healthier environment for the fetus.

- Other drugs: Using certain drugs during pregnancy can cause health problems for a woman and the fetus. If you are pregnant or trying to get pregnant and can't stop using drugs, get help. A healthcare provider can help you with counseling, treatment, and other support services.

Chapter 4

Understanding Fertility

Chapter Contents

Section 4.1

Fertility Basics

This section includes text excerpted from "Understanding Fertility: The Basics," U.S. Department of Health and Human Services (HHS), January 29, 2019.

Understanding the Body and Fertility

It is important to understand what happens to the body during puberty and a woman's menstrual cycle, how a woman's reproductive system works, and how overall health and wellness are connected to fertility and the reproductive system.

Understanding the body and the biology of reproduction can inform decisions about preventing pregnancy and deciding whether and when to become pregnant. The next sections describe the basics of puberty, the menstrual cycle, and what it means to have fertility awareness.

- **Puberty.** Puberty is the time in life when a child reaches sexual maturity. This means that the hormone levels in the body—estrogen and progesterone in girls and testosterone in boys—increase and cause physical and emotional changes to occur. Puberty usually happens between ages 8 and 13 for girls and ages 10 and 15 for boys, and the process affects boys and girls differently. When girls enter puberty, they typically start their menstrual cycle.

- **Menstrual cycle.** The menstrual cycle refers to the monthly process that happens in a woman's body to prepare for a possible pregnancy. It includes the release of an egg from the ovaries (called "ovulation"), changes in the cervix and thickening of the uterine wall, several hormonal changes, and shedding of the thickened uterine wall through bleeding (called "menstruation," also known as the "period" or "menses"). Hormonal fluctuations drive the changes that occur during the menstrual cycle. If pregnancy does not occur, the body sheds the extra lining of the uterus. The blood and tissue leave the uterus through the cervix and exit the body through the vagina. The length of the menstrual cycle is the number of days starting from the first day when bleeding begins until the first day of the next month when bleeding begins again. Regular menstrual periods occurring in the years between puberty and menopause are usually a sign that the female body is working normally. Some women experience period problems, such as irregular periods or heavy, painful periods—which may be a sign of a health problem. Many women also get premenstrual syndrome (PMS) symptoms. Women with period problems or PMS should talk to a healthcare provider about ways to treat these issues.

- **How to chart menstrual cycles.** To chart her menstrual cycle, a woman can simply record the day her period starts and when it ends on a paper or electronic calendar. Smartphone and computer applications that chart menstrual cycles are also available. Over time, this tracking will help a woman see what the typical amount of time between periods is, which can help her predict when her next period will start. Tracking the menstrual cycle can provide useful information for conversations with healthcare providers. For example, a patient may want to discuss the length of her cycle or her experiences with pain or extreme bleeding during her cycle. In addition, tracking the cycle is key to predicting ovulation, which can inform decisions about when to have sex, whether the intent is to avoid pregnancy or become pregnant.

Fertility Awareness

"Fertility awareness" means being aware of the menstrual cycle and the changes in a woman's body that happen during this time, and understanding when a woman is most likely to get pregnant. Women and couples become more familiar with the signs of ovulation and the pattern of the menstrual cycle to understand how to plan sexual activity to avoid pregnancy or become pregnant.

Section 4.2

Age and Fertility

This section contains text excerpted from the following sources: Text beginning with the heading "What Types of Things Can Cause or Contribute to Infertility?" is excerpted from "What You Need to Know about Sinus Disorders," *Eunice Kennedy Shriver* National Institute of Child Health and Human Development (NICHD), January 5, 2018; Text under the heading "A Molecular Explanation for Age-Related Fertility Decline in Women" is excerpted from "A Molecular Explanation for Age-Related Fertility Decline in Women," National Institutes of Health (NIH), May 21, 2013. Reviewed February 2019.

What Types of Things Can Cause or Contribute to Infertility?

Health conditions and behaviors, age, genetics, and other factors can all cause or contribute to infertility in men and women.

Health Conditions and Behaviors
Women

- Gynecological disorders, such as polycystic ovary syndrome (PCOS), primary ovarian insufficiency (POI), endometriosis, and uterine fibroids

- Problems with anatomy of the reproductive organs

Men

- Certain medications, such as testosterone gels/patches to treat "low T"
- Testicular injury or overheating

Men and Women

- Exposure to chemicals
- Cancer and/or exposure to radiation or chemotherapy
- Stress
- Conditions such as diabetes, heart disease, obesity, high blood pressure, and autoimmune disorders
- Smoking and/or alcohol and drug abuse
- Sexually transmitted infections (STIs)

What's Age Got to Do with It?

People are waiting longer than ever before to start families. Women are now eight times more likely to have their first child after age 35 than they were in 1970. But waiting too long can cause problems.

As age increases, so does the likelihood of infertility.

* Older men produce fewer sperm and lower-quality sperm.
* Older women have fewer eggs and lower-quality eggs.
* The risk of some health conditions associated with infertility increases with age.
* Age-related declines in sperm and egg quality increase the risk of health conditions, such as Down syndrome, autism, and schizophrenia, in future generations.

After age 30, a woman's fertility decreases rapidly every year until menopause, usually around age 50. In the decade before menopause, her fertility is also greatly reduced. Male fertility also declines with age, but more gradually.

A Molecular Explanation for Age-Related Fertility Decline in Women

Scientists supported by the National Institutes of Health (NIH) have a new theory as to why a woman's fertility declines after her mid-30s. They also suggest an approach that might help slow the process, enhancing and prolonging fertility.

They found that, as women age, their egg cells become riddled with deoxyribonucleic acid (DNA) damage and die off because their DNA repair systems wear out. Defects in one of the DNA repair genes— *BRCA1*—have long been linked with breast cancer, and now also appear to cause early menopause.

"We all know that a woman's fertility declines in her 40s. This study provides a molecular explanation for why that happens," said Dr. Susan Taymans, Ph.D., of the Fertility and Infertility Branch of the *Eunice Kennedy Shriver* National Institute of Child Health and Human Development (NICHD), the NIH institute that funded the study. "Eventually, such insights might help us find ways to improve and extend a woman's reproductive life."

The findings appear in *Science Translational Medicine*.

In general, a woman's ability to conceive and maintain a pregnancy is linked to the number and health of her egg cells. Before a baby girl is born, her ovaries contain her lifetime supply of egg cells (known as "primordial follicle oocytes") until they are more mature. As she enters her late 30s, the number of oocytes—and fertility—dips precipitously. By the time she reaches her early 50s, her original ovarian supply of about one million cells drops virtually to zero.

Only a small proportion of oocytes—about 500—are released via ovulation during the woman's reproductive life. The remaining 99.9 percent are eliminated by the woman's body, primarily through cellular suicide, a normal process that prevents the spread or inheritance of damaged cells.

The scientists suspect that most aging oocytes self-destruct because they have accumulated a dangerous type of DNA damage called "double-stranded breaks." According to the study, older oocytes have more of this sort of damage than do younger ones. The researchers also found that older oocytes are less able to fix DNA breaks due to their dwindling supply of repair molecules.

Examining oocytes from mice, and from women 24 to 41 years old, the researchers found that the activity of four DNA repair genes (*BRCA1*, MRE11, Rad51, and ATM) declined with age. When the research team experimentally turned off these genes in mouse oocytes, the cells had more DNA breaks and higher death rates than did oocytes with properly working repair systems.

The research team's findings stemmed from their initial focus on *BRCA1*, a DNA repair gene that has been closely studied for nearly 20 years because defective versions of it dramatically increase a woman's risk of breast cancer. Using mice bred to lack the *BRCA1* gene, the NICHD-supported scientists confirmed that a healthy version of *BRCA1* is vital to reproductive health.

BRCA1-deficient mice were less fertile, had fewer oocytes, and had more double-stranded DNA breaks in their remaining oocytes than did normal mice. Abnormal *BRCA1* appears to cause the same problems in humans—the team's studies suggest that if a woman's oocytes contain mutant versions of *BRCA1*, she will exhaust her ovarian supply sooner than women whose oocytes carry the healthy version of *BRCA1*.

Together, these findings show that the ability of oocytes to repair double-stranded DNA breaks is closely linked with ovarian aging and, by extension, a woman's fertility. This molecular-level understanding points to new reproductive therapies. Specifically, the scientists suggest that finding ways to bolster DNA repair systems in the ovaries might lead to treatments that can improve or prolong fertility.

Section 4.3

Fertility Preservation

This section includes text excerpted from "What Is Fertility Preservation?" *Eunice Kennedy Shriver* National Institute of Child Health and Human Development (NICHD), January 31, 2017.

What Is Fertility Preservation?

Fertility preservation is the process of saving or protecting eggs, sperm, or reproductive tissue so that a person can use them to have biological children in the future.

Who Can Benefit from Fertility Preservation?

People with certain diseases, disorders, and life events that affect fertility may benefit from fertility preservation. These include people who:

- Have been exposed to toxic chemicals in the workplace or during military duty

- Have endometriosis

- Have uterine fibroids

- Are about to be treated for cancer

- Are about to be treated for an autoimmune disease, such as lupus

- Have a genetic disease that affects future fertility

- Delay having children

What Fertility-Preserving Options Are Available?

A number of fertility-preserving options are available. Fertility-preserving options for males include:

- **Sperm cryopreservation.** In this process, a male provides samples of his semen. The semen is then frozen and stored for future use in a process called "cryopreservation."

- **Gonadal shielding.** Radiation treatment for cancer and other conditions can harm fertility, especially if it is used in the pelvic area. Some radiation treatments use modern techniques to aim the rays on a very small area. The testicles can also be protected with a lead shield.

Fertility-preserving options for females include:

- **Embryo cryopreservation.** This method, also called "embryo freezing," is the most common and successful option for preserving a female's fertility. First, a healthcare provider removes eggs from the ovaries. The eggs are then fertilized with sperm from her partner or a donor in a lab in a process called "in vitro fertilization." The resulting embryos are frozen and stored for future use.

- **Oocyte cryopreservation.** This option is similar to embryo cryopreservation, except that unfertilized eggs are frozen and stored.

- **Gonadal shielding.** This process is similar to gonadal shielding for males. Steps are taken, such as aiming rays at a small area or covering the pelvic area with a lead shield, to protect the ovaries from radiation.

- **Ovarian transposition.** A healthcare provider performs a minor surgery to move the ovaries and sometimes the fallopian tubes from the area that will receive radiation to an area that will not receive radiation. For example, they may be relocated to an area of the abdomen wall that will not receive radiation.

Some of these options, such as sperm, oocyte, and embryo cryopreservation, are available only to males and females who have gone through puberty and have mature sperm and eggs. However, gonadal shielding and ovarian transposition can be used to preserve fertility in children who have not gone through puberty.

Chapter 5

Trying to Conceive

Chapter Contents

Section 5.1

Steps to Conceive

This section includes text excerpted from "Planning for Pregnancy,"
Centers for Disease Control and Prevention (CDC), January 23, 2018.

If you are trying to have a baby or are just thinking about it, it is not too early to start getting ready for pregnancy. Preconception health and healthcare focus on things you can do before and between pregnancies to increase the chances of having a healthy baby. For some women, getting their body ready for pregnancy takes a few months. For other women, it might take longer. Whether this is your first, second, or sixth baby, the following are important steps to help you get ready for the healthiest pregnancy possible.

1. Make a Plan and Take Action

Whether or not you've written them down, you've probably thought about your goals for having or not having children, and how to achieve those goals. For example, when you didn't want to have a baby, you used effective birth-control methods to achieve your goals. Now that you're thinking about getting pregnant, it's really important to take steps to achieve your goal.

2. See Your Doctor

Before getting pregnant, talk to your doctor about preconception healthcare. Your doctor will want to discuss your health history and any medical conditions you currently have that could affect a pregnancy. She or he also will discuss any previous pregnancy problems, medicines that you currently are taking, vaccinations that you might need, and steps you can take before pregnancy to prevent certain birth defects.

If your doctor has not talked with you about this type of care, ask about it! Take a list of talking points so you don't forget anything.

Be sure to talk to your doctor about:

Medical Conditions

If you currently have any medical conditions, be sure they are under control and being treated. Some of these conditions include sexually transmitted diseases (STDs), diabetes, thyroid disease,

36

phenylketonuria (PKU), seizure disorders, high blood pressure, arthritis, eating disorders, and chronic diseases.

Lifestyle and Behaviors

Talk with your doctor or another health professional if you smoke, drink alcohol, or use street drugs; live in a stressful or abusive environment; or work with or live around toxic substances. Healthcare professionals can help you with counseling, treatment, and other support services.

Medications

Taking certain medicines during pregnancy can cause serious birth defects. These include some prescription and over-the-counter (OTC) medications and dietary or herbal supplements. If you are planning a pregnancy, you should discuss the need for any medication with your doctor before becoming pregnant and make sure you are taking only those medications that are necessary.

Vaccinations (Shots)

Some vaccinations are recommended before you become pregnant, during pregnancy, or right after delivery. Having the right vaccinations at the right time can help keep you healthy and help keep your baby from getting very sick or having lifelong health problems.

3. Take 400 Micrograms of Folic Acid Every Day

Folic acid is a B vitamin. If a woman has enough folic acid in her body at least one month before and during pregnancy, it can help prevent major birth defects of the baby's brain and spine.

4. Stop Drinking Alcohol, Smoking, and Using Street Drugs

Smoking, drinking alcohol, and using street drugs can cause many problems during pregnancy for a woman and her baby, such as premature birth, birth defects, and infant death.

If you are trying to get pregnant and cannot stop drinking, smoking, or using drugs, get help. Contact your doctor or local treatment center.

5. Avoid Toxic Substances and Environmental Contaminants

Avoid toxic substances and other environmental contaminants and harmful materials, such as synthetic chemicals, metals, fertilizer, bug spray, and cat or rodent feces at work or at home. These substances can hurt the reproductive systems of men and women. They can make it more difficult to get pregnant. Exposure to even small amounts during pregnancy, infancy, childhood, or puberty can lead to diseases. Learn how to protect yourself and your loved ones from toxic substances at work and at home.

6. Reach and Maintain a Healthy Weight

People who are overweight or obese have a higher risk for many serious conditions, including complications during pregnancy, heart disease, type 2 diabetes, and certain cancers (endometrial, breast, and colon). People who are underweight are also at risk for serious health problems.

The key to achieving and maintaining a healthy weight isn't about short-term dietary changes. It's about a lifestyle that includes healthy eating and regular physical activity.

If you are underweight, overweight, or obese, talk with your doctor about ways to reach and maintain a healthy weight before you get pregnant.

7. Get Help for Violence

Violence can lead to injury and death among women at any stage of life, including during pregnancy. The number of violent deaths experienced by women tells only part of the story. Many more survive violence and are left with lifelong physical and emotional scars.

If someone is violent toward you or you are violent toward your loved ones, get help. Violence destroys relationships and families.

8. Learn Your Family History

Collecting your family's health history can be important for your child's health. You might not realize that your sister's heart defect or your cousin's sickle cell disease (SCD) could affect your child, but sharing this family history information with your doctor can be important.

Based on your family history, your doctor might refer you for genetic counseling. Other reasons people go for genetic counseling include having had several miscarriages, infant deaths, or trouble getting pregnant (infertility), or a genetic condition or birth defect that occurred during a previous pregnancy.

9. Get Mentally Healthy

Mental health is how we think, feel, and act as we cope with life. To be at your best, you need to feel good about your life and value yourself. Everyone feels worried, anxious, sad, or stressed sometimes. However, if these feelings do not go away and they interfere with your daily life, get help. Talk with your doctor or another health professional about your feelings and treatment options.

10. Have a Healthy Pregnancy

Once you are pregnant, be sure to continue all of your new healthy habits and see your doctor regularly for prenatal care.

Section 5.2

Using Ovulation Predictor Kits

This section contains text excerpted from the following sources: Text
under the heading "Charting Your Fertility Pattern" is excerpted
from "Trying to Conceive," Office on Women's Health (OWH), U.S.
Department of Health and Human Services (HHS), June 6, 2018;
Text under the heading "Ovulation Saliva Test" is excerpted from
"Ovulation (Saliva Test)," U.S. Food and Drug Administration (FDA),
February 6, 2018; Text under the heading "Ovulation Urine Test"
is excerpted from "Ovulation (Urine Test)," U.S. Food and Drug
Administration (FDA), February 4, 2018.

Charting Your Fertility Pattern

Knowing when you're most fertile will help you plan pregnancy.
There are three ways you can keep track of your fertile times. They are:

- **Basal body temperature method**—Basal body temperature is
  your temperature at rest as soon as you awake in the morning.
  A woman's basal body temperature rises slightly with ovulation.
  So by recording this temperature daily for several months, you'll
  be able to predict your most fertile days.

  Basal body temperature differs slightly from woman to woman.
  Anywhere from 96 to 98 degrees Fahrenheit orally is average before
  ovulation. After ovulation, most women have an oral temperature
  between 97 and 99 degrees Fahrenheit. The rise in temperature
  can be a sudden jump or a gradual climb over a few days.

  Usually, a woman's basal body temperature rises by only 0.4 to
  0.8 degrees Fahrenheit. To detect this tiny change, women must
  use a basal body thermometer. These thermometers are very
  sensitive. Most pharmacies sell them for about $10.

  The rise in temperature doesn't show exactly when the egg is
  released. But almost all women have ovulated within three days
  after their temperatures spike. Body temperature stays at the
  higher level until your period starts.

  You are most fertile and most likely to get pregnant:

  - 2 to 3 days before your temperature hits the highest point
    (ovulation), and

  - 12 to 24 hours after ovulation

A man's sperm can live for up to three days in a woman's body. The sperm can fertilize an egg at any point during that time. So if you have unprotected sex a few days before ovulation, you could get pregnant.

Many things can affect basal body temperature. For your chart to be useful, make sure to take your temperature every morning at about the same time. Things that can alter your temperature include:

- Drinking alcohol the night before

- Smoking cigarettes the night before

- Getting a poor night's sleep

- Having a fever

- Doing anything in the morning before you take your temperature—including going to the bathroom and talking on the phone

- **Calendar method**—This involves recording your menstrual cycle on a calendar for 8 to 12 months. The first day of your period is Day 1. Circle Day 1 on the calendar. The length of your cycle may vary from month to month. So write down the total number of days it lasts each time. Using this record, you can find the days you are most fertile in the months ahead:

  1. To find out the first day when you are most fertile, subtract 18 from the total number of days in your shortest cycle. Take this new number and count ahead that many days from the first day of your next period. Draw an X through this date on your calendar. The X marks the first day you're likely to be fertile.

  2. To find out the last day when you are most fertile, subtract 11 from the total number of days in your longest cycle. Take this new number and count ahead that many days from the first day of your next period. Draw an X through this date on your calendar. The time between the two Xs represents your most fertile window.

This method always should be used along with other fertility awareness methods, especially if your cycles are not always the same length.

- **Cervical mucus method** (also known as the "ovulation method")—This involves being aware of the changes in your cervical mucus throughout the month. The hormones that control the menstrual cycle also change the kind and amount of mucus you have before and during ovulation. Right after your period, there are usually a few days when there is no mucus present or "dry days." As the egg starts to mature, white or yellow or cloudy or sticky mucus increases in the vagina and appears at the vaginal opening. The greatest amount of mucus appears just before ovulation. During these "wet days" it becomes clear and slippery, like raw egg whites. Sometimes it can be stretched apart. This is when you are most fertile. About four days after the wet days begin, the mucus changes again. There is much less of it and it becomes sticky and cloudy. You might have a few more dry days before your period returns. Describe these mucosal changes on a calendar. Label the days, "Sticky," "Dry," or "Wet." You are most fertile at the first sign of wetness after your period or a day or two before wetness begins.

  The cervical mucus method is less reliable for some women. Women who are breastfeeding, taking hormonal birth control (such as the pill), using feminine-hygiene products, have vaginitis or sexually transmitted infections (STIs), or have had surgery on the cervix should not rely on this method.

- To most accurately track your fertility, use a combination of all three methods. This is called the "symptothermal method." You can also purchase over-the-counter (OTC) ovulation kits or fertility monitors to help find the best time to conceive. These kits work by detecting surges in a specific hormone called "luteinizing hormone" (LH), which triggers ovulation.

Ovulation Saliva Test
What Does This Test Do?

This is a home-use test kit to predict ovulation by looking at patterns formed by your saliva. When estrogen increases near your time of ovulation, your dried saliva may form a fern-shaped pattern.

What Type of Test Is This?

This is a qualitative test designed to determine whether you may be near your ovulation time, not if you will definitely become pregnant.

Why Should You Do This Test?

You should do this test if you want to know when you expect to ovulate and be in the most fertile part of your menstrual cycle. This test can be used to help you plan to become pregnant. You should not use this test to help prevent pregnancy, because it is not reliable for that purpose.

How Accurate Is This Test?

This test may not work well for you. Some of the reasons are

- Not all women fern
- You may not be able to see the fern
- Women who fern on some days of their fertile period don't necessarily fern on all of their fertile days
- Ferning may be disrupted by:
  - Smoking
  - Eating
  - Drinking
  - Brushing your teeth
  - How you put your saliva on the slide
  - Where you were when you did the test

How Do You Do This Test?

In this test, you get a small microscope with built-in or removable slides. You put some of your saliva on a glass slide, allow it to dry, and look at the pattern it makes. You will see dots and circles, a fern (full or partial), or a combination depending on where you are in your monthly cycle.

You will get your best results when you use the test within the five-day period around your expected ovulation. This period includes the two days before and the two days after your expected day of ovulation. The test is not perfect, though, and you might fern outside of this time period or when you are pregnant. Even some men will fern.

Is This Test Similar to the One My Doctor Uses?

The fertility tests your doctor uses are automated, and they may give more consistent results. Your doctor may use other tests that are not yet available for home use (i.e., blood and urine laboratory tests) and information about your history to get a better view of your fertility status.

Does a Positive Test Mean You Are Ovulating?

A positive test indicates that you may be near ovulation. It does not mean that you will definitely become pregnant.

Do Negative Test Results Mean That You Are Not Ovulating?

No, there may be many reasons why you did not detect your time of ovulation. You should not use this test to help prevent pregnancy, because it is not reliable for that purpose.

Ovulation Urine Test
What Does This Test Do?

This is a home-use test kit to measure luteinizing hormone (LH) in your urine. This helps detect the LH surge that happens in the middle of your menstrual cycle, about 1 to 1½ days before ovulation. Some tests also measure another hormone—estrone-3-glucuronide (E3G).

What Is Luteinizing Hormone?

Luteinizing hormone (LH) is a hormone produced by your pituitary gland. Your body always makes a small amount of LH, but just before you ovulate, you make much more LH. This test can detect this LH surge, which usually happens 1 to 1½ days before you ovulate.

What Is Estrone-3-Glucuronide?

Estrone-3-glucuronide (E3G) is produced when estrogen breaks down in your body. It accumulates in your urine around the time of ovulation and causes your cervical mucus to become thin and slippery. Sperm may swim more easily in your thin and slippery cervical mucus, increasing your chances of getting pregnant.

What Type of Test Is This?

This is a qualitative test designed to help you find out whether or not you have elevated LH or E3G levels. The test will not indicate if you will definitely become pregnant.

Why Should You Do This Test?

You should do this test if you want to know when you expect to ovulate and be in the most fertile part of your menstrual cycle. This test can be used to help you plan to become pregnant. You should not use this test to help prevent pregnancy, because it is not reliable for that purpose.

How Accurate Is This Test?

How well this test will predict your fertile period depends on how well you follow the instructions. These tests can detect LH and E3G reliably about 9 times out of 10, but you must do the test carefully.

How Do You Do This Test?

You add a few drops of your urine to the test, hold the tip of the test in your urine stream, or dip the test in a cup of your urine. You either read the test by looking for colored lines on the test or you put the test device into a monitor. You can get results in about five minutes. The details of what the color looks like, or how to use the monitor varies among the different brands.

Most kits come with multiple tests to allow you to take measurements over several days. This can help you find your most fertile period, the time during your cycle when you can expect to ovulate based on your hormone levels. Follow the instructions carefully to ensure good results. You will need to start your testing at the proper time during your cycle; otherwise, the test will be unreliable, and you will not find your hormonal surges or your fertile period.

Is This Test Similar to the One My Doctor Uses?

The fertility tests your doctor uses are automated, and they may give more consistent results. Your doctor may use other tests that are not yet available for home use (i.e., blood and urine laboratory tests) and information about your history to get a better view of your fertility status.

Chapter 6

Preventing Unintended Pregnancies

Chapter Contents

Section 6.1

Unintended Pregnancies

This section contains text excerpted from the following
sources: Text in this section begins with excerpts from "Unintended
Pregnancy," Centers for Disease Control and Prevention (CDC),
September 15, 2017; Text beginning with the heading "Unintended
Pregnancy Prevention" is excerpted from "Unintended Pregnancy
Prevention," Centers for Disease Control and Prevention (CDC),
December 20, 2016.

Unintended pregnancies are either mistimed (the woman didn't
plan to become pregnant until later in life) or unwanted (the woman
had no plan to ever become pregnant). This pervasive public-health
problem occurs regardless of age, marital status, socioeconomic status,
race, or ethnicity. Studies show unintended pregnancy may lead to
delayed start of prenatal care, increased risk of premature birth, and
increased physical violence against the mother. Almost all induced
abortions are related to unintended pregnancy.

Almost one-half (49%) of the approximately 6 million pregnancies
in the United States in 1995 were unintended, and approximately
one-third (31%), resulting in an estimated 1.22 million births, are
unintended.

Who's at Risk?

Most unintended pregnancies occur in women who are older than
19 years of age. About half of unintended pregnancies occur among
couples using no contraceptive method and half are due to incorrect
use of contraceptives or contraceptive failures. Twenty-one percent of
births among married couples are unintended. The proportion of all
unintended pregnancies varies by age, with teenagers younger than
18 and women 40 and older having the highest percentage. About 48
percent of all women aged 15 to 44 have had an unintended pregnancy
(either an unplanned birth, an abortion, or both).

Can It Be Prevented?

Most unintended pregnancies can be prevented. Approximately
8 to 10 contraceptive methods are available to prevent unintended
pregnancy.

Even so, there are many obstacles to consistently preventing unwanted pregnancy. Abstinence is the only method that is 100 percent effective—some other methods reach 98 to 99 percent.

- Some people believe using contraception or planning ahead to use contraception is "not romantic."

- Some women may have misconceptions about side effects and long-term risks of certain contraceptive methods.

- A contraceptive may be used, but not consistently and correctly.

- There are stigmas associated with contraception, abortion, pregnancy, being unmarried and pregnant, etc.

- Some people believe it will not happen to them.

- Some people believe using contraception is unhealthy, sinful, or makes them appear "loose."

- The financial cost associated with using some contraceptive methods (physical examination, routine laboratory tests, time away from work, transportation, cost of method, maintenance costs, etc.) may be too expensive for some people.

- A woman may not want to be pregnant, but her partner may want a baby.

- Some contraceptive methods may have disadvantages or side effects that may discourage use, and

- Some unintended pregnancies are caused by rape or forced sex.

Unintended Pregnancy Prevention

Unintended pregnancy is associated with an increased risk of problems for the mother and baby. If a pregnancy is not planned before conception, a woman may not be in optimal health for childbearing. For example, women with an unintended pregnancy could delay prenatal care that may affect the health of the baby. Therefore, it is important for all women of reproductive age to adopt healthy behaviors such as:

- Taking folic acid

- Maintaining a healthy diet and weight

- Being physically active regularly

- Quitting tobacco use

- Abstaining from alcohol and drugs

- Talking to their healthcare provider about screening and proper management of chronic diseases

- Visiting their healthcare provider at the recommended scheduled time periods for their age and discuss if or when they are considering becoming pregnant

- Using effective contraception correctly and consistently if they are sexually active but wish to delay or avoid pregnancy

In the United States

According to a study published in 2016:

- In 2011, 45 percent of pregnancies were unintended—a decline from 51 percent in 2008.

- Progress was made in almost every demographic group from 2008 to 2011.

  - The rate of unintended pregnancies decreased 18 percent— from 54 to 45 unintended pregnancies per 1,000 women aged 15 to 44 years.

  - Some of the largest declines occurred among teens aged 15 to 17 years (44%), women who had not completed high school (32%), and Hispanic women (26%).

- Despite this progress, differences persist across groups.

  - Among teens 15 to 19 years of age, 3 out of every 4 pregnancies were unintended.

  - Unintended pregnancy rates per 1,000 women were highest among women age 18 to 24, had low incomes (<100% of the federal poverty level), had not graduated from high school, were non-Hispanic Black, and those cohabiting women who had never been married.

The United States has established family-planning goals in Healthy People 2020 aimed at improving pregnancy planning, spacing, and preventing unintended pregnancy. Family-planning efforts that can help reduce unintended pregnancy include increasing access to contraception (particularly to the more effective and longer acting reversible forms of contraception) and increasing correct and consistent use of contraceptive methods overall among those who are sexually active but wish to delay or avoid pregnancy.

Section 6.2

Understanding Birth Control and Contraception

This section includes text excerpted from "Contraception and Birth Control" is excerpted from "Contraception and Birth Control," *Eunice Kennedy Shriver* National Institute of Child Health and Human Development (NICHD), January 31, 2017.

Contraception allows for the prevention of pregnancy and for planning the timing of pregnancy. Some methods can also protect against infections. Modern methods of contraception include oral contraceptives (such as birth control pills), contraceptive vaginal rings, condoms, intrauterine devices (also called "IUDs"), injectable and implantable products, and sterilization.

About Contraception and Birth Control

Contraception is the prevention of pregnancy. Contraception, or birth control, also allows couples to plan the timing of pregnancy. Some methods can also protect against infections. Choosing a particular method of birth control depends on many factors, including a woman's overall health, age, frequency of sexual activity, number of sexual partners, desire to have children in the future, and family medical history. Individuals should work with their healthcare provider to choose a method that is best for them. It is also important to discuss birth-control methods with one's sexual partner.

General methods of contraception include:

- **Barrier**—physically interferes with conception by keeping the egg and sperm apart

- **Hormonal**—regulates ovulation by changing the balance of hormones related to development and release of the egg; changes cervical mucus to impair sperm function or transport

- **Intrauterine devices**—small devices inserted into the uterus that change the conditions in the cervix and uterus to prevent pregnancy, as well as inhibiting the transit of sperm from the cervix to the fallopian tubes

- **Sterilization**—surgical procedures that make a woman permanently unable to get pregnant and a man unable to get a woman pregnant

Some forms of birth control combine methods, such as IUDs that also release hormones. Some types of birth control may carry serious risks for some individuals. For specific information about birth control, individuals should talk to their healthcare providers.

What Are the Different Types of Contraception?

There are many different types of contraception, but not all types are appropriate for all situations. The most appropriate method of birth control depends on an individual's overall health, age, frequency of sexual activity, number of sexual partners, desire to have children in the future, and family history of certain diseases.

Long-Acting Reversible Contraception
Intrauterine Methods

An intrauterine device (IUD), also known as an "intrauterine system" (IUS), is a small, T-shaped device that is inserted into the uterus to prevent pregnancy. A healthcare provider inserts the device. An IUD can remain in place and function effectively for many years at a time. After the recommended length of time, or when the woman no longer needs or desires contraception, a healthcare provider replaces or removes the device.

- A hormonal IUD, or IUS, releases a progestin hormone (levonorgestrel) into the uterus. The released hormone causes thickening of the cervical mucus, inhibits sperm from reaching or fertilizing the egg, thins the uterine lining, and may prevent the ovaries from releasing eggs. The failure rate of a hormonal IUS is less than 1 percent; however, a small percentage of women may experience expulsion of the device and have to have it reinserted. Some research also suggests that these IUDs maintain their effectiveness up to a year beyond their recommended use period. This method may also be used to treat heavy menstrual bleeding because the hormone often reduces or eliminates uterine bleeding.

- A copper IUD prevents sperm from reaching and fertilizing the egg, and it may prevent the egg from attaching in the womb. If fertilization of the egg does occur, the physical presence of the device prevents the fertilized egg from implanting into the lining of the uterus. The failure and expulsion/reinsertion rates of a copper IUD are similar to those of a hormonal IUD. Copper IUDs may remain in the body for 10 years. A copper IUD is not recommended for women who may be pregnant, have pelvic infections, or had uterine perforations during previous IUD insertions. It also is not recommended for women who have cervical cancer or cancer of the uterus, unexplained vaginal bleeding, or pelvic tuberculosis. Currently, ParaGard® is the only U.S. Food and Drug Administration (FDA)-approved copper IUD.

Implants

Implants are implantable rods. Each rod is matchstick-sized, flexible, and plastic. The method has a failure rate of less than one percent. A physician surgically inserts the rod under the skin of the woman's upper arm.

The rod releases a progestin and can remain implanted for up to five years. Currently, Implanon® and Nexplanon®, which release etonogestrel, are the only implantable rods available in the United States. A two-rod method, Jadelle®, which releases levonorgestrel, is FDA approved but not currently distributed in America. A new levonorgestrel-releasing, two-rod method, Sino-implant (II)®, is in clinical development.

Hormonal Methods
Short-Acting Hormonal Methods

Hormonal methods of birth control use hormones to regulate or stop ovulation and prevent pregnancy. Ovulation is the biological process in which the ovary releases an egg, making it available for fertilization. Hormones can be introduced into the body through various methods, including pills, injections, skin patches, transdermal gels, vaginal rings, intrauterine systems, and implantable rods. Depending on the types of hormones that are used, these methods can prevent ovulation; thicken cervical mucus, which helps block sperm from reaching the egg; or thin the lining of the uterus. Healthcare providers prescribe and monitor hormonal contraceptives.

Short-acting hormonal methods (e.g., injectables, pills, patches, rings) are highly effective if used perfectly, but in typical use, they have a range of failure rates.

- **Injectable birth control.** This method involves injection of a progestin, Depo-Provera® (depot medroxyprogesterone acetate [DMPA]), given in the arm or buttocks once every three months. This method of birth control can cause a temporary loss of bone density, particularly in adolescents. However, this bone loss is generally regained after discontinuing use of DMPA. Most patients using injectable birth control should eat a diet rich in calcium and vitamin D or take vitamin supplements while using this medication. A new self-injectable formulation of DMPA, Sayana® Press, is approved in the United Kingdom and is expected to be approved more widely in the near future. This subcutaneous injectable product has a lower amount of hormone and may be more acceptable for some users.

- **Progestin-only pills (POPs).** A woman takes one pill daily, preferably at the same time each day. POPs may interfere with ovulation or with sperm function. POPs thicken cervical mucus, making it difficult for sperm to swim into the uterus or to enter the fallopian tube. POPs alter the normal cyclical changes in the uterine lining and may result in unscheduled or breakthrough bleeding. These hormones do not appear to be associated with an increased risk of blood clots.

Combined Hormonal Methods

Combined hormonal methods contain a synthetic estrogen (ethinyl estradiol) and one of the many progestins approved in the United States. All of the products work by inhibiting ovulation and thickening cervical mucus. The combined estrogen/progestin drugs can be delivered by pills, a patch, or a vaginal ring. The combined hormonal methods have some medical risks, such as blood clots, that are associated with the synthetic estrogen in the product. These risks have not been observed with progestin-only hormonal methods, such as injectable birth control, POPs, or hormonal long-acting reversible contraception (LARCs). Your healthcare provider can discuss your risk factors and help you select the most appropriate contraceptive method for you.

- **Combined oral contraceptives (COCs, "the pill").** COCs contain a synthetic estrogen and a progestin, which function to inhibit ovulation. A woman takes one pill daily, preferably at the same time each day. Many types of oral contraceptives are available, and a healthcare provider helps to determine which type best meets a woman's needs.

- **Contraceptive patch.** This is a thin, plastic patch that sticks to the skin and releases hormones through the skin into the bloodstream. The patch is placed on the lower abdomen, buttocks, outer arm, or upper body. A new patch is applied once a week for three weeks, and no patch is used on the fourth week to enable menstruation. Currently, Ortho Evra® is the only patch that is FDA approved.

- **Vaginal ring.** The ring is thin, flexible, and approximately two inches in diameter. It delivers a combination of ethinyl estradiol and a progestin. The ring is inserted into the vagina, where it continually releases hormones for three weeks. The woman removes it for the fourth week and reinserts a new ring seven days later. Risks for this method of contraception are similar to those for the combined oral contraceptive pills. A vaginal ring may not be recommended for women with certain health conditions, including high blood pressure, heart disease, or certain types of cancer. Currently, the NuvaRing® is the only FDA-approved vaginal ring. A new contraceptive vaginal ring that can be used for 13 cycles is under clinical development.

Barrier Methods

Designed to prevent sperm from entering the uterus, barrier methods are removable and may be an option for women who cannot use hormonal methods of contraception. Failure rates for barrier methods differ depending on the method.

Types of barrier methods that do not require a healthcare provider visit include the following:

- **Male condoms.** This condom is a thin sheath that covers the penis to collect sperm and prevent it from entering the woman's body. Male condoms are generally made of latex or polyurethane, but a natural alternative is lambskin (made from the intestinal membrane of lambs). Latex or polyurethane condoms reduce the risk of spreading sexually transmitted diseases (STDs). Lambskin condoms do not prevent STDs. Male condoms are disposed of after a single use.

- **Female condoms.** These are thin, flexible plastic pouches. A portion of the condom is inserted into a woman's vagina before intercourse to prevent sperm from entering the uterus. The female condom also reduces the risk of STDs. Female condoms are disposed of after a single use.

- **Contraceptive sponges.** These are soft, disposable, spermicide-filled foam sponges. One is inserted into the vagina before intercourse. The sponge helps block sperm from entering the uterus, and the spermicide also kills the sperm cells. The sponge should be left in place for at least six hours after intercourse and then removed within 30 hours after intercourse. Currently, the Today® Vaginal Contraceptive Sponge is the only sponge approved by the U.S. Food and Drug Administration (FDA).

- **Spermicides.** A spermicide can kill sperm cells. A spermicide can be used alone or in combination with a diaphragm or cervical cap. The most common spermicidal agent is a chemical called nonoxynol-9 (N-9). It is available in several concentrations and forms, including foam, jelly, cream, suppository, and film. A spermicide should be inserted into the vagina close to the uterus no more than 30 minutes prior to intercourse and left in place 6 to 8 hours after intercourse to prevent pregnancy. Spermicides do not prevent the transmission of STDs and may cause allergic reactions or vaginitis.

Methods that require a healthcare provider visit include the following:

- **Diaphragms.** Each diaphragm is a shallow, flexible cup made of latex or soft rubber that is inserted into the vagina before intercourse, blocking sperm from entering the uterus. Spermicidal cream or jelly should be used with a diaphragm. The diaphragm should remain in place for 6 to 8 hours after intercourse to prevent pregnancy, but it should be removed within 24 hours. Traditional latex diaphragms must be the correct size to work properly, and a healthcare provider can determine the proper fit.

A diaphragm should be replaced after one or two years. Women also need to be measured for a new diaphragm after giving birth, having pelvic surgery, or gaining or losing more than 15 pounds. Newer diaphragms, such as Caya®, are designed to fit most women and do not require fitting by a healthcare provider.

- **Cervical caps.** These are similar to diaphragms but are smaller and more rigid. The cervical cap is a thin silicone cup that is inserted into the vagina before intercourse to block sperm from entering the uterus. As with a diaphragm, the cervical cap should be used with spermicidal cream or jelly. The cap must remain in place for 6 to 8 hours after intercourse to prevent pregnancy, but it should be removed within 48 hours. Cervical caps come in different sizes, and a healthcare provider determines the proper fit. With proper care, a cervical cap can be used for two years before replacement. Currently, FemCap is the only cervical cap approved by the FDA.

Emergency Contraception

Emergency contraception can be used after unprotected intercourse or if a condom breaks.

- **Copper IUD.** The copper IUD is the most effective method of emergency contraception. The device can be inserted within 120 hours of unprotected intercourse. The method is nearly 100 percent effective at preventing pregnancy and has the added benefit of providing a highly effective method of contraception for as long as the device remains in place. There are very few contraindications to use of the copper IUD, and there are no issues related to weight or obesity associated with the effectiveness of the method.

- **Emergency contraceptive pills (ECPs)** are hormonal pills, taken either as a single dose or two doses 12 hours apart, that are intended for use in the event of unprotected intercourse. If taken prior to ovulation, the pills can delay or inhibit ovulation for at least five days to allow the sperm to become inactive. They also cause thickening of cervical mucus and may interfere with sperm function. ECPs should be taken as soon as possible after semen exposure and should not be used as a regular contraceptive method. Pregnancy can occur if the pills are taken after ovulation or if the woman has unprotected sex in the same cycle.

Sterilization

Sterilization is a permanent form of birth control that either prevents a woman from getting pregnant or prevents a man from releasing sperm. A healthcare provider must perform the sterilization procedure, which usually involves surgery. These procedures usually are not reversible.

- A sterilization implant is a nonsurgical method for permanently blocking the fallopian tubes. A healthcare provider threads a thin tube through the vagina and into the uterus to place a soft, flexible insert into each fallopian tube. No incisions are necessary. During the next three months, scar tissue forms around the inserts and blocks the fallopian tubes so that sperm cannot reach an egg. After three months, a healthcare provider conducts tests to ensure that scar tissue has fully blocked the fallopian tubes. A backup method of contraception is used until the tests show that the tubes are fully blocked.

- Tubal ligation is a surgical procedure in which a doctor cuts, ties, or seals the fallopian tubes. This procedure blocks the path between the ovaries and the uterus. The sperm cannot reach the egg to fertilize it, and the egg cannot reach the uterus.

- Vasectomy is a surgical procedure that cuts, closes, or blocks the vas deferens. This procedure blocks the path between the testes and the urethra. The sperm cannot leave the testes and cannot reach the egg. It can take as long as three months for the procedure to be fully effective. A backup method of contraception is used until tests confirm that there is no sperm in the semen.

Section 6.3

Mifepristone (The Morning-After Pill)

This section includes text excerpted from "Questions and
Answers on Mifeprex," U.S. Food and Drug
Administration (FDA), March 28, 2018.

What Is Mifeprex and How Does It Work?

Mifeprex (mifepristone) is a drug that blocks a hormone called
"progesterone" that is needed for a pregnancy to continue. Mifeprex,
when used together with another medicine called "misoprostol," is
used to end an early pregnancy (70 days or less since the first day of
the last menstrual period).

Who Should Not Take Mifeprex?

Some women should not take Mifeprex. A woman should not take
Mifeprex if it has been more than 70 days since the first day of her
last menstrual period, or if she:

- Has an ectopic pregnancy (a pregnancy outside of the uterus)

- Has problems with the adrenal glands (the glands near the
kidneys)

- Is currently being treated with long-term corticosteroid therapy
(medications)

- Has had an allergic reaction to mifepristone, misoprostol, or
similar drugs

- Has bleeding problems or is taking anticoagulant (blood-
thinning) drug products

- Has inherited porphyria

- Has an intrauterine device (IUD) in place (which must be
removed before taking Mifeprex)

What Changes to the Mifeprex Application Did the U.S. Food and Drug Administration Approve on March 29, 2016?

The U.S. Food and Drug Administration (FDA) first approved
Mifeprex in 2000. In 2016, the agency approved a supplemental

application submitted by the drug company that markets Mifeprex. This approval includes changes in the dose of Mifeprex and the dosing regimen for taking Mifeprex and misoprostol (including the dose of misoprostol and a change in the route of misoprostol administration from oral to buccal (in the cheek pouch), the interval between taking Mifeprex and misoprostol, and the location at which the woman may take misoprostol). The approval also modifies the gestational age up to which Mifeprex has been shown to be safe and effective, as well as the process for follow-up after administration of the drug. In addition, the labeling has been revised to meet the current labeling requirements in FDA regulations. The FDA also approved changes to the existing Risk Evaluation and Mitigation Strategy (REMS) to reflect the changes approved in the supplemental application, and to make the Mifeprex REMS consistent with more recently approved REMS.

Where Can Women Get Mifeprex?

Mifeprex is supplied directly to healthcare providers who meet certain qualifications. It is only available to be dispensed in certain healthcare settings, specifically, clinics, medical offices, and hospitals, by or under the supervision of a certified prescriber. It is not available in retail pharmacies, and it is not legally available over the Internet.

What Qualifications Must Healthcare Providers Have to Obtain and Dispense Mifeprex?

Healthcare providers who would like to become certified to prescribe Mifeprex must have the ability to date pregnancies accurately and to diagnose ectopic pregnancies. Healthcare providers must also be able to provide any necessary surgical intervention, or have made arrangements for others to provide for such care. Healthcare providers must be able to ensure that women have access to medical facilities for emergency care, and must agree to other responsibilities, including reviewing and signing the Patient Agreement Form with the patient and providing each patient with a copy of the signed Patient Agreement Form and the Medication Guide.

Healthcare providers who prescribe and who meet certain qualifications are authorized to order and dispense Mifeprex. Some states allow healthcare providers other than physicians to prescribe medications. Healthcare providers should check their individual state laws.

Are There Restrictions on the Distribution of This Drug?

Yes. When the agency reviewed and approved the original new drug application for Mifeprex, it concluded that certain distribution restrictions were necessary to ensure the safe use of the drug. After reviewing the data and information submitted by the drug company that markets Mifeprex, and after taking into consideration the safety data that have become available since the initial approval of Mifeprex in 2000, the FDA concluded that certain restrictions continue to be necessary to ensure the safe use of the drug.

What Are the Possible Side Effects of Using Mifeprex?

Cramping and vaginal bleeding are expected effects of the treatment regimen. In some cases, very heavy vaginal bleeding will need to be stopped by a surgical procedure, which can often be performed in the office. Other common side effects of the treatment regimen include nausea, weakness, fever/chills, vomiting, headache, diarrhea, and dizziness in the first day or two after taking the two medicines.

The possible side effects are described in the Adverse Reactions section of the labeling and in the Medication Guide for Mifeprex.

What Serious Adverse Events Have Been Reported after Mifeprex Use?

It is not uncommon for the FDA to receive reports of serious adverse events for prescription drugs after they are approved. The FDA has received reports of serious adverse events in women who took Mifeprex. As of December 31, 2017, there were reports of 22 deaths of women associated with Mifeprex since the product was approved in September 2000, including two cases of ectopic pregnancy resulting in death; and several cases of severe systemic infection (also called "sepsis"), including some that were fatal. The adverse events cannot with certainty be causally attributed to mifepristone because of concurrent use of other drugs, other medical or surgical treatments, coexisting medical conditions, and information gaps about patient health status and clinical management of the patient.

As with all approved drugs, when the FDA receives new information regarding adverse events, the agency reviews the new information and, as appropriate, takes necessary action, including providing updates to doctors and their patients so that they have information on how to use the drug safely.

What Should Healthcare Providers Watch for in Women Who Have Taken Mifeprex?

All providers of medical abortion and emergency room healthcare practitioners should investigate the possibility of sepsis in women who are undergoing medical abortion and present with nausea, vomiting, or diarrhea and weakness with or without abdominal pain. These symptoms, even without a fever, may indicate a serious infection. Strong consideration should be given to obtaining a complete blood count in these patients. Significant leukocytosis with a marked left shift and hemoconcentration may be indicative of sepsis.

When Can a Woman Become Pregnant Again If She Takes Mifeprex?

A woman can become pregnant again right after a pregnancy ends. If a woman does not want to become pregnant, she should start using a birth-control method after the pregnancy ends and before she resumes sexual activity.

How Much Does Mifeprex Cost?

A woman can become pregnant again right after a pregnancy ends. If a woman does not want to become pregnant, she should start using a birth-control method after the pregnancy ends and before she resumes sexual activity.

Is Mifeprex Approved in Any Other Countries?

Yes, mifepristone has been approved in France since 1998, and also is approved in the United Kingdom, Sweden and approximately 60 other countries.

Part Two

Understanding Pregnancy-Related Changes and Fetal Development

Chapter 7

Are You Pregnant?

Chapter Contents

Section 7.1

Signs of Pregnancy

This section includes text excerpted from "What Are Some Common Signs of Pregnancy?" *Eunice Kennedy Shriver* National Institute of Child Health and Human Development (NICHD), January 31, 2017.

What Are Some Common Signs of Pregnancy?

The primary sign of pregnancy is missing a menstrual period or two or more consecutive periods, but many women experience other symptoms of pregnancy before they miss a period.

Missing a period does not always mean a woman is pregnant. Menstrual irregularities are common and can have a variety of causes, including taking birth control pills, conditions such as diabetes and polycystic ovary syndrome (PCOS), eating disorders, and certain medications. Women who miss a period should see their healthcare provider to find out whether they are pregnant or whether they have another health problem.

Pregnancy symptoms vary from woman to woman. A woman may experience every symptom, just a few, or none at all. Some signs of early pregnancy include:

- **Slight bleeding.** One study shows as many as 25 percent of pregnant women experience slight bleeding or spotting that is lighter in color than normal menstrual blood. This typically occurs at the time of implantation of the fertilized egg (about 6 to 12 days after conception), but is common in the first 12 weeks of pregnancy.

- **Tender, swollen breasts or nipples.** Women may notice this symptom as early as one to two weeks after conception. Hormonal changes can make the breasts sore or even tingly. The breasts feel fuller or heavier as well.

- **Fatigue.** Many women feel more tired early in pregnancy because their bodies are producing more of a hormone called "progesterone," which helps maintain the pregnancy and encourages the growth of milk-producing glands in the breasts. In addition, the body pumps more blood to carry nutrients to the fetus. Pregnant women may notice fatigue as early as one week after conception.

- **Headaches.** The sudden rise of hormones may trigger headaches early in pregnancy.

- **Nausea and/or vomiting.** This symptom can start anywhere from two to eight weeks after conception and can continue throughout pregnancy. Commonly referred to as "morning sickness," it can actually occur at any time during the day.

- **Food cravings or aversions.** Sudden cravings or developing a dislike of favorite foods are both common throughout pregnancy. A food craving or aversion can last the entire pregnancy or vary throughout this period.

- **Mood swings.** Hormonal changes during pregnancy often cause sharp mood swings. These can occur as early as a few weeks after conception.

- **Frequent urination.** The need to empty the bladder more often is common throughout pregnancy. In the first few weeks of pregnancy, the body produces a hormone called "human chorionic gonadotropin," which increases blood flow to the pelvic region, causing women to have to urinate more often.

Many of these symptoms can also be signs of other conditions, results of changing birth control pills, or effects of stress, so they do not always mean that a woman is pregnant. Women should see their healthcare provider if they suspect they are pregnant.

Section 7.2

Pregnancy Tests

This section includes text excerpted from "Pregnancy Tests," Office on Women's Health (OWH), U.S. Department of Health and Human Services (HHS), January 31, 2019.

If you think you may be pregnant, taking a pregnancy test as soon as the first day of your missed period can help you get the care and support you need. A home pregnancy test can tell whether you are pregnant with almost 99 percent accuracy, depending on how you use it. If a pregnancy test says you are pregnant, you should see your doctor for another test to confirm the pregnancy and talk about the next steps.

How Soon Can I Use a Home Pregnancy Test?

Some home pregnancy tests are more sensitive than others and can be taken before a missed period. But you may get more accurate results if you wait until after the first day of your missed period. This is because the amount of the pregnancy hormone, called "human chorionic gonadotropin" (hCG), in your urine increases with time. The earlier you take the test, the harder it is for the test to detect hCG.

hCG is made when a fertilized egg implants in the uterus. This usually happens about 10 days after conception (when the man's sperm fertilizes the woman's egg).

My Pregnancy Test Says I Am Pregnant. What Should I Do Next?

If a home pregnancy test shows that you are pregnant, you should call your doctor to schedule an appointment.

Your doctor can use a blood test to tell for sure whether you are pregnant. Seeing your doctor early in your pregnancy also means you can begin prenatal care to help you and the fetus stay healthy.

My Pregnancy Test Says I Am Not Pregnant. Could I Still Be Pregnant?

Yes, it is possible you could still be pregnant. It is possible to be pregnant and to have a pregnancy test show that you are not pregnant.

The accuracy of home pregnancy test results varies from woman to woman because:

- Each woman ovulates at a different time in her menstrual cycle.

- The fertilized egg can implant in a woman's uterus at different times.

- Sometimes women get false-negative results when they test too early in the pregnancy. A false negative means that a test says you are not pregnant when you are.

- Problems with the pregnancy can affect the amount of hCG in the urine.

If a test says you are not pregnant, take another pregnancy test in a few days. If you are pregnant, your hCG levels should double every 48 hours. If you think you are pregnant but numerous tests say you are not, call your doctor.

What If I Can't Tell Whether My Pregnancy Test Is Positive or Negative?

Sometimes it can be hard to tell whether the test is positive or negative. The line may be faint, or you may worry whether you peed too much or too little on the stick.

No matter how faint the line or plus sign, if you see it, you are most likely pregnant. The faintness of the line can indicate that you are early in your pregnancy and hCG levels are still low.

A pregnancy test should also have a control line that tells you whether the test was done correctly. If the control line is blank, then the test did not work, and you should take another test.

What Should I Consider When Buying a Pregnancy Test?

- **Cost.** Home pregnancy tests come in many different types. Most stores sell them over-the-counter (OTC) (without a doctor's prescription). The cost varies depending on the brand and how many tests come in the box.

- **Accuracy.** Most tests can be taken as soon as you miss your period. Some newer, more expensive tests say they can be used four or five days before your period. Even so, tests report with the best accuracy only after the date of your expected period.

What Are the Different Types of Pregnancy Tests?

Pregnancy tests check for the hCG hormone in two ways:

- **Urine test.** This type of pregnancy test can be done at home or at a doctor's office.

- **Blood test.** This type of pregnancy test can only be done at a doctor's office. It takes longer than a urine test to get results, but it can detect a pregnancy earlier than a urine test (about 10 days after conception, compared to 2 weeks or more for a urine test). Your doctor may use one or both types of blood tests:

  - A quantitative blood test (also called a "beta hCG test") that measures the exact amount of hCG in your blood. It can even find tiny amounts of hCG. It can also tell you and your doctor how many weeks you are pregnant.

69

- A qualitative hCG blood test checks to see whether the pregnancy hormone is present or not. The qualitative hCG blood test is about as accurate as a urine test.

How Do I Use a Home Pregnancy Test?

All home pregnancy tests come with written instructions. Depending on the brand you buy, the instructions may vary:

- You hold a stick in your urine stream.

- You pee into a cup and dip a stick into it.

- You pee into a cup and then use a dropper to put a few drops of the urine into a special container.

Different brands tell you to wait different amounts of time; although most tests call for a wait time of two minutes. Depending on the brand of the test, you may see a line or a plus symbol, or the words "pregnant" or "not pregnant." A line or plus symbol, no matter how faint, means the result is positive.

Most tests also have a control indicator in the result window. This control line or symbol shows whether the test is working properly. If the control line or symbol does not appear, then the test is not working properly.

Look for the toll-free phone number on the package to call in case of questions about use or results.

How Accurate Are Home Pregnancy Tests?

Most home pregnancy tests claim to be up to 99 percent accurate. But the accuracy depends on:

- **How you use them.** Be sure to check the expiration date and follow the instructions. Wait up to 10 minutes after taking the test before checking the results window. Research suggests that waiting 10 minutes will give the most accurate result.

- **When you use them.** The amount of hCG in your urine increases with time. The earlier you take the test, the harder it is for the test to detect the hCG. Most home pregnancy tests can accurately detect pregnancy after a missed period. Also, testing your urine first thing in the morning can boost the accuracy.

- **Who uses them.** Each woman ovulates at a different time in her menstrual cycle, and a fertilized egg can implant in a woman's uterus at different times. Your body makes hCG after implantation occurs. In up to 10 percent of women, implantation does not occur until after the first day of a missed period. This means home pregnancy tests can be accurate for some women as soon as one day after a missed period.

- **The brand of test.** Some home pregnancy tests are more sensitive than others. For that reason, some tests are better than others at detecting hCG early on. Talk to your pharmacist about which brand may be best for you.

I Have Irregular Periods and Don't Know When My Next Period Will Start. When Should I Take a Pregnancy Test?

Most pregnancy tests claim to be the most accurate after a missed period. But irregular periods can make it hard to predict when to take a test.

Periods are considered irregular if:

- The number of days between periods is either shorter than 21 days or longer than 35 days.

- The number of days in the menstrual cycle varies from month to month. For example, your cycle may be 22 days one month and 33 days the next month.

If you have irregular periods, try counting 36 days from the start of your last menstrual cycle, or four weeks from the time you had sex. At this point, if you are pregnant, your levels of hCG should be high enough to detect the pregnancy.

If your test says you are not pregnant, but you still think you may be pregnant, wait a few more days and take another pregnancy test. Or, call your doctor for a blood test.

Can Anything Affect Home Pregnancy Test Results?

Yes. If you take medicine with the pregnancy hormone hCG as an active ingredient, you may get a false-positive test result. A false positive is when a test says you are pregnant when you are not.

Some examples of medicines with hCG include certain medicines for infertility. If you are taking medicine to help you get pregnant, you may want to see your doctor for a pregnancy test.

Most medicines should not affect the results of a home pregnancy test. This includes OTC and prescription medicines, such as birth control and antibiotics. Also, alcohol and illegal drugs do not affect pregnancy test results.

How Do Pregnancy Tests Work?

All pregnancy tests work by detecting hCG, in the urine or blood. This hormone is present only when a woman is pregnant. If the pregnancy test detects hCG, it will say you are pregnant.

hCG is made when a fertilized egg implants in the uterus. This usually happens about 10 days after conception. The amount of hCG builds up quickly in your body with each passing day you are pregnant.

So if you take a home pregnancy test too soon after implantation, your hCG level may not be high enough to detect the pregnancy. If the test says you are not pregnant, take another pregnancy test in a few days.

Chapter 8

Physical Changes during Pregnancy

Chapter Contents

Section 8.1

Common Pregnancy Discomforts

This section includes text excerpted from "Body Changes and Discomforts," Office on Women's Health (OWH), U.S. Department of Health and Human Services (HHS), January 30, 2019.

Everyone expects pregnancy to bring an expanding waistline. But many women are surprised by the other body changes that also occur.

Body Aches

As your uterus expands, you may feel aches and pains in the back, abdomen, groin area, and thighs. Many women also have backaches and aching near the pelvic bone due to the pressure of the fetus's head, increased weight, and loosening joints. Some pregnant women complain of pain that runs from the lower back, down the back of one leg, and to the knee or foot. This is called "sciatica." It is thought to occur when the uterus puts pressure on the sciatic nerve.

What Might Help?

- Lie down
- Rest
- Apply heat

Call the doctor if pain does not improve.

Breast Changes

A woman's breasts increase in size and fullness during pregnancy. As the due date approaches, hormone changes will cause your breasts to grow in preparation of breastfeeding. Your breasts may feel full, heavy, or tender.

In the third trimester, some pregnant women begin to leak colostrum from their breasts. Colostrum is the first milk that your breasts produce for the baby. It is a thick, yellowish fluid containing antibodies that protect newborns from infection.

What Might Help?

- Wear a maternity bra with good support.
- Put pads in your bra to absorb leakage.

Tell your doctor if you feel a lump or have nipple changes or discharge (that is not colostrum) or skin changes.

Constipation

Many pregnant women complain of constipation. Signs of constipation include having hard, dry stools; fewer than three bowel movements per week; and painful bowel movements.

Higher levels of hormones due to pregnancy slow down digestion and relax muscles in the bowels, leaving many women constipated. The pressure of the expanding uterus on the bowels can also contribute to constipation.

What Might Help?

- Drink eight to ten glasses of water daily.

- Do not drink caffeine.

- Eat fiber-rich foods, such as fresh or dried fruit, raw vegetables, and whole-grain cereals and breads.

- Try mild physical activity.

Tell your doctor if constipation does not go away.

Dizziness

Many pregnant women complain of dizziness and lightheadedness throughout their pregnancies. Fainting is rare but can even occur in healthy pregnant women. There are many reasons for these symptoms. The growth of more blood vessels in early pregnancy, the pressure of the expanding uterus on blood vessels, and the body's increased need for food can all make a pregnant woman feel lightheaded and dizzy.

What Might Help?

- Stand up slowly.

- Avoid standing for too long.

- Do not skip meals.

- Lie on your left side.

- Wear loose clothing.

Call your doctor if you feel faint and have vaginal bleeding or abdominal pain.

Fatigue, Sleep Problems

During your pregnancy, you might feel tired even after a lot of sleep. Many women find they are exhausted in the first trimester. Don't worry, this is normal. This is your body's way of telling you that you need more rest. In the second trimester, tiredness is usually replaced with a feeling of well-being and energy. But in the third trimester, exhaustion often sets in again. As the fetus grows, sleeping may become more difficult. Bathroom runs, an increase in the body's metabolism, and the fetus's movements might interrupt or disturb sleep. Leg cramping can also interfere with a good night's sleep.

What Might Help?

- Lie on your left side.

- Use pillows for support, such as behind your back, tucked between your knees, and under your stomach.

- Practice good sleep habits, such as going to bed and getting up at the same time each day and using your bed only for sleep and sex.

- Go to bed a little earlier.

- Nap if you are not able to get enough sleep at night.

- Drink needed fluids earlier in the day, so you can drink less in the hours before bed.

Heartburn and Indigestion

Hormones and the pressure of the growing uterus cause indigestion and heartburn. Pregnancy hormones slow down the muscles of the digestive tract, so food tends to move more slowly, and digestion is sluggish. This causes many pregnant women to feel bloated.

Hormones also relax the valve that separates the esophagus from the stomach. This allows food and acids to come back up from the stomach and into the esophagus. The food and acid causes the burning feeling of heartburn. As the fetus gets bigger, the uterus pushes on the stomach making heartburn more common in later pregnancy.

What Might Help?

- Eat several small meals instead of three large meals, and eat slowly.

- Drink fluids between meals, not with meals.

- Do not eat greasy and fried foods.

- Avoid citrus fruits or juices and spicy foods.

- Do not eat or drink within a few hours of bedtime.

- Do not lie down right after meals.

Call your doctor if symptoms do not improve after trying these suggestions. Ask your doctor about using an antacid.

Hemorrhoids

Hemorrhoids are swollen and bulging veins in the rectum. They can cause itching, pain, and bleeding. Up to 50 percent of pregnant women get hemorrhoids. Hemorrhoids are common during pregnancy for many reasons. During pregnancy, blood volume increases greatly, which can cause veins to enlarge. The expanding uterus also puts pressure on the veins in the rectum. Plus, constipation can worsen hemorrhoids. Hemorrhoids usually improve after delivery.

What Might Help?

- Drink lots of fluids.

- Eat fiber-rich foods, like whole grains, raw or cooked leafy green vegetables, and fruits.

- Try not to strain with bowel movements.

- Talk to your doctor about using products, such as witch hazel, to soothe hemorrhoids.

Itching

About 20 percent of pregnant women feel itchy during pregnancy, usually in the abdomen. But red, itchy palms and soles of the feet are also common complaints. Pregnancy hormones and stretching skin are probably to blame for most of this discomfort. The itchy feeling typically goes away after delivery.

What Might Help?

- Use gentle soaps and moisturizing creams.

- Avoid hot showers and baths.

- Avoid itchy fabrics.

  Call your doctor if symptoms do not improve after a week of self-care.

Leg Cramps

At different times during your pregnancy, you might have sudden muscle spasms in your legs or feet. They usually occur at night. This is due to a change in the way your body processes calcium.

What Might Help?

- Gently stretch muscles.

- Get mild exercise.

- For sudden cramps, flex your foot forward.

- Eat calcium-rich foods.

- Ask your doctor about calcium supplements.

Morning Sickness

In the first trimester, hormone changes can cause nausea and vomiting. This is called "morning sickness," although it can occur at any time of the day. Morning sickness usually tapers off by the second trimester.

What Might Help?

- Eat several small meals instead of three large meals to keep your stomach from being empty.

- Do not lie down after meals.

- Eat dry toast, saltines, or dry cereals before getting out of bed in the morning.

- Eat bland foods that are low in fat and easy to digest, such as cereal, rice, and bananas.

- Sip on water, weak tea, clear soft drinks, or eat ice chips.

- Avoid smells that upset your stomach.

Call your doctor if you have flu-like symptoms, which may signal a more serious condition.

Call your doctor if you have severe, constant nausea and/or vomiting several times every day.

Nasal Problems

Nosebleeds and nasal stuffiness are common during pregnancy. They are caused by the increased amount of blood in your body and hormones acting on the tissues of your nose.

What Might Help?

- Blow your nose gently.

- Drink fluids, and use a cool mist humidifier.

- To stop a nosebleed, squeeze your nose between your thumb and forefinger for a few minutes.

Call your doctor if nosebleeds are frequent and do not stop after a few minutes.

Numb or Tingling Hands

Feelings of swelling, tingling, and numbness in fingers and hands, called "carpal tunnel syndrome," can occur during pregnancy. These symptoms are due to swelling of tissues in the narrow passages in your wrists, and they should disappear after delivery.

What Might Help?

- Take frequent breaks to rest hands.

- Ask your doctor about fitting you for a splint to keep wrists straight.

Stretch Marks, Skin Changes

Stretch marks are red, pink, or brown streaks on the skin. Most often they appear on the thighs, buttocks, abdomen, and breasts. These scars are caused by the stretching of the skin, and usually appear in the second half of pregnancy.

Some women notice other skin changes during pregnancy. For many women, the nipples become darker and browner during pregnancy. Many pregnant women also develop a dark line (called the "linea nigra") on the skin that runs from the belly button down to the pubic hairline. Patches of darker skin over the cheeks, forehead, nose, or upper lip are also common. Patches often match on both sides of the face. These spots are called "melasma" or "chloasma" and are more common in darker-skinned women.

What Might Help?

- Be patient—stretch marks and other changes usually fade after delivery.

Swelling

Many women develop mild swelling in the face, hands, or ankles at some point in their pregnancies. As the due date approaches, swelling often becomes more noticeable.

What Might Help?

- Drink 8 to 10 glasses of fluids daily.
- Do not drink caffeine or eat salty foods.
- Rest and elevate your feet.
- Ask your doctor about support hose.

Call your doctor if your hands or feet swell suddenly or you rapidly gain weight, as this may be preeclampsia.

Urinary Frequency and Leaking

Temporary bladder control problems are common during pregnancy. The fetus pushes down on the bladder, urethra, and pelvic-floor muscles. This pressure can lead a more frequent need to urinate, as well as leaking of urine when sneezing, coughing, or laughing.

What Might Help?

- Take frequent bathroom breaks.
- Drink plenty of fluids to avoid dehydration.

- Do Kegel exercises to tone pelvic muscles.

Call your doctor if you experience burning along with frequency of urination, as this may be an infection.

Varicose Veins

During pregnancy, blood volume increases greatly. This can cause veins to enlarge. Plus, pressure on the large veins behind the uterus causes the blood to slow upon returning to the heart. For these reasons, varicose veins in the legs and anus (hemorrhoids) are more common in pregnancy.

Varicose veins look like swollen veins raised above the surface of the skin. They can be twisted or bulging, and are dark purple or blue in color. They are found most often on the backs of the calves or on the inside of the leg.

What Might Help?

- Avoid tight knee-highs.

- Sit with your legs and feet raised.

Section 8.2

Back Pain during Pregnancy

"Back Pain during Pregnancy," © 2019 Omnigraphics.
Reviewed February 2019.

During pregnancy, a woman can expect some degree of discomfort in her back. Back pain is prevalent in almost 50 to 70 percent of all pregnant women and can be experienced at any point of the pregnancy. However, it occurs most commonly in the later stages of pregnancy. This pain may persist after delivery (postpartum)—but usually resolves after some months—and can sometimes be intense enough to disrupt daily activities and interfere with good night's sleep.

The types of back pain that occur during pregnancy are:

- **Lumbar or lower-back pain** generally occurs in the center of the back, at and above the waist. It is similar to the lower-back pain experienced by nonpregnant woman. Lumbar or lower-back pain that radiates into the legs or feet is called "sciatica." Lower-back pain during pregnancy may or may not be concurrent with sciatica.

- **Posterior pelvic pain** is a deep pain felt below and at the side of the waistline and across the tailbone on either side. This kind of a pain in the back or pelvis can sometimes radiate down to the buttocks region and further down to the upper posterior portion of the thighs (the back of the thighs), but does not extend below the knees. Posterior pelvic pain can sometimes be associated with pubic pain and morning stiffness.

Risk factors for back pain during pregnancy include obesity and a prior history of back pain.

Some of the potential causes of back pain or discomfort during pregnancy are:

- **Hormonal changes.** Hormones released during pregnancy allow the softening and relaxation of ligaments attached to the pelvic bones and spine and loosen the joints in preparation for birth. These changes affect back support and cause pain while walking, climbing stairs, sitting for prolonged periods of time, rolling over in bed, getting out of a low chair or the tub, bending, and lifting.

- **Muscle separation.** As the uterus expands during pregnancy, rectal abdominis muscles (two parallel sheets of muscles that run from the ribcage to the pubic bone) separate to create space for the fetus to grow. This can worsen the back pain or discomfort.

- **Center of gravity.** An expectant mother's center of gravity shifts forward as a result of significant weight gain in the abdominal region. This postural change can trigger back pain.

- **Additional weight.** As the fetus grows, the back is responsible for managing the additional weight, which can contribute to some amount of discomfort.

- **Posture or position.** Poor posture while walking, sitting for prolonged periods of time, excessive standing, and inappropriate bending can escalate the back pain.

- **Increased stress.** Stress increases muscle stiffness and pain, especially in weak areas, which contributes to pain.

Tips for Reducing Back Pain throughout the Pregnancy

- Avoid excessive weight gain. Gain a healthy amount of weight by maintaining a healthy diet.
- Maintain good posture. Stand straight with a high chest and relaxed shoulders and back.
- Avoid standing for long periods of time.
- Wear supportive footwear and avoid high-heels. Move your feet while turning to avoid twisting your spine. Balance your weight on both sides when completing activities.
- Ensure that the chairs that you sit in provide good back support, and use a lumbar pillow for additional support.
- Elevate your feet while resting.
- When bending down, bend at your knees and try to keep your back straight (squat) as you pick things up.
- Avoid heavy lifting.
- Avoid sleeping on your back. Try to sleep on your side instead, with pillows tucked under your abdomen and between your knees for support.
- Avoid tight clothing. Wearing comfortable, loose garments may relieve back pressure to some extent.
- Include pregnancy-safe exercise in your daily routine. Pregnancy-safe exercise includes swimming, relaxed walking, and pelvic tilts, and is designed to support and strengthen the abdomen and back.
- If the back pain seems to be related to stress, then prenatal yoga, meditation, and extra rest may be helpful.
- Use cold compresses (ice packs) and prenatal massage to relax and soothe an aching back.
- Get plenty of rest.
- Contact a local chiropractor who specializes in pregnancy-related care and learn how small adjustments can help ease the back pain.

- If the pain is unbearable, then contact your doctor. Don't take any pain-relief medication without prior approval from your doctor.

References

1. "Back Pain in Pregnancy," WebMD, August 4, 2018.

2. "Back Pain during Pregnancy," Mayoclinic, April 5, 2016.

3. "Types of Back Pain in Pregnancy," SPINE-health, May 28, 2008.

Section 8.3

Carpal Tunnel Syndrome

This section includes text excerpted from "Carpal Tunnel Syndrome," Office on Women's Health (OWH), U.S. Department of Health and Human Services (HHS), January 31, 2019.

What Is Carpal Tunnel Syndrome?

Carpal tunnel syndrome (CTS) is the name for a group of problems that includes swelling, pain, tingling, and loss of strength in your wrist and hand. Your wrist is made of small bones that form a narrow groove or carpal tunnel. Tendons and a nerve called the "median nerve" must pass through this tunnel from your forearm into your hand. The median nerve controls the feelings and sensations in the palm side of your thumb and fingers. Sometimes swelling and irritation of the tendons can put pressure on the wrist nerve, causing the symptoms of CTS. A person's dominant hand is the one that is usually affected. However, nearly half of CTS sufferers have symptoms in both hands.

CTS has become more common in the United States and is quite costly in terms of time lost from work and expensive medical treatment.

The U.S. Department of Labor (DOL) reported that in 2015 the average number of missed days of work due to CTS was 28 days.

What Are the Symptoms of Carpal Tunnel Syndrome?

Typically, CTS begins slowly with feelings of burning, tingling, and numbness in the wrist and hand. The areas most affected are the thumb, index, and middle fingers. At first, symptoms may happen more often at night. Many CTS sufferers do not make the connection between a daytime activity that might be causing the CTS and the delayed symptoms. Also, many people sleep with their wrist bent, which may cause more pain and symptoms at night. As CTS gets worse, the tingling may be felt during the daytime too, along with pain moving from the wrist to your arm or down to your fingers. Pain is usually felt more on the palm side of the hand.

Another symptom of CTS is weakness of the hands that gets worse over time. Some people with CTS find it difficult to grasp an object, make a fist, or hold onto something small. The fingers may even feel like they are swollen even though they are not. Over time, this feeling will usually happen more often.

If left untreated, those with CTS can have a loss of feeling in some fingers and permanent weakness of the thumb. Thumb muscles can actually waste away over time. Eventually, CTS sufferers may have trouble telling the difference between hot and cold temperatures by touch.

What Causes Carpal Tunnel Syndrome and Who Is More Likely to Develop It?

Women are three times more likely to have CTS than men. Although there is limited research on why this is the case, scientists have several ideas. It may be that the wrist bones are naturally smaller in most women, creating a tighter space through which the nerves and tendons must pass. Other researchers are looking at genetic links that make it more likely for women to have musculoskeletal injuries, such as CTS. Women also deal with strong hormonal changes during pregnancy and menopause that make them more likely to suffer from CTS. Generally, women are at higher risk of CTS between the ages of 45 and 54. Then, the risk increases for both men and women as they age.

There are other factors that can cause CTS, including certain health problems and, in some cases, the cause is unknown.

These are some of the risk factors that might increase your chances of developing CTS:

- **Genetic predisposition.** The carpal tunnel is smaller in some people than others.

- **Repetitive movements.** People who do the same movements with their wrists and hands over and over may be more likely to develop CTS. People with certain types of jobs are more likely to have CTS, including manufacturing and assembly line workers, grocery store checkers, violinists, and carpenters. Some hobbies and sports that use repetitive hand movements can also cause CTS, such as golfing, knitting, and gardening. Whether or not long-term typing or computer use causes CTS is still being debated. Limited research points to a weak link, but more research is needed.

- **Injury or trauma.** A sprain or a fracture of the wrist can cause swelling and pressure on the nerve, increasing the risk of CTS. Forceful and stressful movements of the hand and wrist can also cause trauma, such as strong vibrations caused by heavy machinery or power tools.

- **Pregnancy.** Hormonal changes during pregnancy and buildup of fluid can put pregnant women at greater risk of getting CTS, especially during the last few months. Most doctors treat CTS in pregnant women with wrist splints or rest, rather than surgery, as CTS almost always goes away following childbirth.

- **Menopause.** Hormonal changes during menopause can put women at greater risk of getting CTS. Also, in some postmenopausal women, the wrist structures become enlarged and can press on the wrist nerve.

- **Breast cancer.** Some women who have a mastectomy get lymphedema, the buildup of fluids that go beyond the lymph system's ability to drain it. In mastectomy patients, this causes pain and swelling of the arm. Although rare, some of these women will get CTS due to pressure on the nerve from this swelling.

- **Medical conditions.** People who have diabetes, hypothyroidism, lupus, obesity, and rheumatoid arthritis are more likely to get CTS. In some of these patients, the normal structures in the wrist can become enlarged and lead to CTS.

Also, smokers with CTS usually have worse symptoms and recover more slowly than nonsmokers.

How Is Carpal Tunnel Syndrome Treated?

It is important to be treated by a doctor for CTS in order to avoid permanent damage to the wrist nerve and muscles of the hand and thumb. Underlying causes, such as diabetes or a thyroid problem, should be addressed first. Left untreated, CTS can cause nerve damage that leads to loss of feeling and hand strength. Over time, the muscles of the thumb can become weak and damaged. You can even lose the ability to feel hot and cold by touch. Permanent injury occurs in about one percent of those with CTS.

CTS is much easier to treat early on. Most CTS patients get better after first-step treatments and the following tips for protecting the wrist. Treatments for CTS include the following:

- **Wrist splint.** A splint can be worn to support and brace your wrist in a neutral position so that the nerves and tendons can recover. A splint can be worn 24 hours a day or only at night. Sometimes, wearing a splint at night helps to reduce the pain. Splinting can work the best when done within three months of having any symptoms of CTS.

- **Rest.** For people with mild CTS, stopping or doing less of a repetitive movement may be all that is needed. Your doctor will likely talk to you about steps that you should take to prevent CTS from coming back.

- **Medication.** The short-term use of nonsteroidal anti-inflammatory drugs (NSAIDs) may be helpful to control CTS pain. NSAIDs include aspirin, ibuprofen, and other nonprescription pain relievers. In severe cases, an injection of cortisone may help to reduce swelling. Your doctor may also give you corticosteroids in a pill form. But, these treatments only relieve symptoms temporarily. If CTS is caused by another health problem, your doctor will probably treat that problem first. If you have diabetes, it is important to know that long-term corticosteroid use can make it hard to control insulin levels.

- **Physical therapy.** A physical therapist can help you do special exercises to make your wrist and hand stronger. There are also many different kinds of treatments that can make CTS better and help relieve symptoms. Massage, yoga, ultrasound, chiropractic manipulation, and acupuncture are just a few such options that have been found to be helpful. You should talk with your doctor before trying these alternative treatments.

- **Surgery.** CTS surgery is one of the most common surgeries done in the United States. Generally, surgery is only an option for severe cases of CTS and/or after other treatments have failed for a period of at least six months. Open-release surgery is a common approach to CTS surgery and involves making a small incision in the wrist or palm and cutting the ligament to enlarge the carpal tunnel. This surgery is done under a local anesthetic to numb the wrist and hand area and is an outpatient procedure.

What Is the Best Way to Prevent Carpal Tunnel Syndrome?

Current research is focused on figuring out what causes CTS and how to prevent it. The National Institute of Neurological Disorders and Stroke (NINDS) and the National Institute of Arthritis and Musculo-skeletal and Skin Diseases (NIAMS) support research on work-related factors that may cause CTS. Scientists are also researching better ways to detect and treat CTS, including alternative treatments, such as acupuncture.

The following steps can help to prevent CTS:

- **Prevent workplace musculoskeletal injury.** Make sure that your workspace and equipment are at the right height and distance for your hands and wrist to work with less strain. If you are working on a computer, the keyboard should be at a height that allows your wrist to rest comfortably without having to bend at an angle. Desk or table workspace should be about 27 to 29 inches above the floor for most people. It also helps to keep your elbows close to your sides as you type to reduce the strain on your forearm. Keeping good posture and wrist position can lower your risk of getting CTS.

- **Take breaks.** Allowing your hand and wrist to rest and recover every so often will lower your risk of swelling. Experts believe that taking a 10 to 15 minute break every hour is a good way to prevent CTS.

- **Vary tasks.** Avoid repetitive movements without changing up your routine. Try to do tasks that use different muscle movements during each hour. Break up tasks that require repetitive wrist and hand motion with those that do not.

- **Relax your grip.** Sometimes, people get into a habit of tensing muscles without needing to. Practice doing hand and wrist motion tasks more gently and less tightly. Stress and tension play a role in muscle strain and irritation.

- **Do exercises.** After doing repetitive movements for a while, you can sometimes cancel out the effects of those movements by flexing and bending your wrists and hands in the opposite direction. For example, after typing with your wrist and hand extended, it is helpful to make a tight fist and hold it for a second, then stretch out the fingers and hold for a few seconds. Try repeating this several times.

- **Stay warm.** Muscles that are warm are less likely to get hurt, and the risk of getting CTS is greater in a cold environment. It is important to keep your hands warm while you work, even if you must wear fingerless gloves.

Chapter 9

Pregnancy, Pelvic-Floor Disorders, and Bladder Control

Chapter Contents

91

Section 9.1

Pregnancy and Pelvic-Floor Disorders

This section includes text excerpted from "Pelvic Floor
Disorders: Condition Information," *Eunice Kennedy Shriver*
National Institute of Child Health and Human
Development (NICHD), December 1, 2016.

What Is the Pelvic-Floor?

The term "pelvic floor" refers to the group of muscles that form a sling or hammock across the pelvis. Together with their surrounding tissues, these muscles hold the pelvic organs, such as the uterus, bladder, or bowel, in place so that they can function correctly. The pelvic organs include the bladder, urethra, small intestine, and rectum. A woman's pelvic organs also include the uterus, cervix, and vagina.

What Is a Pelvic-Floor Disorder?

A pelvic-floor disorder (PFD) occurs when the pelvic muscles and connective tissue weaken or are injured. The most common types of PFDs are the following:

- **Pelvic-organ prolapse.** A "prolapse" occurs in women when the pelvic muscles and tissue can no longer support one or more pelvic organs, causing them to drop or press into the vagina. For instance, in uterine prolapse, the cervix and uterus can descend into the vagina and even come out of the vaginal opening. In vaginal prolapse, the top of the vagina loses support and can drop through the vaginal opening. Prolapse can also cause a kink in the urethra, the tube that brings urine from the bladder to the outside of the body.

- **Bladder-control problems.** The leaking of urine, a problem called "urinary incontinence," can occur in women or men when the bladder falls from its proper place. Other symptoms include a sudden, strong urge to urinate.

- **Bowel-control problems.** The leaking of liquid or solid stool from the rectum, called "fecal incontinence," can occur in women and men when the rectum is out of place. It can also occur if there is damage to the anal sphincter, the ring of muscles that keep the anus closed.

What Causes Pelvic-Floor Disorders?

The complete picture about what contributes to the development of pelvic-floor problems is not clear, but the following conditions are being studied as possible contributors:

- **Pregnancy and childbirth.** Going through pregnancy and childbirth and the relation to pelvic-floor problems has been an active area of research, but the contribution is not clear. In some studies, the risk increases with the number of children a woman has. The risk may be greater if forceps or a vacuum device is used during delivery. However, because pelvic problems also affect women who have never been pregnant, and because delivering via cesarean section (C-section) does not eliminate the risk of pelvic floor problems, the relationship among pregnancy, childbirth, and PFDs remains unknown.

- **Factors that put pressure on the pelvic floor.** These factors include being overweight or obese, chronic constipation and straining during bowel movements, and chronic coughing from smoking or health problems.

- **Getting older.** The pelvic floor can weaken as women age. However, this weakening does not occur for all women, leading many researchers to believe it may not be a natural part of aging, but rather due to other contributors.

- **Having weaker tissues.** Genes and race influence the strength of a woman's bones, muscles, and connective tissues. Women born with genetically weaker tissues are more likely to have pelvic-organ prolapse. African American women may have a lower risk of pelvic organ prolapse than women of other races.

- **Radiation treatment.** Radiation therapy for endometrial, cervical, or other types of cancer in a woman's pelvic region can damage pelvic-floor muscles and tissues.

- **Surgery.** Hysterectomy and prior surgery to correct prolapse increase the risk of PFDs.

How Many Women Have Pelvic-Floor Disorders?

More than one-third of U.S. women have a PFD, and nearly one-quarter of women in the United States have one or more PFDs that cause symptoms. PFDs are more likely to occur as a woman gets older. An estimated 377,000 women underwent surgery in 2010 to correct a bladder control problem or pelvic-organ prolapse, and this number is projected to rise sharply over the next several decades.

Section 9.2

Pregnancy and Bladder Control

This section includes text excerpted from "Urinary Incontinence," Office on Women's Health (OWH), U.S. Department of Health and Human Services (HHS), January 31, 2019.

Urinary incontinence is the loss of bladder control. The two most common types of urinary incontinence that affect women are stress incontinence and urge incontinence, also called "overactive bladder." Incontinence affects twice as many women as men. This may be because pregnancy, childbirth, and menopause may make urinary incontinence more likely. Urinary incontinence is not a normal part of aging and can be treated.

What Is Urinary Incontinence?

Urine is made by the kidneys and stored in the bladder. The bladder has muscles that tighten when you need to urinate. When the bladder muscles tighten, urine is forced out of your bladder through a tube called the "urethra." At the same time, sphincter muscles around the urethra relax to let the urine out of your body.

Incontinence can happen when the bladder muscles suddenly tighten, and the sphincter muscles are not strong enough to pinch the urethra shut. This causes a sudden, strong, and uncontrollable urge to urinate. Pressure caused by laughing, sneezing, or exercising can cause you to leak urine. Urinary incontinence may also happen if there is a problem with the nerves that control the bladder muscles and urethra. Urinary incontinence can mean you leak a small amount of urine or release a lot of urine all at once.

Who Gets Urinary Incontinence?

Urinary incontinence affects twice as many women as men. This is because reproductive health events unique to women, like pregnancy, childbirth, and menopause, affect the bladder, urethra, and other muscles that support these organs.

Urinary incontinence can happen to women at any age, but it is more common in older women. This is most likely due to hormonal changes during menopause. More than 4 in 10 women 65 years of age and older have urinary incontinence.

Why Does Urinary Incontinence Affect More Women Than Men?

Women have unique health events, such as pregnancy, childbirth, and menopause, that may affect the urinary tract and the surrounding muscles. The pelvic-floor muscles that support the bladder, urethra, uterus (womb), and bowels may become weakened or damaged. When the muscles that support the urinary tract are weak, the muscles in the urinary tract must work harder to hold urine until you are ready to urinate. This extra stress or pressure on the bladder and urethra can cause urinary incontinence or leakage.

The female urethra is also shorter than the male urethra. Any weakness or damage to the urethra in a woman is more likely to cause urinary incontinence. This is because there is less muscle keeping the urine in until you are ready to urinate.

What Are the Symptoms of Urinary Incontinence?

Urinary incontinence is not a disease by itself. Urinary incontinence is a symptom of another health problem, usually weak pelvic-floor muscles. In addition to urinary incontinence, some women have other urinary symptoms:

- Pressure or spasms in the pelvic area that causes a strong urge to urinate

- Going to the bathroom more than usual (more than eight times a day or more than twice at night)

- Urinating while sleeping (bedwetting)

What Causes Urinary Incontinence

Urinary incontinence is usually caused by problems with the muscles and nerves that help the bladder hold or pass urine. Certain health events unique to women, such as pregnancy, childbirth, and menopause, can cause problems with these muscles and nerves.

Other causes of urinary incontinence include:

- **Being overweight.** Being overweight puts pressure on the bladder, which can weaken the muscles over time. A weak bladder cannot hold as much urine.

- **Constipation.** Problems with bladder control can happen to people with long-term (chronic) constipation. Constipation, or straining to have a bowel movement, can put stress or pressure on the bladder and pelvic-floor muscles. This weakens the muscles and can cause urinary incontinence or leaking.

- **Nerve damage.** Damaged nerves may send signals to the bladder at the wrong time or not at all. Childbirth and health problems, such as diabetes and multiple sclerosis, can cause nerve damage in the bladder, urethra, or pelvic-floor muscles.

- **Surgery.** Any surgery that involves a woman's reproductive organs, such as a hysterectomy, can damage the supporting pelvic-floor muscles, especially if the uterus is removed. If the pelvic-floor muscles are damaged, a woman's bladder muscles may not work like they should. This can cause urinary incontinence.

Sometimes urinary incontinence lasts only for a short time and happens because of other reasons, including:

- **Certain medicines.** Urinary incontinence may be a side effect of medicines, such as diuretics ("water pills" used to treat heart failure, liver cirrhosis, hypertension, and certain kidney diseases). The incontinence often goes away when you stop taking the medicine.

- **Caffeine.** Drinks with caffeine can cause the bladder to fill quickly, which can cause you to leak urine. Studies suggest that women who drink more than two cups of drinks with caffeine per day may be more likely to have problems with incontinence. Limiting caffeine may help with incontinence because there is less strain on your bladder.

- **Infection.** Infections of the urinary tract and bladder may cause incontinence for a short time. Bladder control often returns when the infection goes away.

How Does Pregnancy Cause Urinary Incontinence?

As many as 4 in 10 women get urinary incontinence during pregnancy. During pregnancy, as the fetus grows, she or he pushes down on your bladder, urethra, and pelvic-floor muscles. Over time, this pressure may weaken the pelvic-floor muscles and lead to leaks or problems passing urine.

Most problems with bladder control during pregnancy go away after childbirth when the muscles have had some time to heal. If you are still having bladder problems six weeks after childbirth, talk to your doctor, nurse, or midwife.

How Does Childbirth Cause Urinary Incontinence?

Problems during labor and childbirth, especially vaginal birth, can weaken pelvic-floor muscles and damage the nerves that control the bladder. Most problems with bladder control that are a result of labor and delivery go away after the muscles have had some time to heal. If you are still having bladder problems six weeks after childbirth, talk to your doctor, nurse, or midwife.

How Does Menopause Cause Urinary Incontinence?

Some women have bladder-control problems after they stop having periods. Researchers think that having low levels of the estrogen hormone after menopause may weaken the urethra. The urethra helps keep urine in the bladder until you are ready to urinate.

Also, like all muscles, the bladder and urethra muscles lose some of their strength as you get older. This means you may not be able to hold as much urine as you get older.

What Type of Doctor or Nurse Should I Go to for Help with Urinary Incontinence?

If you have urinary incontinence, you can make an appointment with your primary care provider, your obstetrician-gynecologist (OB-GYN), or a nurse practitioner. Your doctor or nurse will work with you to treat your urinary incontinence or refer you to a specialist if you need different treatment.

The specialist may be a urologist, who treats urinary problems in both men and women, or a urogynecologist, who has special training in the female urinary system. You might also need to see a pelvic-floor specialist, a type of physical therapist, who will work with you to strengthen your pelvic-floor muscles that support the urinary tract.

How Is Urinary Incontinence Diagnosed?

Your doctor or nurse will ask you about your symptoms and your medical history, including:

- How often you empty your bladder

- How and when you leak urine

- How much urine you leak

- When your symptoms started

- What medicines you take

- If you have ever been pregnant and what your labor and delivery experience was like

Your doctor or nurse will do a physical exam to look for signs of health problems that can cause incontinence.

Your doctor or nurse also may do other tests such as:

- **Urine test.** After you urinate into a cup, the doctor or nurse will send your urine to a lab. At the lab, your urine will be checked for an infection or other causes of incontinence.

- **Ultrasound.** Your doctor will use an ultrasound wand on the outside of your abdomen to take pictures of the kidneys, bladder, and urethra. Your doctor will look for anything unusual that may be causing urinary incontinence.

- **Bladder stress test.** During this test, you will cough or bear down as if pushing during childbirth as your doctor watches for loss of urine.

- **Cystoscopy.** Your doctor inserts a thin tube with a tiny camera into your urethra and bladder to look for damaged tissue. Depending on the type of cystoscopy you need, your doctor may use medicine to numb your skin and urinary organs while you are still awake, or you may be fully sedated.

- **Urodynamics.** Your doctor inserts a thin tube into your bladder and fills your bladder with water. This allows your doctor to measure the pressure in your bladder to see how much fluid your bladder can hold.

Your doctor or nurse may ask you to keep a diary for two to three days to track when you empty your bladder or leak urine. The diary may help your doctor or nurse see patterns in the incontinence which will give clues about the possible cause and treatments that might work for you.

How Is Urinary Incontinence Treated?

You and your doctor or nurse will work together to create a treatment plan. You may start with steps that can be taken at home. If these steps do not improve your symptoms, your doctor or nurse may recommend other treatments depending on whether you have stress incontinence, urge incontinence, or both.

Be patient as you work with your doctor or nurse on a treatment plan. It may take a month or longer for different treatments to begin working.

What Steps Can I Take at Home to Treat Urinary Incontinence?

Your doctor or nurse may suggest some things you can do at home to help treat urinary incontinence. Some people do not think that such simple actions can treat urinary incontinence. But for many women, these steps make urinary incontinence go away entirely, or help them leak less urine. These steps may include:

- **Doing Kegel exercises.** If you have stress incontinence, Kegel exercises to strengthen your pelvic-floor muscles may help. Some women have urinary symptoms because the pelvic-floor muscles are always tightened. In this situation, Kegel exercises will not help your urinary symptoms and may cause more problems. Talk to your doctor or nurse about your urinary symptoms before doing Kegel exercises.

- **Training your bladder.** You can help control overactive bladder or urge incontinence by going to the bathroom at set times. Start by tracking how often you go to the bathroom each day in a bladder diary. Then slowly add about 15 minutes between bathroom visits. Urinate each time, even if you do not feel the urge to go. By gradually increasing the amount of time between visits, your bladder learns to hold more urine before it signals the need to go again.

- **Losing weight.** Extra weight puts more pressure on your bladder and nearby muscles, which can lead to problems with bladder control. If you are overweight, your doctor or nurse can help you create a plan to lose weight by choosing healthy foods and getting regular physical activity. Your doctor or nurse may refer you to a dietitian or physical therapist to create a healthy eating and exercise plan.

- **Changing your eating habits.** Drinks with caffeine, carbonation (such as sodas), or alcohol may make bladder leakage or urinary incontinence worse. Your doctor might suggest that you stop drinking these drinks for a while to see if that helps.

- **Quitting smoking.** Smoking can make many health problems, including urinary incontinence, worse.

- **Treating constipation.** Your doctor may recommend that you eat more fiber, since constipation can make urinary incontinence worse. Eating foods with a lot of fiber can make you less constipated.

You can also buy pads or protective underwear while you take other steps to treat urinary incontinence. These are sold in many stores that also sell feminine hygiene products, such as tampons and pads.

What Are Kegel Exercises?

Kegel exercises, also called Kegels or pelvic-floor muscle training, are exercises for your pelvic-floor muscles to help prevent or reduce stress urinary incontinence. Your pelvic-floor muscles support your uterus, bladder, small intestine, and rectum.

4 in 10 women improved their symptoms after trying Kegels. Kegels can be done daily and may be especially helpful during pregnancy. They can help prevent the weakening of pelvic-floor muscles, which often happens during pregnancy and childbirth. Your pelvic-floor muscles may also weaken with age and less physical activity.

Some women have urinary symptoms because the pelvic-floor muscles are always tightened. In this situation, Kegel exercises will not help urinary symptoms and may cause more problems. Talk to your doctor or nurse about your urinary symptoms before doing Kegel exercises.

How Do I Do Kegel Exercises?

To do Kegels:

- **Lie down.** It may be easier to learn how to do Kegels correctly while lying down. You don't have to lie down once you learn to do Kegels correctly.

- **Squeeze the muscles in your genital area** as if you were trying to stop the flow of urine or passing gas. Try not to squeeze the muscles in your belly or legs at the same time. Try to squeeze only the pelvic muscles. Be extra careful not to tighten your stomach, legs, or buttocks (because then you will not be using your pelvic-floor muscles).

- **Relax.** Squeeze the muscles again, and hold for three seconds. Then relax for three seconds. Work up to three sets of 10 each day.

- **Practice Kegels anywhere.** When your muscles get stronger, try doing Kegels while sitting or standing. You can do these exercises at any time, such as while sitting at your desk or in the car, waiting in line, or doing the dishes. Don't do Kegel exercises at the same time you are urinating. This can weaken your pelvic-floor muscles over time.

If you are uncomfortable or uncertain about doing Kegel exercises on your own, a doctor or nurse can also teach you how to do Kegels. A pelvic-floor physical therapist or other specialist may also be able to help teach you how to strengthen these muscles.

How Soon after Starting Kegel Exercises Will Urinary Incontinence Get Better?

It may take four to six weeks before you notice any improvement in your symptoms.

Kegel exercises work differently for each person. Your symptoms may go away totally, you may notice an improvement in your symptoms but still have some leakage, or you may not see any improvement at all. But even if your symptoms do not get better, Kegel exercises can help prevent your incontinence from getting worse.

You may need to continue doing Kegel exercises for the rest of your life. Even if your symptoms improve, urinary incontinence can come back if you stop doing the exercises.

Should I Drink Less Water or Other Fluids If I Have Urinary Incontinence?

No. Many people with urinary incontinence think they need to drink less to reduce how much urine leaks out. But you need fluids, especially water, for good health. (But alcohol and caffeine can irritate or stress the bladder and make urinary incontinence worse.)

Women need 91 ounces (about 11 cups) of fluids a day from food and drinks. Getting enough fluids helps keep your kidneys and bladder healthy, prevents urinary tract infections, and prevents constipation, which may make urinary incontinence worse.

After age 60, people are less likely to get enough water, putting them at risk for dehydration and conditions that make urinary incontinence worse.

What Are Some Medical Treatments for Stress Incontinence?

If steps you take at home do not work to improve your stress incontinence, your doctor may talk to you about other options:

- **Medicine.** After menopause, applying vaginal creams, rings, or patches with estrogen (called "topical estrogen") can help strengthen the muscles and tissues in the urethra and vaginal areas. A stronger urethra will help with bladder control.

- **Vaginal pessary.** A reusable pessary is a small plastic or silicone device (shaped like a ring or small donut) that you put into your vagina. The pessary pushes up against the wall of the vagina and the urethra to support the pelvic-floor muscles and help reduce stress incontinence. Pessaries come in different sizes, so your doctor or nurse must write a prescription for the size that will fit you. Another type of pessary looks like a tampon and is used once before being thrown away. You can get this type of pessary at a store that also sells feminine hygiene products.

- **Bulking agents.** Your doctor can inject a bulking agent, such as collagen, into tissues around the bladder and urethra to cause them to thicken. This helps keep the bladder opening closed and reduces the amount of urine that can leak out.

- **Surgery.** Surgery for urinary incontinence is not recommended if you plan to get pregnant in the future. Pregnancy and childbirth can cause leakage to happen again. The two most common types of surgery for urinary incontinence are:

  - **Sling procedures.** The mid-urethral sling is the most common type of surgery to treat stress incontinence. The sling is either a narrow piece of synthetic (man-made) mesh or a piece of tissue from your own body that your doctor places under your urethra. The sling acts like a hammock to support the urethra and hold the bladder in place. Serious complications from the sling procedure include pain, infection, pain during sex, and damage to nearby organs, such as the bladder. The U.S. Food and Drug Administration (FDA) reports that in 1 out of every 50 patients who have synthetic mesh for urinary incontinence, the mesh moves after surgery and stick outs, into the vagina, causing pain. The FDA recommends discussing treatment options with your doctor before surgery, and asking specific questions about side effects.

  - **Colposuspension.** This surgery also helps hold the bladder in place with stitches on either side of the urethra. This is often referred to as a "Burch procedure."

What Are Some Nonsurgical Treatments for Urge Incontinence?

If steps you take at home do not work to improve your urge incontinence, your doctor may suggest one or more of the following treatments:

- **Medicines.** Medicines to treat urge incontinence help relax the bladder muscle and increase the amount of urine your bladder can hold. Common side effects of these medicines include constipation and dry eyes and mouth.

- **Botox.** Botox injections in the bladder can help if other treatments do not work. Botox helps relax the bladder and increases the amount of urine your bladder can hold. You may need to get Botox treatments about once every three months.

- **Nerve stimulation.** This treatment uses mild electric pulses to stimulate nerves in the bladder. The pulses may increase blood flow to the bladder and strengthen the muscles that help control the bladder. Talk to your doctor about the different types of nerve stimulation.

- **Biofeedback.** Biofeedback helps you see how your bladder responds on a screen. A therapist puts an electrical patch on the skin over your bladder and urethral muscles. A wire connected to the patch is linked to a screen. You and your therapist watch the screen to see when these muscles contract, so you can learn to control them.

- **Surgery.** If you have severe urge incontinence, your doctor may recommend surgery to help increase the amount of urine your bladder can hold or to remove your bladder. Removing your bladder is a serious surgery and is only an option when no other treatments work and the quality of your life is seriously affected.

How Can I Prevent Urinary Incontinence?

Although you cannot always prevent urinary incontinence, you can take steps to lower your risk:

- Practice Kegels daily, especially during pregnancy, after talking to your doctor, nurse, or midwife.

- Reach or stay at a healthy weight.

- Eat foods with fiber to help prevent constipation.

Chapter 10

Pregnancy, Breastfeeding, and Bone Health

Both pregnancy and breastfeeding cause changes in, and place extra demands on, women's bodies. Some of these changes may affect their bones. The good news is that most women do not experience bone problems during pregnancy and breastfeeding. If their bones are affected during these times, the problem is often corrected easily. Nevertheless, taking care of one's bone health is especially important during pregnancy and breastfeeding, for the good health of both the mother and her baby.

Pregnancy and Bone Health

During pregnancy, the fetus needs plenty of calcium to develop its skeleton. This need is especially great during the last three months of pregnancy. If the mother does not get enough calcium, the fetus will draw what it needs from the mother's bones. Fortunately, pregnancy appears to help protect most women's calcium reserves in several ways:

- Pregnant women absorb calcium from food and supplements better than women who are not pregnant. This is especially

This chapter includes text excerpted from "Pregnancy, Breastfeeding and Bone Health," NIH Osteoporosis and Related Bone Diseases—National Resource Center (NIH ORBD—NRC), May 2015. Reviewed February 2019.

true during the last half of pregnancy when the baby is growing quickly and has the greatest need for calcium.

• During pregnancy, women produce more estrogen, a hormone that protects bones.

• Any bone mass lost during pregnancy is typically restored within several months after delivery (or several months after breastfeeding is stopped).

Some studies suggest that pregnancy may be good for overall bone health. Some evidence suggests that the more times a woman has been pregnant (for at least 28 weeks), the greater her bone density and the lower her risk of fracture.

In some cases, women develop osteoporosis during pregnancy or breastfeeding, although this is rare. Osteoporosis is bone loss that is serious enough to result in fragile bones and an increased risk of fracture.

In many cases, women who develop osteoporosis during pregnancy or breastfeeding will recover lost bone after childbirth or after they stop breastfeeding. It is less clear whether teenage mothers can recover lost bone and go on to optimize their bone mass.

Teen Pregnancy and Bone Health

Teenage mothers may be at an especially high risk for bone loss during pregnancy and for osteoporosis later in life. Unlike older women, teenage mothers are still building much of their own total bone mass. The fetus's need to develop its skeleton may compete with the young mother's need for calcium to build her own bones, compromising her ability to achieve optimal bone mass that will help protect her from osteoporosis later in life. To minimize any bone loss, pregnant teens should be especially careful to get enough calcium during pregnancy and breastfeeding.

Breastfeeding and Bone Health

Breastfeeding also affects a mother's bones. Studies have shown that women often lose three to five percent of their bone mass during breastfeeding, although they recover it rapidly after weaning. This bone loss may be caused by the fetus's increased need for calcium, which is drawn from the mother's bones. The amount of calcium the mother needs depends on the amount of breast milk produced and how long breastfeeding continues. Women may also lose bone mass during breastfeeding because they are producing less estrogen, which is the hormone that protects bones. The good news is that, like bone lost during pregnancy, bone lost during breastfeeding is usually recovered within six months after breastfeeding ends.

Tips to Keep Bones Healthy during Pregnancy, Breastfeeding, and Beyond

Taking care of your bones is important throughout life, including before, during, and after pregnancy and breastfeeding. A balanced diet with adequate calcium, regular exercise, and a healthy lifestyle are good for mothers and their children.

Calcium

Although this important mineral is important throughout your lifetime, your body's demand for calcium is greater during pregnancy and breastfeeding because both you and the fetus need it. The National Academy of Sciences (NAS) recommends that women who are pregnant or breastfeeding consume 1,000 mg (milligrams) of calcium each day. For pregnant teens, the recommended intake is even higher: 1,300 mg of calcium a day.

Good sources of calcium include:

- Low-fat dairy products, such as milk, yogurt, cheese, and ice cream

- Dark green, leafy vegetables, such as broccoli, collard greens, and bok choy

- Canned sardines and salmon with bones

- Tofu, almonds, and corn tortillas

- Foods fortified with calcium, such as orange juice, cereals, and breads.

In addition, your doctor will probably prescribe a vitamin and mineral supplement to take during pregnancy and breastfeeding to ensure that you absorb enough calcium.

Exercise

Like muscles, bones respond to exercise by becoming stronger. Regular exercise, especially weight-bearing exercise that forces you to work against gravity, helps build and maintain strong bones. Examples of weight-bearing exercise include walking, climbing stairs, dancing, and weight training. Exercising during pregnancy can benefit your health in other ways too. According to the American College of Obstetricians and Gynecologists (ACOG), being active during pregnancy can:

- Help reduce backaches, constipation, bloating, and swelling
- Help prevent or treat gestational diabetes (a type of diabetes that starts during pregnancy)
- Increase energy
- Improve mood
- Improve posture
- Promote muscle tone, strength, and endurance
- Help you sleep better
- Help you get back in shape after your baby is born

Before you begin or resume an exercise program, talk to your doctor about your plans.

Healthy Lifestyle

Smoking is bad for a fetus, bad for your bones, and bad for your heart and lungs. If you smoke, talk to your doctor about quitting. He or she can suggest resources to help you. Alcohol is also bad for pregnant and breastfeeding women and their babies, and excess alcohol is bad for bones. Be sure to follow your doctor's orders to avoid alcohol during this important time.

Chapter 11

Vision and Oral Changes

Chapter Contents

Section 11.1

Pregnancy and Your Vision

During pregnancy, a woman's body undergoes many physical changes in order to support a growing fetus. Natural fluctuations in hormone levels, metabolism, circulation, and fluid retention can affect the eyes just as they affect other organs. As a result, many pregnant women experience changes in their eyes or vision. Although most pregnancy-related eye issues are minor and disappear on their own after delivery, a few types of vision changes can indicate a health condition that requires medical attention. Experts recommend that expectant mothers check with their doctors if they experience any of the following symptoms:

- Double vision
- Temporary loss of vision
- Sensitivity to light
- Seeing spots, auras, or blinking lights

Normal Vision Changes during Pregnancy

Most of the vision changes that occur during pregnancy are temporary. Although they can be annoying, they are usually not a cause for concern. They occur due to changing hormone levels and fluid retention, which are a normal part of pregnancy. Some of the common eye changes that occur during pregnancy include blurry vision, dry eyes, and puffy eyelids.

Blurry Vision

The fluid retention that most women experience during pregnancy can temporarily change the thickness and shape of the cornea, the transparent layer that helps focus light as it enters the eye. These changes can affect the power of corrective lenses the woman needs, resulting in blurry vision. Since the cornea will likely return to normal following delivery, experts generally recommend against getting a new prescription for corrective lenses during pregnancy. Many eye doctors can provide a temporary lens if the blurry vision makes it difficult to drive a car or perform other everyday tasks safely.

Dry Eyes

Many expectant mothers find that their eyes become dry and irritated during pregnancy and breastfeeding. This problem can be uncomfortable and make it difficult to wear contact lenses. Experts suggest using over-the-counter (OTC) lubricating or rewetting eye drops to soothe dry eyes and relieve discomfort. Pregnant women may also switch to glasses temporarily and take frequent breaks while working at a computer to avoid eyestrain.

Puffy Eyelids

Many women experience swollen ankles during pregnancy as a result of water retention. A lesser known effect of pregnancy hormones is swelling around the eyes and puffy eyelids, which can interfere with peripheral vision. To limit fluid retention, experts recommend drinking lots of water and eating a healthy diet low in sodium and caffeine.

Vision Changes of Concern during Pregnancy

A few vision changes that may occur during pregnancy can be symptoms of a serious medical condition, such as preeclampsia or gestational diabetes. Expectant mothers who experience sudden or severe vision disruptions should seek medical attention.

Preeclampsia

Preeclampsia is a complication that occurs in five percent to eight percent of all pregnancies. The main symptoms are high blood pressure, swelling of the hands and feet, and protein in the urine. Many women who develop preeclampsia experience vision problems, such as double vision, temporary loss of vision, sensitivity to light, or seeing spots, auras, or blinking lights. Preeclampsia can progress quickly to cause bleeding, organ damage, and retina detachment in the eyes. Expectant mothers that experience symptoms of preeclampsia should seek medical attention and have their blood pressure checked immediately.

Diabetes and Gestational Diabetes

Diabetes is a disease that affects the body's ability to metabolize carbohydrates, resulting in high levels of sugar in the blood. High blood sugar can damage the blood vessels in the retina, causing a serious eye condition called "diabetic retinopathy." Women who are diabetic need to monitor their blood sugar closely and get regular eye screenings to check for damage to the retina. This is especially important during pregnancy, which increases the risk of vision loss associated with diabetes.

Gestational diabetes is a form of diabetes that develops during pregnancy. Expectant mothers that develop the condition should be examined by an eye doctor for signs of retinopathy. Pregnant women with either form of diabetes should also seek medical attention if they experience blurry vision, which can be a sign of elevated blood sugar levels.

References

1. "Can Pregnancy Affect Your Eyes?" WebMD, 2017.

2. "How Pregnancy Affects Vision," Northwest Vision, August 30, 2015.

3. "Pregnancy and Your Vision," Prevent Blindness, 2017.

4. "Vision Changes during Pregnancy," BabyCenter, 2017.

Section 11.2

Pregnancy and Oral Health

This section includes text excerpted from "Oral Health," Office on Women's Health (OWH), U.S. Department of Health and Human Services (HHS), January 31, 2019.

What Is Oral Health?

Oral health is the health of your mouth, including your teeth, gums, throat, and the bones around the mouth.

Oral health problems, such as gum disease, might be a sign that you have other health problems. Gum diseases are infections caused by plaque, which is a sticky film of bacteria that forms on your teeth. If left untreated, the bacteria in plaque can destroy the tissue and bone around your teeth, leading to tooth loss. The bacteria can then travel throughout your body and make you sick. Infections in your mouth can also affect your fetus if you are pregnant.

How Do Women's Hormones Affect Oral Health?

Changing hormone levels at different stages of a woman's life can affect oral health. When your hormone levels change, your gums can become swollen and irritated. Your gums may also bleed, especially during pregnancy, when your body's immune system is more sensitive than usual. This can cause inflammation (redness, swelling, and sometimes pain) in the gums. Regular, careful brushing and flossing can lessen gum irritation and bleeding.

Other causes of changing hormone levels that may affect your oral health include:

- Your menstrual cycle

- Hormonal birth control

- Menopause

How Does Pregnancy Affect Oral Health?

Pregnancy can make brushing difficult. Some women experience nausea from strongly flavored toothpastes. Switching to a neutral-flavored toothpaste may help. During pregnancy, your hormone levels can increase and decrease. This raises your risk for several oral health problems:

- **Severe gum disease (periodontitis).** Changing hormone levels during pregnancy can make gum disease worse or lead to severe gum disease in as many as two in five pregnant women. Periodontitis is an infection of the tissues that hold your teeth in place. It's usually caused by not brushing and flossing, or brushing and flossing in away that allows plaque to build up on the teeth and harden. Periodontitis can cause sore, bleeding gums, painful chewing, and tooth loss. Women who do not get regular dental care and women who smoke are more likely to have periodontitis.

- **Loose teeth.** The tissue supporting your teeth may loosen during pregnancy since many of your joints and tissues loosen in preparation for childbirth. Taking good care of your mouth can help prevent tooth loss.

- **Wearing down of your tooth enamel.** If you have morning sickness that causes vomiting, the stomach acid that comes up during vomiting can erode tooth enamel (the hard, protective coating on the outside of your teeth). Heartburn, another common pregnancy discomfort, can also wear down your tooth enamel over time if stomach acid is coming up into your throat and mouth. To prevent this erosion, the American Dental Association (ADA) recommends rinsing your mouth with one teaspoon of baking soda mixed in a cup of water 30 minutes before brushing your teeth.

I'm Pregnant. Is It Safe for Me to Get a Dental Checkup?

Yes. You need to continue your regular dental visits to help protect your teeth during pregnancy.

- **Tell your doctor you are pregnant.** Because you are pregnant, your dentist might not take routine X-rays. But the health risk to the fetus is very small. If you need emergency treatment or specific dental X-rays to treat a serious problem, your doctor can take extra care to protect the fetus.

- **Schedule your dental exam early in your pregnancy.** After your 20th week of pregnancy, you may be uncomfortable sitting in a dental chair.

- **Have all needed dental treatments.** If you avoid treatment, you may risk your own health and the fetus's health.

How Can I Prevent Oral Health Problems?

You can help prevent oral health problems by taking the following steps:

- **Visit your dentist once or twice a year.** Your dentist may recommend more or fewer visits depending on your oral health. At most routine visits, the dentist and a dental hygienist (assistant) will treat you. During regular checkups, dentists look for signs of disease, infections, and injuries.

- **Choose healthy foods.** Limit the amount of sugary foods and drinks you have. Lower your risk for tooth decay by brushing after meals and flossing once a day.

- **Do not smoke.** Smoking raises your risk of gum disease and mouth and throat cancers. It can also stain your teeth and cause bad breath.

- **Drink less soda.** If you drink soda, try to drink less, and replace it with water. Even diet soda has acids that can erode tooth enamel.

Chapter 12

Emotional Concerns and Pregnancy

Chapter Contents

Section 12.1

Depression and Pregnancy

This section includes text excerpted from "Medicines to Help You—
Depression," U.S. Food and Drug Administration (FDA), July 18,
2006. Reviewed February 2019.

Some women become depressed when they are pregnant or after
they give birth. Other women notice that their depression gets worse
during pregnancy.

No one knows the exact cause of depression during or after pregnancy, but it may be caused by:

- Stress

- Hormones—After a woman has a baby, her hormone levels drop
  quickly

- Having depression before you get pregnant

- Lack of support from family and friends

- Young age—The younger you are when you have your baby, the
  more likely you are to become depressed

Women should talk to their doctor about the risks of taking depression medicines during pregnancy.

Depression can make it hard for a woman to take care of herself
and the fetus. It is important to talk to your doctor about your feelings.
Also, try to get some help from your family, friends, or a support group.

- Ask a relative to watch your baby for a few hours.

- Join a group for new mothers.

- Ask a friend to cook a meal for your family or to help with
  chores.

Medicines for Depression

There are many different kinds of medicine for depression.

- Selective serotonin reuptake inhibitors (SSRIs)

- Monoamine oxidase inhibitors (MAOIs)

- Tricyclic antidepressants (TCAs)

- Atypical antidepressants

- Selective serotonin and norepinephrine reuptake inhibitors (SNRIs)

Tell your doctor about any medicines that you are taking. Do not forget about cold medicines and herbs, such as St. John's Wort. Some medicines will make you very sick if you take them while you are taking antidepressants.

Like any drug, depression medications may cause some side effects. Do not stop taking your medicines without first talking to your doctor. Tell your doctor about any problems you are having. Your doctor will help find the medicine that is best for you.

Section 12.2

Postpartum Depression

This section includes text excerpted from "Postpartum Depression," Office on Women's Health (OWH), U.S. Department of Health and Human Services (HHS), October 18, 2018.

Your body and mind go through many changes during and after pregnancy. If you feel empty, emotionless, or sad all or most of the time for longer than two weeks during or after pregnancy, reach out for help. If you feel like you do not love or care for your baby, you might have postpartum depression. Treatment for depression, such as therapy or medicine, works and will help you and your baby be as healthy as possible in the future.

What Is Postpartum Depression?

"Postpartum" means the time after childbirth. Most women get the "baby blues," or feel sad or empty, within a few days of giving birth. For many women, the baby blues go away in three to five days. If your baby blues do not go away or you feel sad, hopeless, or empty for longer than two weeks, you may have postpartum depression. Feeling hopeless or empty after childbirth is not a regular or expected part of being a mother.

Postpartum depression is a serious mental illness that involves the brain and affects your behavior and physical health. If you have depression, then the sad, flat, or empty feelings do not go away and can interfere with your day-to-day life. You might feel unconnected to your baby, as if you are not the baby's mother, or you might not love or care for the baby. These feelings can be mild to severe.

Mothers can also experience anxiety disorders during or after pregnancy.

How Common Is Postpartum Depression?

Depression is a common problem after pregnancy. One in nine new mothers has postpartum depression.

How Do I Know If I Have Postpartum Depression?

Some normal changes after pregnancy can cause symptoms similar to those of depression. Many mothers feel overwhelmed when a new baby comes home. But if you have any of the following symptoms of depression for more than two weeks, call your doctor, nurse, or midwife:

- Feeling restless or moody

- Feeling sad, hopeless, or overwhelmed

- Crying a lot

- Having thoughts of hurting the baby

- Having thoughts of hurting yourself

- Not having any interest in the baby, not feeling connected to the baby, or feeling as if your baby is someone else's baby

- Having no energy or motivation

- Eating too little or too much

- Sleeping too little or too much

- Having trouble focusing or making decisions

- Having memory problems

- Feeling worthless, guilty, or like a bad mother

- Losing interest or pleasure in activities you used to enjoy

- Withdrawing from friends and family

- Having headaches, aches and pains, or stomach problems that do not go away

Some women do not tell anyone about their symptoms. New mothers may feel embarrassed, ashamed, or guilty about feeling depressed when they are supposed to be happy. They may also worry that they will be seen as bad mothers. Any woman can become depressed during pregnancy or after having a baby. It does not mean that you are a bad mom. You and your baby do not have to suffer. There is help. Your doctor can help you figure out whether your symptoms are caused by depression or something else.

What Causes Postpartum Depression

Hormonal changes may trigger symptoms of postpartum depression. When you are pregnant, levels of the female hormones estrogen and progesterone are the highest they will ever be. In the first 24 hours after childbirth, hormone levels quickly drop back to normal, prepregnancy levels. Researchers think this sudden change in hormone levels may lead to depression. This is similar to hormone changes before a woman's period but involves much more extreme swings in hormone levels.

Levels of thyroid hormones may also drop after giving birth. The thyroid is a small gland in the neck that helps regulate how your body uses and stores energy from food. Low levels of thyroid hormones can cause symptoms of depression. A simple blood test can tell whether this condition is causing your symptoms. If so, your doctor can prescribe thyroid medicine.

Other feelings may contribute to postpartum depression. Many new mothers say they feel:

- Tired after labor and delivery

- Tired from a lack of sleep or broken sleep

- Overwhelmed with a new baby

- Doubtful about their ability to be a good mother

- Stressed from changes in work and home routines

- An unrealistic need to be a perfect mom

- Grief about loss of who they were before having the baby

- Less attractive

- A lack of free time

These feelings are common among new mothers. But postpartum depression is a serious health condition and can be treated. Postpartum depression is not a regular or expected part of being a new mother.

Are Some Women More at Risk of Postpartum Depression?

Yes. You may be more at risk of postpartum depression if you:

- Have a personal history of depression or bipolar disorder

- Have a family history of depression or bipolar disorder

- Do not have support from family and friends

- Were depressed during pregnancy

- Had problems with a previous pregnancy or birth

- Have relationship or money problems

- Are younger than 20

- Have an alcohol- or substance-use disorder

- Have a baby with special needs

- Have difficulty breastfeeding

- Had an unplanned or unwanted pregnancy

The U.S. Preventive Services Task Force (USPSTF) recommends that doctors look for and ask about symptoms of depression during and after pregnancy, regardless of a woman's risk of depression.

What Is the Difference between the "Baby Blues" and Postpartum Depression?

Many women have the baby blues in the days after childbirth. If you have the baby blues, you may:

- Have mood swings

- Feel sad, anxious, or overwhelmed

- Have crying spells

- Lose your appetite

- Have trouble sleeping

The baby blues usually go away in three to five days after they start. The symptoms of postpartum depression last longer and are more severe. Postpartum depression usually begins within the first month after childbirth, but it can begin during pregnancy and can last up to a year after birth.

Postpartum depression needs to be treated by a doctor or nurse.

What Should I Do If I Have Symptoms of Postpartum Depression?

Call your doctor, nurse, midwife, or pediatrician if:

- Your baby blues do not go away after two weeks

- Symptoms of depression get more and more intense

- Symptoms of depression begin within one year of delivery and last more than two weeks

- It is difficult to work or get things done at home

- You cannot care for yourself or your baby (e.g., eating, sleeping, bathing)

- You have thoughts about hurting yourself or your baby

Ask your partner or a loved one to call a healthcare professional for you if necessary. Your doctor, nurse, or midwife can ask you questions to test for depression. They can also refer you to a mental health professional for help and treatment.

What Can I Do at Home to Feel Better While Seeing a Doctor for Postpartum Depression?

Here are some ways to begin feeling better or getting more rest, in addition to talking to a healthcare professional:

- Rest as much as you can. Sleep when the baby is sleeping.

- Do not try to do too much or to do everything by yourself. Ask your partner, family, and friends for help.

- Make time to go out, visit friends, or spend time alone with your partner.

- Talk about your feelings with your partner, supportive family members, and friends.

- Talk with other mothers so that you can learn from their experiences.

- Join a support group. Ask your doctor or nurse about groups in your area.

- Do not make any major life changes right after giving birth. More major life changes in addition to a new baby can cause unneeded stress. Sometimes big changes cannot be avoided. When that happens, try to arrange support and help in your new situation ahead of time.

It can also help to have a partner, a friend, or another caregiver who can help take care of the baby while you are depressed. If you are feeling depressed during pregnancy or after having a baby, do not suffer alone. Tell a loved one, and call your doctor right away.

How Is Postpartum Depression Treated?

The common types of treatment for postpartum depression are:

- **Talk therapy.** This involves talking to a therapist, psychologist, or social worker to learn strategies to change how depression makes you think, feel, and act.

- **Medicine.** Your doctor or nurse can prescribe an antidepressant medicine. These medicines can help relieve symptoms of depression, and some can be taken while you are breastfeeding. You can enter a medicine into the LactMed® database to find out whether the medicine passes through breast milk and, if so, whether it has any possible side effects for your nursing baby.

- **Electroconvulsive therapy (ECT).** This can be used in extreme cases to treat postpartum depression.

These treatments can be used alone or together. Your depression can affect your baby. Getting treatment is important for you and your baby. Taking medicines for depression or going to therapy does not make you a bad mother or a failure. Getting help is a sign of strength. Talk with your doctor or nurse about the benefits and risks of taking medicine to treat depression when you are pregnant or breastfeeding.

What Can Happen If Postpartum Depression Is Not Treated?

Untreated postpartum depression can affect your ability to parent. You may:

- Not have enough energy
- Have trouble focusing on the baby's needs and your own needs
- Feel moody
- Not be able to care for your baby
- Have a higher risk of attempting suicide

Feeling like a bad mother can make depression worse. It is important to reach out for help if you feel depressed.

Researchers believe postpartum depression in a mother can affect her child throughout childhood, causing:

- Delays in language development and problems learning
- Problems with mother-child bonding
- Behavior problems
- More crying or agitation
- Shorter height and higher risk of obesity in preschoolers
- Problems dealing with stress and adjusting to school and other social situations

What Is Postpartum Psychosis?

Postpartum psychosis is rare. It happens in up to four new mothers out of every 1,000 births. It usually begins in the first two weeks after childbirth, and is a medical emergency. Women who have bipolar disorder or another mental health condition called "schizoaffective disorder" have a higher risk of postpartum psychosis. Symptoms may include:

- Seeing or hearing things that are not there
- Feeling confused most of the time
- Having rapid mood swings within several minutes (for example, crying hysterically, then laughing a lot, followed by extreme sadness)

125

- Trying to hurt yourself or your baby
- Paranoia (thinking that others are focused on harming you)
- Restlessness or agitation
- Behaving recklessly or in a way that is not normal for you

Chapter 13

The Three Trimesters of Pregnancy: You and Your Baby

Pregnancy lasts about 40 weeks, counting from the first day of your last normal period. The weeks are grouped into three trimesters. Find out what's happening with you and your baby in these three stages.

First Trimester (Week 1–Week 12)

During the first trimester, your body undergoes many changes. Hormonal changes affect almost every organ system in your body. These changes can even trigger symptoms in the very first weeks of pregnancy. Your period stopping is a clear sign that you are pregnant. Other changes may include:

- Extreme tiredness

- Tender, swollen breasts. Your nipples might also stick out.

- Upset stomach with or without throwing up (morning sickness)

- Cravings or distaste for certain foods

This chapter includes text excerpted from "Stages of Pregnancy," Office on Women's Health (OWH), U.S. Department of Health and Human Services (HHS), January 30, 2019.

- Mood swings
- Constipation (trouble having bowel movements)
- Need to pass urine more often
- Headache
- Heartburn
- Weight gain or loss

As your body changes, you may need to make changes to your daily routine, such as going to bed earlier or eating frequent, small meals. Fortunately, most of these discomforts will go away as your pregnancy progresses, and some women might not feel any discomfort at all. If you have been pregnant before, you may feel different this time around. Just as each woman is different, so is each pregnancy.

Second Trimester (Week 13–Week 28)

Most women find the second trimester of pregnancy easier than the first, but it is just as important to stay informed about your pregnancy during these months.

You might notice that symptoms such as nausea and fatigue are going away. But other new, more noticeable changes to your body are now happening. Your abdomen will expand as the fetus continues to grow. And before this trimester is over, you will feel the fetus beginning to move.

As your body changes to make room for the developing fetus, you may have:

- Body aches, such as back, abdomen, groin, or thigh pain
- Stretch marks on your abdomen, breasts, thighs, or buttocks
- Darkening of the skin around your nipples
- A line on the skin running from the belly button to the pubic hairline
- Patches of darker skin, usually over the cheeks, forehead, nose, or upper lip. Patches often match on both sides of the face. This is sometimes called the "mask of pregnancy."
- Numb or tingling hands, called "carpal tunnel syndrome"
- Itching on the abdomen, palms, and soles of the feet. (Call your doctor if you have nausea, loss of appetite, vomiting, jaundice or

fatigue combined with itching. These can be signs of a serious liver problem.)

- Swelling of the ankles, fingers, and face. (If you notice any sudden or extreme swelling or if you gain a lot of weight really quickly, call your doctor right away. This could be a sign of preeclampsia.)

Third Trimester (Week 29–Week 40)

Some of the same discomforts you had in your second trimester will continue in the third trimester. Plus, many women find breathing difficult and notice they have to go to the bathroom even more often. This is because the fetus is getting bigger, and it is putting more pressure on your organs. Do not worry, these problems will lessen once you give birth.

Some new body changes you may notice in the third trimester include:

- Shortness of breath

- Heartburn

- Swelling of the ankles, fingers, and face. (If you notice any sudden or extreme swelling or if you gain a lot of weight really quickly, call your doctor right away. This could be a sign of preeclampsia.)

- Hemorrhoids

- Tender breasts, which may leak a watery premilk called "colostrum"

- Your belly button may stick out

- Trouble sleeping

- The baby "dropping," or moving lower in your abdomen

- Contractions, which can be a sign of real or false labor

As you near your due date, your cervix becomes thinner and softer (called "effacing.") This is a normal, natural process that helps the birth canal (vagina) open during the birthing process. Your doctor will check your progress with a vaginal exam as you near your due date.

Part Three

Staying Healthy during Pregnancy

Chapter 14

Choosing a Prenatal Care Provider

You will see your prenatal-care provider many times before you deliver, so you want to be sure that the person you choose has a good reputation, and listens to and respects you. You will want to find out if the doctor or midwife can deliver in the place you want to give birth, such as a specific hospital or birthing center. Your provider should also be willing and able to provide the information and support you need to make an informed choice about whether to breastfeed or bottle-feed.

Healthcare providers that care for women during pregnancy include:

- **Obstetricians (OB)** are medical doctors that specialize in the care of pregnant women and in delivering babies. OBs also have special training in surgery so they are also able to do a cesarean delivery. Women who have health problems or are at risk for pregnancy complications should see an obstetrician. Women with the highest risk pregnancies might need special care from a maternal-fetal medicine specialist.

- **Family practice doctors** are medical doctors that provide care for the whole family through all stages of life. This includes care during pregnancy and delivery, and following birth. Most family practice doctors cannot perform cesarean deliveries.

This chapter includes text excerpted from "Prenatal Care and Tests," Office on Women's Health (OWH), U.S. Department of Health and Human Services (HHS), January 30, 2019.

- **A certified nurse-midwife (CNM) and certified professional midwife (CPM)** are trained to provide pregnancy and postpartum care. Midwives can be a good option for healthy women at low risk for problems during pregnancy, labor, or delivery. A CNM is educated in both nursing and midwifery. Most CNMs practice in hospitals and birth centers. A CPM is required to have experience delivering babies in home settings, because most CPMs practice in homes and birthing centers. All midwives should have a back-up plan with an obstetrician in case of a problem or emergency.

Ask your primary care doctor, friends, and family members for provider recommendations. When making your choice, think about:

- Reputation

- Personality and bedside manner

- The provider's gender and age

- Office location and hours

- Whether you will always be seen by the same provider during office checkups and delivery

- Who covers for the provider when she or he is not available

- Where you want to deliver

- How the provider handles phone consultations and after-hour calls

What Is a Doula?

A doula is a professional labor coach that gives physical and emotional support to women during labor and delivery. They offer advice on breathing, relaxation, movement, and positioning. Doulas also give emotional support and comfort to women and their partners during labor and birth. Doulas and midwives often work together during a woman's labor. A study shows that continuous doula support during labor was linked to shorter labors and much lower use of:

- Pain medicines

- Oxytocin (medicine to help labor progress)

- Cesarean delivery

Check with your health insurance company to find out if they will cover the cost of a doula. When choosing a doula, find out if they are certified by Doulas of North America (DONA) or another professional group.

Places to Deliver Your Baby

Many women have strong views about where and how they would like to deliver. In general, women can choose to deliver at a hospital, birth center, or at home. You will need to contact your health-insurance provider to find out what options are available. Also, find out if the doctor or midwife you are considering can deliver your baby in the place you want to give birth.

- **Hospitals** are a good choice for women with health problems, pregnancy complications, or those who are at risk for problems during labor and delivery. Hospitals offer the most advanced medical equipment and highly trained doctors for pregnant women and their babies. In a hospital, doctors can do a cesarean delivery if you or your baby is in danger during labor. Women can receive epidurals or many other pain-relief options. More hospitals now offer on-site birth centers, which aim to offer a style of care similar to stand alone birth centers.

Questions to ask when choosing a hospital:

- Is it close to your home?
- Is a doctor who can give pain relief, such as an epidural, at the hospital 24 hours a day?
- Do you like the feel of the labor and delivery rooms?
- Are private rooms available?
- How many support people can be in the room with you?
- Does it have a neonatal intensive care unit (NICU) in case of serious problems with the baby?
- Can the baby stay in the room with you?
- Does the hospital have the staff and set-up to support successful breastfeeding?
- Does it have an on-site birth center?

Birth or birthing centers give women a "homey" environment for labor and birth. They try to make labor and delivery a natural and personal process by doing away with most high-tech equipment and routine procedures. So, you will not automatically be hooked up to an intravenous (IV). Likewise, you won't have an electronic fetal monitor around your midsection the whole time. Instead, the midwife or nurse will check in on your baby from time to time with a handheld machine. Once the baby is born, all exams and care will occur in your room. Usually certified nurse-midwives, not obstetricians, deliver babies at birth centers. Healthy women who are at low risk for problems during pregnancy, labor, and delivery may choose to deliver at a birth center.

Women cannot receive epidurals at a birth center, although some pain medicines may be available. If a cesarean delivery becomes necessary, women must be moved to a hospital for the procedure. After delivery, babies with problems can receive basic emergency care while being moved to a hospital.

Many birthing centers have showers or tubs in their rooms for laboring women. They also tend to have comforts of home like large beds and rocking chairs. In general, birth centers allow more people in the delivery room than hospitals do.

Birth centers can be inside of hospitals, a part of a hospital, or completely separate facilities. If you want to deliver at a birth center, make sure it meets the standards of the Accreditation Association for Ambulatory Health Care (AAAHC), The Joint Commission, or the American Association of Birth Centers (AABC). Accredited birth centers must have doctors that can work at a nearby hospital in case of difficulties with the mom or baby. Also, make sure the birth center has the staff and set-up to support successful breastfeeding.

Homebirth is an option for healthy pregnant women with no risk factors for complications during pregnancy, labor, or delivery. It is also important for women to have a strong aftercare support system at home. Some certified nurse-midwives and doctors will deliver babies at home. Many health-insurance companies do not cover the cost of care for homebirths, so check with your plan if you would like to deliver at home.

Homebirths are common in many countries in Europe. But in the United States, planned homebirths are not supported by the American Congress of Obstetricians and Gynecologists (ACOG). The ACOG states that hospitals are the safest place to deliver a baby, and, in case of an emergency, a hospital's equipment and highly trained doctors can provide the best care for a woman and her baby.

If you are thinking about a homebirth, you need to weigh the pros and cons. The main advantage is that you will be able to experience labor and delivery in the privacy and comfort of your own home. Since there will be no routine medical procedures, you will have control of your experience.

The main disadvantage of a homebirth is that in case of a problem, immediate hospital/medical care is unavailable. A problem will have to wait until you are transferred to the hospital. Plus, women who deliver at home have no options for pain relief.

To ensure your safety and that of your baby, you must have a highly trained and experienced midwife along with a fail-safe back-up plan. You will need fast, reliable transportation to a hospital. If you live far away from a hospital, a homebirth may not be the best choice. Your midwife must be experienced and have the necessary skills and supplies to start emergency care for you and your baby if need be. Your midwife should also have access to a doctor 24 hours a day.

Chapter 15

Prenatal Medical Tests and Care during Pregnancy

What Is Prenatal Care and Why Is It Important?

Having a healthy pregnancy is one of the best ways to promote a healthy birth. Getting early and regular prenatal care improves the chances of a healthy pregnancy. This care can begin even before pregnancy with a preconception care visit to a healthcare provider.

Preconception Care

A preconception care visit can help women take steps toward a healthy pregnancy even before they are pregnant. Women can help to promote a healthy pregnancy and birth by taking the following steps before they become pregnant:

- Develop a plan for their reproductive life

- Increase their daily intake of folic acid (one of the B vitamins) to at least 400 micrograms

This chapter contains text excerpted from the following sources: Text under the heading "What Is Prenatal Care and Why Is It Important?" is excerpted from "What Is Prenatal Care and Why Is It Important?" *Eunice Kennedy Shriver* National Institute of Child Health and Human Development (NICHD), January 31, 2017; Text beginning with the heading "Prenatal Checkups" is excerpted from "Prenatal Care and Tests," Office on Women's Health (OWH), U.S. Department of Health and Human Services (HHS), January 30, 2019.

- Make sure their immunizations are up to date

- Control diabetes and other medical conditions

- Avoid smoking, drinking alcohol, and using drugs

- Attain a healthy weight

- Learn about their family health history and that of their partner

- Seek help for depression, anxiety, or other mental-health issues

Prenatal Care

Women who suspect they may be pregnant should schedule a visit with their healthcare provider to begin prenatal care. Prenatal visits with a healthcare provider usually include a physical exam, weight checks, and providing a urine sample. Depending on the stage of the pregnancy, healthcare providers may also conduct blood tests and imaging tests, such as ultrasound exams. These visits also include discussions about the mother's health, the fetus's health, and any questions about the pregnancy.

Preconception and prenatal care can help prevent complications and inform women about important steps they can take to protect the fetus and ensure a healthy pregnancy. With regular prenatal care women can:

- Reduce the risk of pregnancy complications. Following a healthy, safe diet; getting regular exercise as advised by a healthcare provider; and avoiding exposure to potentially harmful substances, such as lead and radiation can help reduce the risk for problems during pregnancy and promote fetal health and development. Controlling existing conditions, such as high blood pressure and diabetes, is important to prevent serious complications and their effects.

- Reduce the fetus's risk for complications. Tobacco smoke and alcohol use during pregnancy have been shown to increase the risk for sudden infant death syndrome (SIDS). Alcohol use also increases the risk for fetal alcohol spectrum disorders (FASDs), which can cause a variety of problems, such as abnormal facial features, having a small head, poor coordination, poor memory, intellectual disability, and problems with the heart, kidneys, or bones. According to a study supported by the National Institutes of Health (NIH), these and other long-term problems can occur even with low levels of prenatal-alcohol exposure.

In addition, taking 400 micrograms of folic acid daily reduces the risk for neural-tube defects by 70 percent. Most prenatal vitamins contain the recommended 400 micrograms of folic acid, as well as other vitamins that a pregnant woman and their developing fetus need. Folic acid has been added to foods such as cereals, breads, pasta, and other grain-based foods. Although a related form (called "folate") is present in orange juice and leafy, green vegetables (such as kale and spinach), folate is not absorbed as well as folic acid.

- Help ensure that the medications women take are safe.
  Women should not take certain medications, including some acne treatments and dietary and herbal supplements, during pregnancy because they can harm the fetus.

Prenatal Checkups

During pregnancy, regular checkups are very important. This consistent care can help keep you and the fetus healthy, spot problems if they occur, and prevent problems during delivery. Typically, routine checkups occur:

- Once a month for weeks 4 through 28
- Twice a month for weeks 28 through 36
- Weekly for weeks 36 to birth

Women with high-risk pregnancies need to see their doctors more often.

At your first visit, your doctor will perform a full physical exam, take your blood for lab tests, and calculate your due date. Your doctor may also conduct a breast exam, a pelvic exam to check your uterus (womb), and a cervical exam, including a Pap test. During this first visit, your doctor will ask a lot of questions about your lifestyle, relationships, and health habits. It is important to be honest with your doctor.

After the first visit, most prenatal visits will include:

- Checking your blood pressure and weight
- Checking the fetus's heart rate
- Measuring your abdomen to check the fetus's growth

You also will have some routine tests throughout your pregnancy, such as tests that look for anemia, tests that measure risk of gestational diabetes, and tests that look for harmful infections.

Become a partner with your doctor to manage your care, and keep all of your appointments. Ask questions and read to educate yourself about this time.

Monitor Activity

After 28 weeks, keep track of the fetus's movement. This will help you to notice if the fetus is moving less than normal, which could be a sign that of distress and require a doctor's care. An easy way to do this is the "count-to-10" approach. Count movements in the evening—the time of day when the fetus tends to be most active. Lie down if you have trouble feeling the fetus move. Most women count 10 movements within about 20 minutes. But it is rare for a woman to count less than 10 movements within two hours at times when the fetus is active. Count the movements every day so you know what is normal for you. Call your doctor if you count less than 10 movements within two hours, or if you notice that the fetus is moving less than normal. If there is no movement at all, call your doctor right away.

Prenatal Tests

Tests are used during pregnancy to check the health of both you and the fetus. At your first prenatal visit, your doctor will use tests to check for a number of things, such as:

- Your blood type and Rh factor
- Anemia
- Infections, such as toxoplasmosis and sexually transmitted infections (STIs), including hepatitis B, syphilis, chlamydia, and human immunodeficiency virus (HIV)
- Signs that you are immune to rubella (German measles) and chicken pox

Throughout your pregnancy, your doctor or midwife may suggest a number of other tests too. Some tests are suggested for all women, such as screenings for gestational diabetes, Down syndrome (DS), and HIV. Other tests might be offered based on your:

- Age
- Personal or family health history
- Ethnic background

- Results of routine tests

Some tests are screening tests. They detect risks for or signs of possible health problems in you or the fetus. Based on screening test results, your doctor might suggest diagnostic tests. Diagnostic tests confirm or rule out health problems in you or the fetus.

Understanding Prenatal Tests and Test Results

If your doctor suggests certain prenatal tests, do not be afraid to ask a lot of questions. Learning about the test, why your doctor is suggesting it for you, and what the test results could mean can help you cope with any worries or fears you may have. Keep in mind that screening tests do not diagnose problems; they evaluate risk. So if a screening test comes back abnormal, this does not mean there is a problem with the fetus. More information is needed. Your doctor can explain what test results mean and possible next steps.

Avoid Keepsake Ultrasounds

You might think a keepsake ultrasound is a must-have for your scrapbook. But, doctors advise against ultrasound when there is no medical need to do so. Some companies sell "keepsake" ultrasound videos and images. Although ultrasound is considered safe for medical purposes, exposure to ultrasound energy for a keepsake video or image may put a mother and the fetus at risk. Do not take that chance.

High-Risk Pregnancy

Pregnancies with a greater chance of complications are called "high-risk," but this does not mean there will be problems. The following factors may increase the risk of problems during pregnancy:

- Very young age or older than 35

- Overweight or underweight

- Problems in previous pregnancy

- Health conditions you have before you become pregnant, such as high blood pressure, diabetes, autoimmune disorders, cancer, and HIV

- Pregnancy with twins or other multiples

Table 15.1. Common Prenatal Tests

Test	What It Is	How It Is Done
Amniocentesis	This test can diagnose certain birth defects, including • Down syndrome • Cystic fibrosis • Spina bifida It is performed at 14 to 20 weeks. It may be suggested for couples at a higher risk for genetic disorders. It also provides DNA for paternity testing.	A thin needle is used to draw out a small amount of amniotic fluid and cells from the sac surrounding the fetus. The sample is sent to a lab for testing.
Biophysical profile (BPP)	This test is used in the third trimester to monitor the overall health of the fetus and to help decide if early delivery is necessary.	BPP involves an ultrasound exam along with a nonstress test. The BPP looks at the fetus's breathing, movement, muscle tone, heart rate, and the amount of amniotic fluid.
Chorionic villus sampling (CVS)	A test done at 10 to 13 weeks to diagnose certain birth defects, including: • Chromosomal disorders, including Down syndrome • Genetic disorders, such as cystic fibrosis CVS may be suggested for couples at a higher risk for genetic disorders. It also provides DNA for paternity testing.	A needle removes a small sample of cells from the placenta to be tested.
First-trimester screen	A screening test done at 11 to 14 weeks to detect higher risk of: • Chromosomal disorders, including Down syndrome and trisomy 18 • Other problems, such as heart defects It also can reveal multiple births. Based on test results, your doctor may suggest other tests to diagnose a disorder.	This test involves both a blood test and an ultrasound exam called "nuchal translucency (NOO-kuhl trans-LOO-sent-see) screening." The blood test measures the levels of certain substances in the mother's blood. The ultrasound exam measures the thickness at the back of the fetus's neck. This information, combined with the mother's age, help doctors determine potential risk to the fetus.

Table 15.1. Continued

Test	What It Is	How It Is Done
Glucose challenge screening	A screening test done at 26 to 28 weeks to determine the mother's risk of gestational diabetes. Based on test results, your doctor may suggest a glucose tolerance test.	First, you consume a special sugary drink from your doctor. A blood sample is taken one hour later to look for high blood sugar levels.
Glucose tolerance test	This test is done at 26 to 28 weeks to diagnose gestational diabetes.	Your doctor will tell you what to eat a few days before the test. Then, you cannot eat or drink anything but sips of water for 14 hours before the test. Your blood is drawn to test your "fasting blood glucose level." Then, you will consume a sugary drink. Your blood will be tested every hour for three hours to see how well your body processes sugar.
Group B streptococcus infection	This test is done at 36 to 37 weeks to look for bacteria that can cause pneumonia or serious infection in newborn.	A swab is used to take cells from your vagina and rectum to be tested.
Maternal serum screen (also called quad screen, triple test, triple screen, multiple marker screen, or AFP)	A screening test done at 15 to 20 weeks to detect higher risk of: • Chromosomal disorders, including Down syndrome and trisomy 18 • Neural tube defects, such as spina bifida Based on test results, your doctor may suggest other tests to diagnose a disorder.	Blood is drawn to measure the levels of certain substances in the mother's blood.
Nonstress test (NST)	This test is performed after 28 weeks to monitor your fetus's health. It can show signs of fetal distress, such as a lack of oxygen.	A belt is placed around the mother's belly to measure the fetus's heart rate in response to its own movements.

Table 15.1. Continued

Test	What It Is	How It Is Done
Ultrasound exam	An ultrasound exam can be performed at any point during the pregnancy. Ultrasound exams are not routine, but it is not uncommon for women to have a standard ultrasound exam between 18 and 20 weeks to look for signs of problems with the fetus's organs and body systems and confirm the age of the fetus and proper growth. It also might be able to tell the sex of the fetus. An ultrasound exam is also used as part of the first trimester screen and biophysical profile (BPP). Based on exam results, your doctor may suggest other tests or other types of ultrasound to help detect a problem.	Ultrasound uses sound waves to create a "picture" of your baby on a monitor. With a standard ultrasound, a gel is spread on your abdomen. A special tool is moved over your abdomen, which allows your doctor and you to view the fetus on a monitor.
Urine test	A urine sample can look for signs of health problems, such as: • Urinary tract infection • Diabetes • Preeclampsia If your doctor suspects a problem, the sample might be sent to a lab for more in-depth testing.	You will collect a small sample of clean, midstream urine in a sterile plastic cup. Testing strips that look for certain substances in your urine are dipped in the sample. The sample also can be looked at under a microscope.

Health problems may also develop during a pregnancy that make it high-risk, such as gestational diabetes or preeclampsia.

Women with high-risk pregnancies need prenatal care more often and sometimes from a specially-trained doctor. A maternal-fetal medicine specialist is a medical doctor that cares for high-risk pregnancies.

If your pregnancy is considered high-risk, you might worry about the fetus's health and have trouble enjoying your pregnancy. Share your concerns with your doctor. Your doctor can explain the risks and the chances of a real problem. Also, be sure to follow your doctor's advice. For example, if your doctor tells you to take it easy, then ask your partner, family members, and friends to help you out in the months ahead. You will feel better knowing that you are doing all you can to care for the fetus.

Chapter 16

Immunization for Pregnant Women

Vaccines can help protect both you and the fetus from vaccine-preventable diseases. During pregnancy, vaccinated mothers pass on infection-fighting proteins called "antibodies" to the fetus.

Antibodies provide some immunity (protection) against certain diseases during a baby's first few months of life when they are still too young to get vaccinated. It also helps provide important protection for you throughout your pregnancy.

To protect yourself and your baby, it is important to understand which vaccines you may need before, during, and after your pregnancy.

Which Vaccines Do I Need before I Get Pregnant?

If you are planning to get pregnant, it is important to make sure you are up to date on all of your adult vaccines. The Centers for Disease Control and Prevention (CDC) offers an easy-to-read vaccine schedule that allow you to find routine vaccine recommendations by age.

This chapter contains text excerpted from the following sources: Text in this chapter begins with excerpts from "Vaccines for Pregnant Women," Vaccines. gov, U.S. Department of Health and Human Services (HHS), December 2017; Text beginning with the heading "Can a Vaccine Harm My Developing Baby?" is excerpted from "Questions and Answers about Vaccines during Pregnancy," Centers for Disease Control and Prevention (CDC), August 28, 2015. Reviewed February 2019.

Before your pregnancy, talk with your doctor about your vaccine history. You may need vaccines that protect against:

- **Rubella:** Rubella during pregnancy can cause serious birth defects that can lead to death before birth or lifelong illness for your child. To find out if you are protected from rubella, you can check with your doctor or have a prepregnancy blood test. It is important to wait one month after getting the vaccine before you try to get pregnant.

- **Hepatitis B:** If you have hepatitis B infection during pregnancy, it can pass to your baby during birth. Hepatitis B can lead to serious, ongoing health problems for your child. Talk with your doctor about getting tested for hepatitis B and whether or not you need to get vaccinated.

Which Vaccines Do I Need during Pregnancy?

All pregnant women need to get vaccinated against the flu and whooping cough during each pregnancy.

The Flu Shot

Getting vaccinated against the flu is important because pregnant women are at an increased risk for serious complications from the flu. The flu can also cause serious problems like early labor and delivery, which can affect your baby's health.

In addition to protecting you and the fetus, getting the flu shot during pregnancy makes it less likely that newborns will get the flu for several months after they are born, which lowers their risk of serious complications, such as pneumonia (lung infection).

You can get the flu shot during any trimester of your pregnancy.

The Whooping Cough Vaccine

Getting vaccinated against whooping cough helps protect young babies from whooping cough before they are old enough to get vaccinated themselves. About half of babies who get whooping cough end up in the hospital, and the disease can be life-threatening.

The vaccine can be given any time during pregnancy, but experts recommend getting the vaccine as early as possible in the third trimester (between 27 and 36 weeks of pregnancy). The whooping cough vaccine is also recommended for other adults who spend time with your baby.

Is It Safe to Get Vaccines during Pregnancy?

Yes. It is safe to get the vaccines recommended during pregnancy. Research shows that whooping cough and flu vaccines help provide important-disease protection for pregnant women, and experts closely monitor the safety of vaccines.

Like any medicine, vaccines can have side effects. But these side effects are usually mild and go away on their own. The side effects of vaccines that protect against the flu and whooping cough include:

- Pain, redness, or swelling where the shot was given

- Muscle aches

- Feeling tired

- Fever

Many people experience these side effects, not just pregnant women.

Which Vaccines Do I Need after My Baby Is Born?

After your baby is born, you may need to get vaccines to protect against:

- **Whooping cough:** If you did not get the whooping cough vaccine when you were pregnant, you will need to get vaccinated right after delivery. Other people who spend time with the baby may also need to get the whooping cough vaccine.

- **Measles, mumps, and rubella, and chickenpox:** If you are not already protected from measles, mumps, rubella, or chickenpox, you will need to get vaccinated before you leave the hospital.

All routinely-recommended vaccines are safe for breastfeeding women.

Are You Planning to Travel? Make Sure You Are Protected

Many vaccine-preventable diseases that are rare in the United States are still common in other parts of the world. If you are pregnant and planning to travel outside the United States, talk with your doctor about vaccines that may be recommended for you.

Can a Vaccine Harm My Developing Baby?

Some vaccines, especially vaccines made using live strains of a virus, should not be given to pregnant women because they may be harmful to the fetus. The recommendations for which vaccines to get during pregnancy, and in which trimester, are developed with highest concern for the safety of both mothers and babies in mind.

What If I Receive a Vaccine and Then Learn That I Am Pregnant?

Some vaccines are not recommended during pregnancy, such as:

• Human papillomavirus (HPV)

• Measles, mumps, and rubella (MMR)

• Some kinds of flu vaccines

• Varicella (chicken pox)

If you receive any of these vaccines and then find out that you are pregnant, talk to your doctor. In most cases, there is no cause for concern.

The CDC's Immunization and Pregnancy chart (www.cdc.gov/vaccines/pregnancy/downloads/immunizations-preg-chart.pdf) shows all recommended vaccines and whether or not they are recommended during pregnancy.

Chapter 17

Taking Medicines during Pregnancy

Chapter Contents

Section 17.1

Is It Safe to Use Medicines during Pregnancy?

This section includes text excerpted from "Pregnancy and Medicines,"
Office on Women's Health (OWH), U.S. Department of Health and
Human Services (HHS), January 31, 2019.

When deciding whether or not to use a medicine during pregnancy, you and your doctor need to talk about the medicine's benefits and risks. Before you start or stop any medicine while you are pregnant, it is always best to speak with your doctor.

Is It Safe to Use Medicine While I Am Pregnant?

There is no clear-cut answer to this question. Before you start or stop any medicine, it is always best to speak with the doctor who is caring for you while you are pregnant.

How Should I Decide Whether to Use a Medicine While I Am Pregnant?

When deciding whether or not to use a medicine in pregnancy, you and your doctor need to talk about the medicine's benefits and risks.

- **Benefits:** What are the good things the medicine can do for me and the fetus?

- **Risks:** What are the ways the medicine might harm me or the fetus?

There may be times during pregnancy when using medicine is a choice. Some of the medicine choices you and your doctor make while you are pregnant may differ from the choices you make when you are not pregnant. For example, if you get a cold, you may decide to deal your stuffy nose instead of using the medicine you use when you are not pregnant.

Other times, using medicine is not a choice—it is needed. Some women need to use medicines while they are pregnant. Sometimes, women need medicine for a few days or a couple of weeks to treat a problem, such as a bladder infection or strep throat. Other women need to use medicine every day to control long-term health problems, such as asthma, diabetes, depression, or seizures. Also, some women have a pregnancy problem that needs medicinal treatment. These problems might include severe nausea and vomiting, earlier pregnancy losses, or preterm labor.

Where Do Doctors and Nurses Find out about Using Medicines during Pregnancy?

Doctors and nurses get information from medicine labels and packages, textbooks, and research journals. They also share knowledge with other doctors and nurses, and talk to the people who make and sell medicines.

The U.S. Food and Drug Administration (FDA) is the part of our country's government that controls the medicines that can and cannot be sold in the United States. The FDA lets a company sell a medicine in the United States if it is safe to use and works for a certain health problem. Companies that make medicines usually have to show the FDA doctors and scientists whether birth defects or other problems occur in baby animals when the medicine is given to pregnant animals. Most of the time, drugs are not studied in pregnant women.

The FDA works with the drug companies to make clear and complete medicine labels. But in most cases, there is not much information about how a medicine affects pregnant women and fetuses. Many prescription medicine labels include the results of studies done in pregnant animals, but a medicine does not always affect fetuses and animals in the same way. Here is an example:

A medicine is given to pregnant rats. If the medicine causes problems in some of the rat babies, it may or may not cause problems in human babies. If there are no problems in the rat babies, it does not prove that the medicine will not cause problems in human babies.

The FDA asks for studies in two different kinds of animals. This improves the chance that the studies can predict what may happen in pregnant women and fetuses.

There is a lot that FDA doctors and scientists do not know about using medicine during pregnancy. In a perfect world, every medicine label would include helpful information about the medicine's effects on pregnant women and their fetuses. Unfortunately, this is not the case.

How Do Prescription and Over-the-Counter Medicine Labels Help My Doctor Choose the Right Medicine for Me When I Am Pregnant?

Doctors use information from many sources when they choose medicine for a patient, including medicine labels. To help doctors, the FDA created pregnancy-letter categories to help explain what is known about using medicine during pregnancy. This system assigns letter categories to all prescription medicines. The letter category is listed in the label of a prescription medicine. The label states whether studies were done in pregnant women or pregnant animals and if so, what happened. Over-the-counter (OTC) medicines do not have a pregnancy letter category. Some OTC medicines were originally prescription medicines and used to have a letter category. Talk to your doctor and follow the instructions on the label before taking OTC medicines.

Prescription Medicines

The FDA chooses a medicine's letter category based on what is known about the medicine when used in pregnant women and animals.

Table 17.1. Definition of Medicine Categories

Pregnancy Category	Definition	Examples of Drugs
A	In human studies, pregnant women used the medicine and the fetuses did not have any problems related to using the medicine.	Folic acid levothyroxine (thyroid hormone medicine)
B	In humans, there are no good studies. But in animal studies, pregnant animals received the medicine, and the fetus did not show any problems related to the medicine. Or In animal studies, pregnant animals received the medicine, and some fetuses had problems. But in human studies, pregnant women used the medicine and fetuses did not have any problems related to using the medicine.	Some antibiotics like amoxicillin. Zofran (ondansetron) for nausea Glucophage (metformin) for diabetes Some insulins used to treat diabetes such as regular and NPH insulin.

Table 17.1. Continued

Pregnancy Category	Definition	Examples of Drugs
C	In humans, there are no good studies. In animals, pregnant animals treated with the medicine had some fetuses with problems. However, sometimes the medicine may still help the human mothers and fetuses more than it might harm. Or No animal studies have been done, and there are no good studies in pregnant women.	Diflucan (fluconazole) for yeast infections Ventolin (albuterol) for asthma Zoloft (sertraline) and Prozac (fluoxetine) for depression
D	Studies in humans and other reports show that when pregnant women use the medicine, some babies are born with problems related to the medicine. However, in some serious situations, the medicine may still help the mother and the baby more than it might harm.	Paxil (paroxetine) for depression Lithium for bipolar disorder Dilantin (phenytoin) for epileptic seizures Some cancer chemotherapy
X	Studies or reports in humans or animals show that mothers using the medicine during pregnancy may have fetuses with problems related to the medicine. There are no situations where the medicine can help the mother or the fetus enough to make the risk of problems worth it. These medicines should never be used by pregnant women.	Accutane (isotretinoin) for cystic acne Thalomid (thalidomide) for a type of skin disease

The FDA is working hard to gather more knowledge about using medicine during pregnancy. The FDA is also trying to make medicine labels more helpful to doctors. Medicine-label information for prescription medicines is now changing, and the pregnancy part of the label will change over the next few years. As this prescription information is updated, it is added to an online information clearinghouse called "DailyMed" that gives up-to-date, free information to consumers and healthcare providers.

Over-the-Counter Medicines

All over-the-counter (OTC) medicines have a drug facts label. The Drug Facts label is arranged the same way on all OTC medicines, making information about using the medicine easier to find. One section of the Drug Facts label is for pregnant women. With OTC medicines, the label usually tells a pregnant woman to speak with her doctor before using the medicine. Some OTC medicines are known to cause certain problems in pregnancy. The labels for these medicines give pregnant women facts about why and when they should not use the medicine. Here are some examples:

- Nonsteroidal anti-inflammatory drugs (NSAIDs), such as ibuprofen (Advil, Motrin), naproxen (Aleve), and aspirin (acetylsalicylate), can cause serious blood-flow problems in the fetus if used during the last three months of pregnancy (after 28 weeks). Also, aspirin may increase the chance for bleeding problems in the mother and the fetus during pregnancy or at delivery.

- The labels for nicotine therapy drugs, such as the nicotine patch and lozenge, remind women that smoking can harm an unborn child. While the medicine is thought to be safer than smoking, the risks of the medicine are not yet fully known. Pregnant smokers are told to try quitting without the medicine first.

What If I Am Thinking about Getting Pregnant?

If you are not pregnant yet, you can help your chances for having a healthy baby by planning ahead. Schedule a prepregnancy checkup. At this visit, you can talk to your doctor about the medicines, vitamins, and herbs you use. It is very important that you keep treating your health problems while you are pregnant. Your doctor can tell you if you need to switch your medicine. Ask about vitamins for women who are trying to get pregnant. All women who can get pregnant should take a daily vitamin with folic acid (a B vitamin) to prevent birth defects of the brain and spinal cord. You should begin taking these vitamins before you become pregnant or if you could become pregnant. It is also a good idea to discuss smoking, and caffeine and alcohol consumption with your doctor at this time.

Is It Safe to Use Medicine While I Am Trying to Become Pregnant?

It is hard to know exactly when you will get pregnant. Once you do get pregnant, you may not know you are pregnant for 10 to 14 days or longer. Before you start trying to get pregnant, it is wise to schedule a meeting with your doctor to discuss medicines that you use daily or every now and then. Sometimes, medicines should be changed, and sometimes they should be stopped before a woman gets pregnant. Each woman is different. So you should discuss your medicines with your doctor rather than making medicine changes on your own.

If you are pregnant or thinking about becoming pregnant:

- Do not stop any prescribed medicines without first talking to your doctor.
- Talk to your doctor before using any OTC medicine.

What If I Get Sick and Need to Use Medicine While I Am Pregnant?

Whether or not you should use medicine during pregnancy is a serious question to discuss with your doctor. Some health problems need treatment. Not using a medicine that you need could harm you and the fetus. For example, a urinary tract infection (UTI) that is not treated may become a kidney infection. Kidney infections can cause preterm labor and low-birth weight. You need an antibiotic to cure a UTI. Ask your doctor whether the benefits of taking a certain medicine outweigh the risks for you and the fetus.

I Have a Health Problem. Should I Stop Using My Medicine While I Am Pregnant?

If you are pregnant or thinking about becoming pregnant, you should talk to your doctor about your medicines. Do not stop or change them on your own. This includes medicines for depression, asthma, diabetes, seizures (epilepsy), and other health problems. Not using medicine that you need may be more harmful to you and the fetus than using the medicine.

For women living with human immunodeficiency virus (HIV), the Centers for Disease Control and Prevention (CDC) recommends using zidovudine (AZT) during pregnancy. Studies show that HIV positive women who use AZT during pregnancy greatly lower the risk of passing HIV to their babies. If a diabetic woman does not use her medicine during pregnancy, she raises her risk for miscarriage, stillbirth, and some birth defects. If asthma and high blood pressure are not controlled during pregnancy, problems with the fetus may result.

Are Vitamins Safe for Me While I Am Pregnant?

Women who are pregnant should not take regular vitamins. They can contain doses that are too high. Ask about special vitamins for pregnant women that can help keep you and the fetus healthy. These prenatal vitamins should contain at least 400 to 800 micrograms (μg) of folic acid. It is best to start taking these vitamins before you become pregnant or if you could become pregnant. Folic acid reduces the chance of a baby having a neural-tube defect, such as spina bifida, where the spine or brain does not form the right way. Iron can help prevent a low red blood cell count (anemia). It is important to take the vitamin dose prescribed by your doctor. Too many vitamins can harm a fetus. For example, very high levels of vitamin A have been linked with severe birth defects.

Are Herbs, Minerals, or Amino Acids Safe for Me While I Am Pregnant?

No one is sure if these are safe for pregnant women, so it is best not to use them. Even some natural products may not be good for women who are pregnant or breastfeeding. Except for some vitamins, little is known about using dietary supplements while pregnant. Some herbal remedy labels claim that they will help with pregnancy, but, most often there are no good studies to show if these claims are true or if the herb can cause harm. Talk with your doctor before using any herbal product or dietary supplement. These products may contain things that could harm you or the fetus during your pregnancy.

In the United States, there are different laws for medicines and for dietary supplements. The part of the FDA that controls dietary supplements is the same part that controls foods sold in the United States. Only dietary supplements containing new dietary ingredients that were not marketed before October 15, 1994, submit safety information for review by the FDA. However, unlike medicines, the FDA does not approve herbal remedies and natural products for safety or for what they say they will do. Most have not even been evaluated for their potential to cause harm to you or the growing fetus, let alone shown to be safe for use in pregnancy. Before a company can sell a medicine, the company must complete many studies and send the results to the FDA. Many scientists and doctors at the FDA check the study results. The FDA allows the medicine to be sold only if the studies show that the medicine works and is safe to use.

Are Vaccines Safe for Me While I Am Pregnant?

Vaccines protect your body against dangerous diseases. Some vaccines are not safe to receive during pregnancy. For some vaccines, the decision to use it during pregnancy depends on the woman's own situation. Her doctor may consider these questions before giving a vaccine:

- Is there a high chance she will be exposed to the disease?
- Would the infection pose a risk to the mother or fetus?
- Is the vaccine unlikely to cause harm?

The Advisory Committee on Immunization Practices (ACIP) recommends that a Hepatitis B vaccination should be considered when women are at risk for developing Hepatitis B during pregnancy, and an inactivated-influenza vaccine should be considered for women who are pregnant during flu season. On the other hand, a pregnant woman who is not immune to rubella (German measles) is not given a rubella vaccine until after pregnancy. Talk with your doctor to make sure you are fully protected. The Centers for Disease Control and Prevention (CDC) provides vaccine guidelines for pregnant women.

In the Future, Will There Be Better Ways to Know If Medicines Are Safe to Use during Pregnancy?

At this time, drugs are rarely tested for safety in pregnant women for fear of harming the fetus. Until this changes, pregnancy-exposure registries help doctors and researchers learn how medicines affect pregnant mothers and fetuses. A pregnancy-exposure registry is a study that enrolls pregnant women that are using a certain medicine. The women sign up for the study while pregnant and are followed for a certain length of time after the baby is born. Researchers compare babies of mothers who used the medicine while pregnant to babies of mothers who did not use the medicine. This type of study compares large groups of pregnant mothers and babies to look for medicine effects. A woman and her doctor can use registry results to make more informed choices about using medicine while pregnant.

If you are pregnant and are using a medicine or were using one when you got pregnant, check to see if there is a pregnancy-exposure registry for that medicine. The FDA has a list of pregnancy-exposure registries that pregnant women can join.

Section 17.2

Aspirin and Pregnancy

This section contains text excerpted from the following sources: Text in this section begins with excerpts from "An Aspirin a Day for Preeclampsia Prevention," *Eunice Kennedy Shriver* National Institute of Child Health and Human Development (NICHD), August 25, 2014. Reviewed February 2019; Text under the heading "Aspirin May Help Increase Pregnancy Chances in Women with High Inflammation" is excerpted from "Aspirin May Help Increase Pregnancy Chances in Women with High Inflammation, NIH Study Finds," *Eunice Kennedy Shriver* National Institute of Child Health and Human Development (NICHD), February 7, 2017.

Aspirin is generally not recommended during pregnancy, as it can lead to bleeding problems for both the mother and the fetus. But for some women, the benefits of a daily low-dose aspirin after the first trimester may outweigh the risk.

Results from multiple clinical trials showed that using low-dose aspirin lowered the risk of preeclampsia in pregnant women at a high risk for the condition. Preeclampsia happens when a woman's blood pressure suddenly gets too high during pregnancy. If preeclampsia occurs during pregnancy, the only current cure is delivery of the fetus, often prematurely. In fact, preeclampsia is responsible for 15 percent of preterm births in the United States.

The clinical trials also found that low-dose aspirin reduced the risk for premature delivery and low-birth weight of infants. Based on these findings, the U.S. Preventive Services Task Force (USPSTF) issued a recommendation policy that women at a high risk for preeclampsia take a daily low-dose aspirin after 12 weeks of pregnancy to help prevent the condition from developing. The USPSTF recommendation mirrored the 2013 guidelines policy from the American College of Obstetricians and Gynecologists (ACOG).

Determining a Pregnant Woman's Risk for Preeclampsia

Preeclampsia affects three to five percent of pregnancies in the United States each year and is a leading cause of maternal and neonatal morbidity/mortality. Women may be at higher risk for preeclampsia if they:

- Had preeclampsia in a previous pregnancy, especially if they delivered prematurely

- Are obese

- Are younger than age 20 or older than age 35

- Are carrying twins or multiples

- Had high blood pressure or kidney disease before getting pregnant

- Are African American

- Have a family history of preeclampsia

- Have certain health conditions, such as diabetes, lupus, or polycystic ovary syndrome (PCOS)

However, it can be difficult to predict if a woman will develop preeclampsia. Pregnant women with normal blood pressure at 20 weeks of pregnancy can suddenly develop the symptoms, which include high blood pressure, increased swelling, and protein in the urine. Much of the time, preeclampsia has no visible symptoms.

For this reason, it is important for all pregnant women to get regular prenatal care. This will allow their healthcare provider to monitor their health closely and determine if a daily aspirin is needed.

Eunice Kennedy Shriver *National Institute of Child Health and Human Development Research on Preeclampsia*

The *Eunice Kennedy Shriver* National Institute of Child Health and Human Development (NICHD) has supported research on preeclampsia for decades. Scientists seek to understand the causes of preeclampsia and how best to prevent and treat the condition. Some of the research led and supported by the NICHD on preeclampsia includes, but is not limited to, the following:

- **A method to triage and monitor the patient with suspected preeclampsia.** Researchers in NICHD's Program in Perinatal Research and Obstetrics (PPRO) have developed a novel classification system by examining biomarkers in the plasma of patients with preeclampsia to identify those at risk for preterm delivery or adverse maternal/neonatal outcome. The PPRO has identified biomarkers that can be measured in maternal blood in the midtrimester that can be used to predict preterm and term preeclampsia.

- **Treatments to lower blood pressure during pregnancy**. Researchers are studying corin, a newly discovered molecule that regulates blood pressure. In previous studies on mice, those that lacked corin developed high blood pressure and high levels of protein in the urine during pregnancy. This suggests that corin may play a key role in preventing high blood pressure during pregnancy. Researchers hope to develop treatments using corin to help prevent preeclampsia.

- **The use of medications other than aspirin to lower the risk of developing preeclampsia.** Researchers are also studying whether daily use of pravastatin and other statins, which are typically used to lower and manage cholesterol levels, can benefit women at high risk for preeclampsia.

- **Potential treatment of preeclampsia.** Researchers are working to develop a new and safe therapy for preeclampsia. Pregnant women with preeclampsia have higher levels of a certain protein in their blood. In this study, researchers will filter patients' blood to remove these proteins, using a therapy similar to dialysis for kidney patients. Researchers hope this treatment will reverse symptoms of preeclampsia and prolong pregnancy.

- **The effect of obesity on preeclampsia.** Studies on the impact of obesity policy may tell researchers if factors contributing to obesity are related to the development of preeclampsia. Researchers are also evaluating whether these same factors contribute to cardiovascular conditions in nonpregnant women with a history of preeclampsia.

These are just a few of the NICHD's ongoing projects related to preeclampsia.

Aspirin May Help Increase Pregnancy Chances in Women with High Inflammation

A daily low-dose of aspirin may help a subgroup of women that have previously lost a pregnancy to successfully conceive and carry a pregnancy to term, according to an analysis by researchers at the National Institutes of Health (NIH). The women who benefited from the aspirin treatment had high levels of C-reactive protein (CRP), a substance in the blood indicating system-wide inflammation, which aspirin is thought to counteract. The study appears in the Journal of Clinical Endocrinology and Metabolism.

Researchers at NIH's NICHD analyzed data originally obtained from the Effects of Aspirin in Gestation and Reproduction (EAGeR) trial. The trial sought to determine if daily low-dose aspirin could prevent subsequent pregnancy loss among women who had one or two prior losses.

For the current study, researchers classified the women into three groups: low CRP (below .70 mg per liter of blood), mid-CRP (from .70 to 1.95 mg per liter) and high CRP (at or above 1.95 mg per liter). Women within each group received either daily low-dose aspirin or a placebo. In their analysis, researchers found no significant differences in birth rates between those receiving aspirin and those receiving placebo in both the low-CRP and mid-CRP groups. For the high-CRP group, those taking the placebo had the lowest rate of live birth at 44 percent, while those taking daily aspirin had a live-birth rate of 59 percent—a 35-percent increase. Aspirin also appeared to reduce CRP levels in the high-CRP group when measured during weeks 8, 20, and 36 of pregnancy.

Chapter 18

Folic Acid

What Are Folic Acid and Folate?

Folic acid is the human-made form of folate, a B vitamin. Folate is found naturally in certain fruits, vegetables, and nuts. Folic acid is found in vitamins and fortified foods.

Folic acid and folate help the body make new, healthy red blood cells (RBCs). Red blood cells carry oxygen to every part of your body. If your body does not make enough red blood cells, you can develop anemia. Anemia happens when your blood cannot carry enough oxygen to your body, which makes you pale, tired, or weak. Also, if you do not get enough folic acid, you could develop a type of anemia called "folate-deficiency anemia."

If you can get pregnant or are pregnant, folic acid is especially important. Folic acid protects unborn babies against serious birth defects. You can get folic acid from vitamins and fortified foods, such as breads, pastas, and cereals. Folate is found naturally in foods such as leafy green vegetables, oranges, and beans.

This chapter includes text excerpted from "Folic Acid," Office on Women's Health (OWH), U.S. Department of Health and Human Services (HHS), October 18, 2018.

Why Do Women Need Folic Acid?

Everyone needs folic acid to be healthy. But it is especially important for women:

- **Before and during pregnancy.** Folic acid protects the fetus against serious birth defects called "neural-tube defects." These birth defects happen in the first few weeks of pregnancy, often before a woman knows she is pregnant. Folic acid might also help prevent other types of birth defects and early pregnancy loss (miscarriage). Since about half of all pregnancies in the United States are unplanned, experts recommend all women get enough folic acid, even if you are not trying to get pregnant.

- **To keep the blood healthy by helping red blood cells form and grow.** Not getting enough folic acid can lead to a type of anemia called "folate-deficiency anemia." Folate-deficiency anemia is more common in women of childbearing age than in men.

How Do I Get Folic Acid?

You can get folic acid in two ways.

1. **Through the foods you eat.** Folate is found naturally in some foods, including spinach, nuts, and beans. Folic acid is found in fortified foods (called "enriched foods"), such as breads, pastas, and cereals. Look for the term "enriched" on the ingredients list to find out whether the food has added folic acid.

2. **As a vitamin.** Most multivitamins sold in the United States contain 400 micrograms, or 100 percentage of the daily value, of folic acid. Check the label to make sure.

How Much Folic Acid Do Women Need?

All women need 400 micrograms of folic acid every day. Women who can get pregnant should get 400 to 800 micrograms of folic acid from a vitamin or from food that has added folic acid, such as breakfast cereal. This is in addition to the folate you get naturally from food.

Some women may need more folic acid each day. See the table to find out how much folic acid you need.

Table 18.1. Amount of Folic Acid a Women Should Have Daily

If You:	Amount of Folic Acid You May Need Daily
Could get pregnant or are pregnant	400–800 micrograms. Your doctor may prescribe a prenatal vitamin with more.
Had a baby with a neural-tube defect (such as spina bifida) and want to get pregnant again	4,000 micrograms. Your doctor may prescribe this amount. Research shows taking this amount may lower the risk of having another baby with spina bifida.
Have a family member with spina bifida and could get pregnant	4,000 micrograms. Your doctor may prescribe this amount.
Have spina bifida and want to get pregnant	4,000 micrograms. Your doctor may prescribe this amount. Women with spina bifida have a higher risk of having children with the condition.
Take medicines to treat epilepsy, type 2 diabetes, rheumatoid arthritis, or lupus	Talk to your doctor or nurse. Folic acid supplements can interact with these medicines.
Are on dialysis for kidney disease	Talk to your doctor or nurse.
Have a health condition, such as inflammatory bowel disease or celiac disease, that affects how your body absorbs folic acid	Talk to your doctor or nurse.

Are Some Women at Risk for Not Getting Enough Folic Acid?

Yes, certain groups of women do not get enough folic acid each day.

- Women who can get pregnant need more folic acid (400 to 800 micrograms)

- Nearly one in three African American women does not get enough folic acid each day

- Spanish-speaking Mexican American women often do not get enough folic acid. However, Mexican Americans who speak English usually get enough folic acid.

Not getting enough folic acid can cause health problems, including folate-deficiency anemia, and problems during pregnancy for you and the fetus.

What Can Happen If I Do Not Get Enough Folic Acid during Pregnancy?

If you do not get enough folic acid before and during pregnancy, the fetus is at higher risk for neural-tube defects.

Neural-tube defects are serious birth defects that affect the spine, spinal cord, or brain and may cause death. These include:

- **Spina bifida.** This condition happens when a fetus's spinal column does not fully close during development in the womb, leaving the spinal cord exposed. As a result, the nerves that control the legs and other organs do not work. Children with spina bifida often have lifelong disabilities. They may also need many surgeries.

- **Anencephaly.** This means that most or all of the brain and skull does not develop in the womb. Almost all babies with this condition die before or soon after birth.

Do I Need to Take Folic Acid Every Day Even If I'm Not Planning to Get Pregnant?

Yes. All women who can get pregnant need to take 400 to 800 micrograms of folic acid every day, even if you're not planning to get pregnant. There are several reasons why:

- Your birth control may not work or you may not use birth control correctly every time you have sex. In a survey from the Centers for Disease Control and Prevention (CDC), almost 40 percent of women with unplanned pregnancies were using birth control.

- Birth defects of the brain and spine can happen in the first few weeks of pregnancy, often before you know you are pregnant. By the time you find out you are pregnant, it might be too late to prevent the birth defects.

- You need to take folic acid every day because it is a water soluble B-vitamin. Water soluble means that it does not stay in the body for a long time. Your body metabolizes (uses) folic acid quickly, so your body needs folic acid each day to work properly.

What Foods Contain Folic Acid

Folic acid is added to foods that are refined or processed (not whole grain):

- Breakfast cereals (Some have 100 percent of the recommended daily value—or 400 micrograms—of folic acid in each serving.)
- Breads and pasta
- Flours
- Cornmeal
- White rice

Since 1998, the U.S. Food and Drug Administration (FDA) has required food manufacturers to add folic acid to processed breads, cereals, flours, cornmeal, pastas, rice, and other grains. For other foods, check the nutrition facts label on the package to see if it has folic acid. The label will also tell you how much folic acid is in each serving. Sometimes, the label will say "folate" instead of folic acid.

What Foods Contain Folate

Folate is found naturally in some foods. Foods that are naturally high in folate include:

- Spinach and other dark green, leafy vegetables
- Oranges and orange juice
- Nuts
- Beans
- Poultry (chicken, turkey, etc.) and meat
- Whole grains

How Can I Be Sure I Get Enough Folic Acid?

You can get enough folic acid from food alone. Many breakfast cereals have 100 percent of your recommended daily value (400 micrograms) of folic acid.

If you are at risk for not getting enough folic acid, your doctor or nurse may recommend that you take a vitamin with folic acid every day. Most U.S. multivitamins have at least 400 micrograms of folic acid. Check the label on the bottle to be sure. You can also take a pill that contains only folic acid.

If swallowing pills is hard for you, try a chewable or liquid product with folic acid.

Supplement Facts

Serving Size: 1 tablet

Amount Per Serving		% Daily Value
Vitamin A	5000IU	100
Vitamin C	60mg	100
Vitamin D	400IU	100
Vitamin E	30IU	100
Thiamin	1.5mg	100
Riboflavin	1.7mg	100
Niacin	20mg	100
Vitamin B6	2mg	100
Folic Acid	400mcg	100
Vitamin B12	6mcg	100
Biotin	30mg	10
Pantothenic Acid	10mg	100
Calcium	162mg	16
Iron	18mg	100
Iodine	150mcg	100
Magnesium	100mg	25
Zinc	15mg	100
Selenium	20mcg	100
Copper	2mg	100
Manganese	3.5mg	175
Chromium	65mcg	54
Molybdenum	150mcg	200
Chloride	72mg	2
Potassium`	80mg	2

Find **folic acid:** Choose a vitamin that says "400mcg" or "100%" next to folic acid

Figure 18.1. *Supplements Fact Label*

What Should I Look for When Buying Vitamins with Folic Acid?

Look for "United States Pharmacopeia (USP)" or "National Sanitation Foundation (NSF)" on the label when choosing vitamins. These seals of approval mean that the pills are made properly and have the amounts of vitamins it says on the label. Also, make sure the pills have not expired. If the bottle has no expiration date, do not buy it.

Ask your pharmacist for help with selecting a vitamin or folic acid-only pill. If you are pregnant and already take a daily prenatal vitamin, you probably get all the folic acid you need. Check the label to be sure.

Vitamin Label

Check the supplement facts label to be sure you are getting 400 to 800 micrograms (mcg) of folic acid.

Can I Get Enough Folic Acid from Food Alone?

Yes, many people get enough folic acid from food alone. Some foods have high amounts of folic acid. For example, many breakfast cereals have 100 percent of the recommended daily value (400 micrograms) of folic acid in each serving. Check the label to be sure.

Some women, especially women who could get pregnant, may not get enough folic acid from food. African American women and Mexican Americans are also at higher risk for not getting enough folic acid each day. Talk to your doctor or nurse about whether you should take a vitamin to get the 400 micrograms of folic acid you need each day.

What Is Folate-Deficiency Anemia?

Folate-deficiency anemia is a type of anemia that happens when you do not get enough folate. Folate-deficiency anemia is most common during pregnancy. Other causes of folate-deficiency anemia include alcoholism and certain medicines to treat seizures, anxiety, or arthritis.

The symptoms of folate-deficiency anemia include:

- Fatigue
- Headache
- Pale skin
- Sore mouth and tongue

If you have folate-deficiency anemia, your doctor may recommend taking folic acid vitamins and eating more foods with folate.

Can I Get Too Much Folic Acid?

Yes, you can get too much folic acid, but only from man-made products such as multivitamins and fortified foods, such as breakfast cereals. You cannot get too much folic acid from foods that naturally contain folate.

You should not get more than 1,000 micrograms of folic acid a day, unless your doctor prescribes a higher amount. Too much folic acid can hide signs that you lack vitamin B_{12}, which can cause nerve damage.

Do I Need Folic Acid after Menopause?

Yes. Women who have gone through menopause still need 400 micrograms of folic acid every day for good health. Talk to your doctor or nurse about how much folic acid you need.

Are Folic Acid Pills Covered under Insurance?

Yes. Under the Affordable Care Act (ACA) (the healthcare law), all health insurance marketplace plans and most other insurance plans cover folic acid pills for women who could get pregnant at no cost to you. Check with your insurance provider to find out what is included in your plan.

Chapter 19

Nutrition and Pregnancy

Chapter Contents

Section 19.1

What to Eat: A Guide for Pregnant Women

This section contains text excerpted from the following sources:
Text beginning with the heading "Eating for Two" is excerpted from
"Staying Healthy and Safe," Office on Women's Health (OWH),
U.S. Department of Health and Human Services (HHS), January 30,
2019; Text under the heading "Healthy Eating" is excerpted
from "Health Tips for Pregnant Women," National Institute
of Diabetes and Digestive and Kidney Diseases (NIDDK),
June 2013. Reviewed February 2019.

Eating for Two

Eating healthy foods is more important now than ever. You need more protein, iron, calcium, and folic acid than you did before pregnancy. You also need more calories. But eating for two does not mean eating twice as much. Rather, it means that the foods you eat are the main source of nutrients for the fetus. Sensible, balanced meals combined with regular physical fitness is still the best recipe for good health during your pregnancy.

Calorie Needs

Your calorie needs will depend on your weight-gain goals. Most women need 300 calories a day more during the last six months of pregnancy than they do prepregnancy. Keep in mind that not all calories are equal. Your baby needs healthy foods that are packed with nutrients, not "empty calories" such as those found in soft drinks, candies, and desserts.

Although you want to be careful not to eat more than necessary for a healthy pregnancy, make sure not to restrict your diet during pregnancy either. If you do not get the calories you need, your baby might not get the right amounts of protein, vitamins, and minerals. Low-calorie diets can break down a pregnant woman's stored fat, which can cause your body to make substances called "ketones." Ketones can be found in the mother's blood and urine and are a sign of starvation. Constant production of ketones can result in a child with mental deficiencies.

Foods Good for the Mother and the Fetus

A pregnant woman needs more of many important vitamins, minerals, and nutrients than she did before pregnancy. Making healthy food choices every day will help you give the fetus what it needs to develop. For pregnant and breastfeeding women, ChooseMyPlate can show you what to eat as well as how much you need to eat from each food group based on your height, weight, and activity level.

Talk to your doctor if you have special diet needs for these reasons:

- **Diabetes.** Make sure you review your meal plan and insulin needs with your doctor. High blood-glucose levels can be harmful to the fetus.

- **Lactose intolerance.** Find out about low-lactose or reduced-lactose products and calcium supplements to ensure you are getting the calcium you need.

- **Vegetarian.** Ensure that you are eating enough protein, iron, vitamin B_{12}, and vitamin D.

- **Phenylketonuria (PKU).** Keep good control of phenylalanine levels in your diet.

Food Safety

Most foods are safe for pregnant women and their babies. But you will need to use caution or avoid eating certain foods. Follow these guidelines:

Clean, Handle, Cook, and Chill Food Properly to Prevent Foodborne Illness, including Listeria and Toxoplasmosis

- Wash hands with soap after touching soil or raw meat

- Keep raw meats, poultry, and seafood away from other foods or surfaces

- Cook meat completely

- Wash produce before eating

- Wash cooking utensils with hot, soapy water

Do Not Eat

- Refrigerated smoked seafood like whitefish, salmon, and mackerel

- Hot dogs or deli meats unless steaming hot

- Refrigerated meat spreads

- Unpasteurized milk or juices

- Store-made salads, such as chicken, egg, or tuna salad

- Unpasteurized-soft cheeses, such as unpasteurized feta, Brie, queso blanco, queso fresco, and blue cheeses

- Shark, swordfish, king mackerel, or tile fish (also called "golden snapper" or "white snapper"); these fish have high levels of mercury

- More than six ounces of white (albacore) tuna per week

- Herbs and plants used as medicines without doctor approval. The safety of herbal and plant therapies is not always known. Some herbs and plants might be harmful during pregnancy, such as bitter melon (karela), noni juice, and unripe papaya.

- Raw sprouts of any kind (including alfalfa, clover, radish, and mung bean)

Don't Forget Fluids

All of your body's systems need water. When you are pregnant, your body needs even more water to stay hydrated and support the fetus. Water also helps prevent constipation, hemorrhoids, excessive swelling, and urinary tract or bladder infections. Not getting enough water can lead to premature or early labor.

Your body gets the water it needs through the fluids you drink and the foods you eat. How much fluid you need to drink each day depends on many factors, such as your activity level, the weather, and your size. Your body needs more fluids when it is hot and when you are physically active. It also needs more water if you have a fever or if you are vomiting or have diarrhea.

The Institute of Medicine (IOM) recommends that pregnant women drink about 10 cups of fluids daily. Water, juices, coffee, tea, and soft drinks all count toward your fluid needs. But keep in mind that some beverages are high in sugar and "empty calories." A good way to tell if your fluid intake is okay is if your urine is pale yellow or colorless and you rarely feel thirsty. Thirst is a sign that your body is on its way to dehydration. Do not wait until you feel thirsty to drink.

Healthy Eating
How Much Should I Eat?

Eating healthy foods and the right amount of calories helps you and fetus gain the proper amount of weight.

How much food you need depends on factors such as your weight before pregnancy, your age, and how fast you gain weight. In the first three months of pregnancy, most women do not need extra calories. You also may not need extra calories during the final weeks of pregnancy.

Check with your doctor about this. If you are not gaining the right amount of weight, your doctor may advise you to eat more calories. If you are gaining too much weight, you may need to cut down on calories. Each woman's needs are different. Your needs depend on if you were underweight, overweight, or obese before you became pregnant, or if you are having more than one baby.

What Kinds of Foods Should I Eat?

A healthy eating plan for pregnancy includes nutrient-rich foods. Current U.S. dietary guidelines advise eating these foods each day:

- Fruits and veggies (provide vitamins and fiber)

- Whole grains, such as oatmeal, whole-wheat bread, and brown rice (provide fiber, B vitamins, and other needed nutrients)

- Fat-free or low-fat milk and milk products or nondairy soy, almond, rice, or other drinks with added calcium and vitamin D

- Protein from healthy sources, such as beans and peas, eggs, lean meats, seafood (8 to 12 ounces per week), and unsalted nuts and seeds

A healthy eating plan also limits salt, solid fats (like butter, lard, and shortening), and sugar-sweetened drinks and foods.

Does your eating plan measure up? How can you improve your eating habits? Try eating fruit like berries or a banana with low-fat yogurt for breakfast, a salad with beans for lunch, and a lean chicken breast and steamed veggies for dinner. Think about things you can try.

179

Do I Have Any Special Nutrition Needs Now That I Am Pregnant?

Yes. During pregnancy, you need more vitamins and minerals, such as folate, iron, and calcium.

Getting the right amount of folate is very important. Folate, a B vitamin also known as folic acid, may help prevent birth defects. Before pregnancy, you need 400 mcg per day. During pregnancy and when breastfeeding, you need 600 mcg per day from foods or vitamins. Foods high in folate include orange juice, strawberries, spinach, broccoli, beans, and fortified breads and breakfast cereals.

Most healthcare providers tell women who are pregnant to take a prenatal vitamin every day and to eat a healthy diet. Ask your doctor about what you should take.

What Other New Eating Habits May Help My Weight Gain?

Pregnancy can create some new food and eating concerns. Meet the needs of your body and be more comfortable with these tips:

- **Eat breakfast every day.** If you feel sick to your stomach in the morning, try dry whole-wheat toast or whole-grain crackers when you first wake up. Eat them even before you get out of bed. Eat the rest of your breakfast (fruit, oatmeal, whole-grain cereal, low-fat milk or yogurt, or other foods) later in the morning.

- **Eat high-fiber foods.** Eating high-fiber foods, drinking plenty of water, and getting daily physical activity may help prevent constipation. Try to eat whole-grain cereals, vegetables, fruits, and beans.

- **If you have heartburn, eat small meals more often.** Try to eat slowly and avoid spicy and fatty foods, such as hot peppers or fried chicken. Have drinks between meals instead of with meals. Do not lie down soon after eating.

What Foods Should I Avoid?

There are certain foods and drinks that can harm the fetus if you have them while you are pregnant. Here is a list of items you should avoid:

- **Alcohol.** Do not drink alcohol, such as wine or beer. Enjoy decaf coffee or tea, nonsugar-sweetened drinks, or water with a dash of juice. Avoid diet drinks and drinks with caffeine.

- **Fish that may have high levels of mercury** (a substance that can build up in fish and harm a fetus). You should eat 8 to 12 ounces of seafood per week, but limit white (albacore) tuna to 6 ounces per week. Do not eat tilefish, shark, swordfish, and king mackerel.

- **Anything that is not food.** Some pregnant women may crave something that is not food, such as laundry starch or clay. This may mean that you are not getting the right amount of a nutrient. Talk to your doctor if you crave something that is not food. He or she can help you get the right amount of nutrients.

Section 19.2

Vegetarian Diets and Pregnancy

This section includes text excerpted from "Vegetarian Eating," Office on Women's Health (OWH), U.S. Department of Health and Human Services (HHS), October 18, 2018.

A vegetarian is someone who does not eat meat. Some vegetarians, called vegans, do not eat any animal products, such as eggs or milk. If you are a vegetarian or vegan, you may need to take a dietary supplement, especially if you are pregnant or breastfeeding.

What Is a Healthy Eating Plan for Women Who Are Vegetarian?

A healthy eating plan for women who are vegetarian is the same as for any woman. Because vegetarians eat mostly plant-based foods, they usually get more fiber-rich foods and low-cholesterol foods than nonvegetarians do. But women who are vegetarians still need to make sure they are eating healthy, which includes foods with calcium and protein.

Do Women Who Are Vegetarian Need to Take a Dietary Supplement?

Not always. You can get all the nutrients you need from a vegetarian eating plan by eating a variety of foods from all of the food groups. But you may need to take extra steps to get enough protein, iron, calcium, vitamin B_{12}, and zinc.

The extra steps you need to take depend on what type of vegetarian you are. For example, low-fat and fat-free milk and milk products are good sources of calcium, vitamin B_{12}, and complete protein. Eggs are a good source of vitamin B_{12}, choline, and complete protein. But if you do not drink milk or eat eggs, you need to get these nutrients from other foods.

Do Vegetarians Need More Nutrients during Pregnancy?

Yes. Just like all women, your body needs more of some nutrients, such as folic acid, during pregnancy to help the fetus grow and develop. In general, though, choosing a variety of healthy foods from each of the food groups will help you get the nutrients you need during pregnancy. Be sure to get enough protein, found in beans, nuts, nut butters, and eggs if you eat them. Get a personalized daily food checklist based on your age, weight, height, and activity level.

A vegetarian eating plan during pregnancy can be healthy. Talk to your healthcare provider to make sure you are getting calcium, iron, protein, vitamin B_{12}, vitamin D, and other needed nutrients. She or he may ask you to meet with a registered dietitian (a nutrition expert who has a degree in diet and nutrition approved by the Academy of Nutrition and Dietetics, has passed a national exam, and is licensed to practice in your state) who can help you plan meals. Your doctor may also tell you to take vitamins and minerals that will help you meet your needs.

Section 19.3

Anemia and Pregnancy

This section includes text excerpted from "Older Adults and Alcohol,"
Office on Women's Health (OWH), U.S. Department of Health and
Human Services (HHS), November 21, 2018.

Iron-deficiency anemia means that your body does not have enough
iron. Your body needs iron to help carry oxygen through your blood to
every part of your body. Iron-deficiency anemia affects more women
than men and is more common during pregnancy.

What Is Iron-Deficiency Anemia?

Iron-deficiency anemia (IDA) is the most common type of anemia, a
condition that happens when your body does not make enough healthy
red-blood cells (RBC) or the blood cells do not work correctly.

Iron-deficiency anemia happens when you don't have enough iron
in your body. Your body needs iron to make hemoglobin, the part of
the red-blood cell that carries oxygen through your blood to all parts
of your body.

Who Gets Iron-Deficiency Anemia

Iron-deficiency anemia affects more women than men. The risk of
iron-deficiency anemia is highest for women who:

- **Are pregnant.** Iron-deficiency anemia affects one in six
  pregnant women. You need more iron during pregnancy to
  support the fetus's development.

- **Have heavy menstrual periods.** Up to five percent of women
  of childbearing age develop iron-deficiency anemia because of
  heavy bleeding during their periods.

Infants, small children, and teens are also at high risk for
iron-deficiency anemia.

What Are the Symptoms of Iron-Deficiency Anemia?

Iron-deficiency anemia often develops slowly. In the beginning, you
may not have any symptoms, or they may be mild. As it gets worse,
you may notice one or more of these symptoms:

- Fatigue (very common)

- Weakness (very common)

- Dizziness

- Headaches

- Low body temperature

- Pale or yellow "sallow" skin

- Rapid or irregular heartbeat

- Shortness of breath or chest pain, especially with physical activity

- Brittle nails

- Pica (unusual cravings for ice, very cold drinks, or nonfood items like dirt or paper)

If you think you may have iron-deficiency anemia, talk to your doctor or nurse.

What Causes Iron-Deficiency Anemia

Women can have low iron levels for several reasons:

- **Iron lost through bleeding.** Bleeding can cause you to lose more blood cells and iron than your body can replace. Women may have low iron levels from bleeding caused by:

  - Digestive system problems, such as ulcers, colon polyps, or colon cancer

  - Regular, long-term use of aspirin and other over-the-counter (OTC) pain relievers

  - Donating blood too often or without enough time in between donations for your body to recover

  - Heavier or longer than normal menstrual periods

  - Uterine fibroids, which are noncancerous growths in the uterus that can cause heavy bleeding

- **Increased need for iron during pregnancy.** During pregnancy, your body needs more iron than normal to support your developing fetus.

- **Not eating enough food that contains iron.** Your body absorbs the iron in animal-based foods, such as meat, chicken, and fish, two to three times better than the iron in plant-based foods. Vegetarians or vegans, who eat little or no animal-based foods, need to choose other good sources of iron to make sure they get enough. Your body also absorbs iron from plant-based foods better when you eat them with foods that have vitamin C, such as oranges and tomatoes. But most people in the United States get enough iron from food.

- **Problems absorbing iron.** Certain health conditions, such as Crohn disease or celiac disease, or having had gastric bypass surgery for weight loss can make it harder for your body to absorb iron from food.

How Is Iron-Deficiency Anemia Diagnosed?

Talk to your doctor if you think you might have iron-deficiency anemia. Your doctor may:

- Ask you questions about your health history, including how regular or heavy your menstrual periods are. Your doctor may also ask you about any digestive-system problems you may have, such as blood in your stool.

- Do a physical exam

- Talk to you about the foods you eat, the medicines you take, and your family health history

- Do blood tests. Your doctor will do a complete blood count (CBC). A CBC measures many parts of your blood. If the CBC test shows that you have anemia, your doctor will likely do another blood test to measure the iron levels in your blood and confirm that you have iron-deficiency anemia.

If you have iron-deficiency anemia, your doctor may want to do other tests to find out what is causing it.

Do I Need to Be Tested for Iron-Deficiency Anemia?

Maybe. Talk to your doctor about getting tested as part of your regular health exam if you have heavy menstrual periods or a health problem, such as Crohn disease or celiac disease.

How Is Iron-Deficiency Anemia Treated?

Treatment for iron-deficiency anemia depends on the cause:

- **Blood loss from a digestive system problem.** If you have an ulcer, your doctor may give you antibiotics or other medicines to treat the ulcer. If your bleeding is caused by a polyp or cancerous tumor, you may need surgery to remove it.

- **Blood loss from heavy menstrual periods.** Your doctor may give you hormonal birth control to help relieve heavy periods. If your heavy bleeding does not get better, your doctor may recommend surgery. Types of surgery to control heavy bleeding include endometrial ablation, which removes or destroys your uterine lining, and a hysterectomy, which removes all or parts of your uterus.

- **Increased need for iron.** If you have problems absorbing iron or have lower iron levels but do not have severe anemia, your doctor may recommend:

  - Iron pills to build up your iron levels as quickly as possible. Do not take any iron pills without first talking to your doctor or nurse.

  - Eating more foods that contain iron. Good sources of iron include meat, fish, eggs, beans, peas, and fortified foods (look for cereals fortified with 100 percentage of the daily value for iron).

  - Eating more foods with vitamin C. Vitamin C helps your body absorb iron. Good sources of vitamin C include oranges, broccoli, and tomatoes.

If you have severe bleeding or symptoms of chest pain or shortness of breath, your doctor may recommend iron or red blood cell transfusions. Transfusions are only for severe iron deficiencies and are much less common.

What Do I Need to Know about Iron Pills?

Your doctor may recommend iron pills to help build up your iron levels. Do not take these pills without talking to your doctor or nurse first. Taking iron pills can cause side effects, including an upset stomach, constipation, and diarrhea. If taken as a liquid, iron supplements may stain your teeth.

You can reduce side effects from iron pills by taking these steps:

- Start with half of the recommended dose. Gradually increase to the full dose.

- Take iron in divided doses. For example, if you take two pills daily, take one in the morning with breakfast and the other after dinner.

- Take iron with food (especially something with vitamin C, such as a glass of orange juice, to help your body absorb the iron).

- If one type of iron pill causes side effects, ask your doctor for another type.

- If you take iron as a liquid instead of as a pill, aim it toward the back of your mouth. This will prevent the liquid from staining your teeth. You can also brush your teeth after taking the medicine to help prevent staining.

What Can Happen If Iron-Deficiency Anemia Is Not Treated?

If left untreated, iron-deficiency anemia can cause serious health problems. Having too little oxygen in the body can damage organs. With anemia, the heart must work harder to make up for the lack of red blood cells or hemoglobin. This extra work can harm the heart.

Iron-deficiency anemia can also cause problems during pregnancy.

How Can I Prevent Iron-Deficiency Anemia?

You can help prevent iron-deficiency anemia with the following steps:

- **Treat the cause of blood loss.** Talk to your doctor if you have heavy menstrual periods or if you have digestive-system problems, such as frequent diarrhea or blood in your stool.

- **Eat foods with iron.** Good sources of iron include lean meat and chicken; dark, leafy vegetables; and beans.

- **Eat and drink foods that help your body absorb iron,** such as orange juice, strawberries, broccoli, or other fruits and vegetables with vitamin C.

- **Make healthy food choices.** Most people who make healthy, balanced food choices get the iron and vitamins their bodies need from the foods they eat.

- **Avoid drinking coffee or tea with meals.** These drinks make it harder for your body to absorb iron.

- **Talk to your doctor if you take calcium pills.** Calcium can make it harder for your body to absorb iron. If you have a hard time getting enough iron, talk to your doctor about the best way to also get enough calcium.

How Much Iron Do I Need Every Day?

The chart below lists how much iron you need every day. The recommended amounts are listed in milligrams (mg).

Table 19.1. Good Sources of Iron

Age	Women	Pregnant Women	Breastfeeding Women	Vegetarian Women*
14–18 years	15 mg	27 mg	10 mg	27 mg
19–50 years	18 mg	27 mg	9 mg	32 mg
51+ years	8 mg	n/a	n/a	14 mg

(Source: Adapted from Institute of Medicine (IOM), Food and Nutrition Board (FNB).)
* Vegetarians need more iron from food than people who eat meat. This is because the body can absorb iron from meat better than from plant-based foods.

What Foods Contain Iron

Food sources of iron include:

- Fortified breakfast cereals (18 milligrams per serving)

- Oysters (8 milligrams per 3-ounce serving)

- Canned white beans (8 milligrams per cup)

- Dark chocolate (7 milligrams per 3-ounce serving)

- Beef liver (5 milligrams per 3-ounce serving)

- Spinach (3 milligrams per ½ cup)

- Tofu, firm (3 milligrams per ½ cup)

- Kidney beans (2 milligrams per ½ cup)

- Canned tomatoes (2 milligrams per ½ cup)
- Lean beef (2 milligrams for a 3-ounce serving)
- Baked potato (2 milligrams for a medium potato)

Do I Need More Iron during Pregnancy?

Yes. During pregnancy, your body needs more iron to support the growing fetus. In fact, pregnant women need almost twice as much iron as women who are not pregnant. Not getting enough iron during pregnancy raises your risk for premature birth or a low-birth-weight baby (less than 5 ½ pounds). Premature birth is the most common cause of infant death. Both premature birth and low birth weight raise your baby's risk for health and developmental problems at birth and during childhood.

If you are pregnant, talk to your doctor about these steps:

- Getting 27 milligrams of iron every day. Take a prenatal vitamin with iron every day, or talk to your doctor about taking an iron supplement (pill).
- Testing for iron-deficiency anemia
- Testing for iron-deficiency anemia four to six weeks after childbirth

Do I Need More Iron If I Am Breastfeeding?

No, you do not need more iron during breastfeeding. In fact, you need less iron than before you were pregnant. The amount of iron women need during breastfeeding is 10 milligrams per day for mothers aged 14 to 18 years, and 9 milligrams per day for breastfeeding women older than 18.

You need less iron while breastfeeding because you likely will not lose a lot through your menstrual cycle. Many breastfeeding women do not have a period or may only have a light period. Also, if you got enough iron during pregnancy (27 milligrams a day), your breastmilk will supply enough iron for your baby.

I Am a Vegetarian. How Can I Make Sure I Get Enough Iron?

You can help make sure you get enough iron by choosing foods that contain iron more often. Vegetarians need more iron from food than people who eat meat, because the body can absorb iron from meat better than from plant-based foods.

Vegetarian sources of iron include:

- Cereals and bread with added iron

- Lentils and beans

- Dark chocolate

- Dark green, leafy vegetables, such as spinach and broccoli

- Tofu

- Chickpeas

- Canned tomatoes

Talk to your doctor or nurse about whether you get enough iron. Most people get enough iron from food.

Can I Get More Iron Than My Body Needs?

Yes, your body can get too much iron. Extra iron can damage the liver, heart, and pancreas. Try to get no more than 45 milligrams of iron a day, unless your doctor prescribes more.

Some people get too much iron because of a condition called "hemochromatosis" that runs in families.

You can also get too much iron from iron pills (if you also get iron from food) or from repeated blood transfusions.

Section 19.4

What You Need to Know about Mercury in Fish and Shellfish

This section contains text excerpted from the following sources:
Text beginning with the heading "Should I Be Concerned about
Eating Fish and Shellfish?" is excerpted from "Should I Be Concerned
About Eating Fish and Shellfish?" U.S. Environmental Protection
Agency (EPA), February 14, 2017; Text under the heading
"Fish Facts" is excerpted from "Staying Healthy and Safe," Office on
Women's Health (OWH), U.S. Department of Health
and Human Services (HHS), January 30, 2019.

Should I Be Concerned about Eating Fish and Shellfish?

For most people, the risk of eating contaminated fish and shellfish is not a health concern. However, some groups of people—such as pregnant women, children, and the elderly—are at a greater health risk than others. Additionally, some individuals are at a higher risk simply because they eat substantially more fish than others.

The U.S. Environmental Protection Agency (EPA) and U.S. Food and Drug Administration (FDA) issue advice on eating fish and shellfish for women about 16 to 49 years old, especially pregnant and breastfeeding women, and young children.

The Interstate Shellfish Sanitation Conference (ISSC) was formed in 1982 to foster and promote shellfish sanitation through the cooperation of state and federal control agencies, the shellfish industry, and the academic community.

Women Who Are Pregnant, May Become Pregnant or Are Nursing

The nutritional value of fish is important during growth and development before birth, in early infancy for breastfed infants, and in childhood. The health risks from mercury in fish and shellfish depend on the amount of fish and shellfish a person eats and the levels of mercury in the specific fish and shellfish. Some fish contain higher levels of mercury that may harm a fetus or young child's developing nervous system.

As a result, women who are pregnant or may become pregnant and women who are nursing risk exposing their children to contamination if they eat these fish.

The EPA and FDA recommend that women who are pregnant, may become pregnant, or are breastfeeding should eat 2 to 3 servings (8 to 12 ounces) of fish each week from choices that are lower in mercury.

Fish Facts

Fish and shellfish can be an important part of a healthy diet. They are a great source of protein and heart-healthy omega-3 fatty acids. What's more, some researchers believe low fish intake may be linked to depression in women during and after pregnancy. Research also suggests that omega-3 fatty acids consumed by pregnant women may aid in a fetus's brain and eye development.

Women who are or may become pregnant and nursing mothers need 12 ounces of fish per week to reap the health benefits. Unfortunately, some pregnant and nursing women do not eat any fish because they worry about mercury in seafood. Mercury is a metal that, at high levels, can harm the brain of the fetus—even before it is conceived. Mercury mainly gets into our bodies by eating large, predatory fish. Yet many types of seafood have little or no mercury at all. So the risk of mercury exposure depends on the amount and type of seafood you eat.

Women who are nursing, pregnant, or who may become pregnant can safely eat a variety of cooked seafood, but should steer clear of fish with high levels of mercury. Keep in mind that removing all fish from your diet will rob you of important omega-3 fatty acids. To reach 12 ounces while limiting exposure to mercury, follow these tips:

- Do not eat these fish that are high in mercury:
  - Swordfish
  - Tilefish
  - King mackerel
  - Shark
- Eat up to 6 ounces (about 1 serving) per week:
  - Canned albacore or chunk white tuna (also sold as tuna steaks), which has more mercury than canned light tuna

- Eat up to 12 ounces (about 2 servings) per week of cooked* fish and shellfish with little or no mercury, such as:

  - Shrimp

  - Crab

  - Clams

  - Oysters

  - Scallops

  - Canned light tuna

  - Salmon

  - Pollock

  - Catfish

  - Cod

  - Tilapia

* Do not eat uncooked fish or shellfish (such as clams, oysters, scallops), which includes refrigerated and uncooked seafood labeled nova-style, lox, kippered, smoked, or jerky.

- Check before eating fish caught in local waters. State health departments have guidelines on fish from local waters. Or get local fish advisories at the EPA. If you are unsure about the safety of a fish from local waters, only eat 6 ounces per week and do not eat any other fish that week.

- Eat a variety of cooked seafood rather than just a few types

Foods supplemented with docosahexaenoic acid (DHA)/EPA (such as "omega-3 eggs") and prenatal vitamins supplemented with DHA are other sources of the type of omega-3 fatty acids found in seafood.

Section 19.5

Caffeine Use during Pregnancy

This section contains text excerpted from the following
sources: Text under the heading "Caffeine" is excerpted from
"Staying Healthy and Safe," Office on Women's Health (OWH), U.S.
Department of Health and Human Services (HHS), January 30, 2019;
Text under the heading "National Institutes of Health Study Finds
Daily Multivitamin before and after Conception Greatly Reduces
Miscarriage Risk" is excerpted from "Couples' Pre-Pregnancy
Caffeine Consumption Linked to Miscarriage Risk," *Eunice
Kennedy Shriver* National Institute of Child Health and
Human Development (NICHD), March 24, 2016.

Caffeine

Moderate amounts of caffeine appear to be safe during pregnancy.
Moderate means less than 200 mg of caffeine per day, which is the
amount in about 12 ounces of coffee. Most caffeinated teas and soft
drinks have much less caffeine. Some studies have shown a link
between higher amounts of caffeine and miscarriage and preterm
birth, but there is no solid proof that caffeine causes these problems.
The effects of too much caffeine are unclear. Ask your doctor whether
drinking a limited amount of caffeine is okay for you.

National Institutes of Health Study Finds Daily Multivitamin before and after Conception Greatly Reduces Miscarriage Risk

A woman is more likely to miscarry if she and her partner drink more
than two caffeinated beverages a day during the weeks leading up to
conception, according to a study from researchers at the National Institutes of Health (NIH) and Ohio State University, Columbus. Similarly,
women who drank more than two daily caffeinated beverages during
the first seven weeks of pregnancy were also more likely to miscarry.

However, women who took a daily multivitamin before conception
and through early pregnancy were less likely to miscarry than women
who did not. The study was published online in Fertility and Sterility.

"Our findings provide useful information for couples who are
planning a pregnancy and who would like to minimize their risk for
early pregnancy loss," said the study's first author, Germaine Buck
Louis, Ph.D., director of the Division of Intramural Population Health

Research at NIH's *Eunice Kennedy Shriver* National Institute of Child Health and Human Development (NICHD).

The researchers analyzed data from the Longitudinal Investigation of Fertility and the Environment (LIFE) Study, which was established to examine the relationship between fertility, lifestyle, and exposure to environmental chemicals. The LIFE Study enrolled 501 couples from four counties in Michigan and 12 counties in Texas, from 2005 to 2009.

For the study, researchers compared such lifestyle factors as cigarette use, caffeinated beverage consumption, and multivitamin use among 344 couples with a singleton pregnancy from the weeks before they conceived through the seventh week of pregnancy.

The researchers reported their results using a statistical concept known as a "hazard ratio," which estimates the chances of a particular health outcome occurring during the time frame of the study. For example, the researchers evaluated caffeinated beverage consumption in terms of the daily likelihood of pregnancy loss over a given time period. A score greater than 1 indicates an increased risk for pregnancy loss each day following conception, and a score less than 1 indicates a reduced daily risk.

Of the 344 pregnancies, 98 ended in miscarriage, or 28 percent. For the preconception period, miscarriage was associated with females 35 years of age or older, for a hazard ratio of 1.96 (nearly twice the miscarriage risk of younger women). The study was not designed to conclusively prove cause and effect. The study's authors cited possible explanations for the higher risk, including advanced age of sperm and egg in older couples or cumulative exposure to substances in the environment, which could be expected to increase as people age.

Both male and female consumption of more than two caffeinated beverages a day was also associated with an increased hazard ratio: 1.74 for females and 1.73 for males. Earlier studies, the authors noted, have documented increased pregnancy loss associated with caffeine consumption in early pregnancy. However, those studies could not rule out whether caffeine consumption contributed to pregnancy loss or was a sign of an unhealthy pregnancy. It is possible, the authors wrote, that these earlier findings could have been the result of a healthy pregnancy, rather than caffeine consumption interfering with pregnancy. For example, the increase in food aversions and vomiting associated with a healthy pregnancy led the women to give up caffeinated beverages.

Because their study found caffeine consumption before pregnancy was associated with a higher risk of miscarriage, it is more likely that caffeinated beverage consumption during this time directly contributes to pregnancy loss.

"Our findings also indicate that the male partner matters, too," Dr. Buck Louis said. "Male preconception consumption of caffeinated beverages was just as strongly associated with pregnancy loss as females."

Finally, the researchers saw a reduction in miscarriage risk for women who took a daily multivitamin. During the preconception period, researchers found a hazard ratio of 0.45—a 55 percent reduction in risk for pregnancy loss. Women who continued to take the vitamins through early pregnancy had a hazard ratio of 0.21, or a risk reduction of 79 percent. The authors cited other studies that found that vitamin B_6 and folic acid—included in preconception and pregnancy vitamin formulations—can reduce miscarriage risk. Folic acid supplements are recommended for women of childbearing age, as their use in the weeks leading up to and following conception reduces the risk for having a child with a neural-tube defect.

Chapter 20

Exercise during Pregnancy

Expecting? Keep Active.

Pregnancy should not keep women from a healthy dose of activity. Both during pregnancy and after delivery, exercise can help the mother through improved cardiovascular fitness and in many other ways. Postpartum benefits also include mood improvement and weight management. Some evidence points toward shortened labor and reduced risk for certain complications. The 2008 *Physical Activity Guidelines for Americans* spell it out, based on solid evidence and in lay terms.

Among the key recommendations:

- Healthy women who are not already highly active or doing vigorously intense activities should get at least 150 minutes

This chapter contains text excerpted from the following sources: Text under the heading "Expecting? Keep Active." is excerpted from "Exercise during Pregnancy: You'll Both Benefit," Office of Disease Prevention and Health Promotion (ODPHP), U.S. Department of Health and Human Services (HHS), February 19, 2019; Text under the heading "Being Physically Active during Pregnancy" is excerpted from "Stay Active during Pregnancy: Quick Tips," Office of Disease Prevention and Health Promotion (ODPHP), U.S. Department of Health and Human Services (HHS), March 26, 2018; Text under the heading "Pelvic Floor Exercises" is excerpted from "Staying Healthy and Safe," Office on Women's Health (OWH), U.S. Department of Health and Human Services (HHS), January 30, 2019; Text beginning with the heading "Benefits of Regular, Moderate Physical Activity during Pregnancy" is excerpted from "Should I Exercise during My Pregnancy?" MedlinePlus, National Institutes of Health (NIH), February 10, 2009. Reviewed February 2019.

(2 hours and 30 minutes) of moderate-intensity aerobic activity per week during pregnancy and the postpartum period. Preferably, this activity should be spread throughout the week.

- Pregnant women who habitually engage in vigorously intense aerobic activity or are highly active can continue physical activity during pregnancy and the postpartum period provided, that they remain healthy and discuss how and when activity should be adjusted over time with their healthcare provider.

Pregnant women should review the recommendations in full, including activities to avoid and the wisdom of seeking a healthcare professional who can provide knowledgeable guidance. Armed with solid information and motivation, pregnant women can remain active through pregnancy and beyond.

Being Physically Active during Pregnancy
Before You Start

Talk to your doctor about getting active during your pregnancy. As long as there isn't a medical reason for you to avoid physical activity during your pregnancy, you can start or keep doing moderate physical activity.

Aim for 2 Hours and 30 Minutes a Week of Moderate Aerobic Activities

- If you weren't exercising before, start slowly. Try breaking your activity up into 10-minute chunks of time.

- Choose aerobic activities—activities that make your heart beat faster—like walking fast, dancing, swimming, or raking leaves. You should still be able to talk during these activities.

- Be sure to drink extra water before, during, and after exercising.

- Take a break if you get short of breath or feel uncomfortable.

Follow These Tips When You Do Strengthening Exercises

- Don't strain to lift heavy weights. Instead, do more repetitions (lifts) with lighter weights. You can also use bottles of water or cans of food as weights.

- Make sure you aren't holding your breath. Breathe out as you lift something, and breathe in as you relax.

- Avoid exercises that could strain your lower back.

Avoid High-Risk Activities

- Avoid exercising while lying on your back after the first trimester (12 weeks).

- Stay away from activities that increase your risk of falling, like downhill skiing or horseback riding.

- Avoid playing sports where you could get hit in the stomach, like basketball or soccer.

- Don't scuba dive while you are pregnant.

Pelvic-Floor Exercises

Your pelvic-floor muscles support the rectum, vagina, and urethra in the pelvis. Toning these muscles with Kegel exercises will help you push during delivery and recover from birth. It also will help control bladder leakage and lower your chance of getting hemorrhoids.

Pelvic muscles are the same ones used to stop the flow of urine. Still, it can be hard to find the right muscles to squeeze. You can be sure you are exercising the right muscles if when you squeeze them you stop urinating. Or you can put a finger into the vagina and squeeze. If you feel pressure around the finger, you've found the pelvic floor muscles. Try not to tighten your stomach, legs, or other muscles.

Kegel Exercises

1. Tighten the pelvic-floor muscles for a count of three, then relax for a count of three.

2. Repeat 10 to 15 times, three times a day.

3. Start Kegel exercises lying down. This is the easiest position. When your muscles get stronger, you can do Kegel exercises sitting or standing as you like.

Benefits of Regular, Moderate Physical Activity during Pregnancy

- Helps you and the fetus gain the proper amounts of weight

- Reduces the discomforts of pregnancy, such as backaches, leg cramps, constipation, bloating, and swelling

- Lowers the risk of gestational diabetes (diabetes that occurs when a woman is pregnant)

- Boosts mood and energy level

- Improves sleep

- Helps with an easier, shorter labor

- Assists faster recovery from delivery and return to a healthy weight

Steps for Safe Exercise during Pregnancy

- Choose moderate activities unlikely to injure, such as walking, water aerobics, swimming, yoga, or using a stationary bike

- Stop exercising when you start to feel tired, and never exercise until you are exhausted or overheated

- Drink plenty of water

- Wear comfortable clothing that fits well and supports and protects your breasts

- Stop exercising if you feel dizzy, become short of breath, feel pain in your back, experience swelling or numbness, feel sick to your stomach, or your heart beats too fast or at an uneven rate

Tips for Initiating Safe Exercise

- Go for a walk around the block or through a shopping mall with your spouse or a friend

- Join a prenatal yoga, water aerobics, or fitness class, letting the instructor know you are pregnant before beginning

- Follow an exercise video for pregnant women

- Sign up for pregnancy fitness session at your gym, community center, Young Men's Christian Association (YMCA) or Young Women's Christian Association (YWCA)

- Stand up, stretch, and move at least once an hour if you sit most of the day, as well as during commercials when watching television

What Shouldn't I Do?

For you and the fetus health and safety, it is best to avoid:

- Being active outside during hot weather

- Steam rooms, hot tubs, and saunas

- Certain yoga poses or other activities that call for lying flat on your back after the twentieth week of pregnancy

- Contact sports such as football and boxing that might injure you

- Sports such as tennis or basketball that make you jump or change directions quickly

- Horseback riding, in-line skating, downhill skiing, and other activities that can result in falls

Chapter 21

Weight Gain during Pregnancy

Chapter Contents

Section 21.1

How Much Weight Should You Gain?

This section includes text excerpted from "Health Tips for Pregnant Women," National Institute of Diabetes and Digestive and Kidney Diseases (NIDDK), June 1, 2013. Reviewed February 2019.

Why Is Gaining a Healthy Amount of Weight during Pregnancy Important?

Gaining the right amount of weight during pregnancy helps the fetus grow to a healthy size. But gaining too much or too little weight may lead to serious health problems for you and the fetus.

Too much weight gain raises your chances for diabetes and high blood pressure during and after pregnancy. If you are overweight when you get pregnant, your chances for health problems may be even higher. It also makes it more likely that you will have a hard delivery and need a cesarean section (C-section).

Gaining a healthy amount of weight helps you have an easier pregnancy and delivery. It may also help make it easier for you to get back to your normal weight after delivery. Research shows that a healthy weight gain can also lower the chances that you or your child will have obesity and weight-related problems later in life.

How Much Weight Should I Gain during My Pregnancy?

How much weight you should gain depends on how much you weighed before pregnancy.

General weight gain advice below refers to weight before pregnancy and is for women having only one baby.

Table 21.1. Weight Gain during Pregnancy

If You Are	You Should Gain About
underweight (BMI* less than 18.5)	28 to 40 pounds
normal weight (BMI of 18.5 to 24.9)	25 to 35 pounds
overweight (BMI of 25 to 29.9)	15 to 25 pounds
obese (BMI of 30+)	11 to 20 pounds

* The body mass index (BMI) measures your weight in relation to your height.

It is important to gain weight very slowly. The old myth that you are eating for two is not true. During the first three months, your baby is only the size of a walnut and does not need very many extra calories. The following rate of weight gain is advised:

- One to four pounds total in the first three months

- Two to four pounds each month from four months until delivery

Talk to your healthcare provider about how much weight you should gain. Work with her or him to set goals for your weight gain. Take into account your age, weight, and health. Track your weight at home or at your provider visits using charts from the Institute of Medicine (IOM).

Do not try to lose weight if you are pregnant. Healthy food is needed to help your baby grow. Some women may lose a small amount of weight at the start of pregnancy. Speak to your healthcare provider if this happens to you.

Section 21.2

Gestational Weight Gain Warnings

This section includes text excerpted from "Researcher Warns about Gestational Weight Gain," National Institute of Environmental Health Sciences (NIEHS), February 21, 2008. Reviewed February 2019.

Nutritional epidemiologist Anna Maria Siega-Riz, Ph.D., had good reason to sound alarmed when she talked about pregnancy and weight gain during her Frontiers of Environmental Sciences lecture in Rodbell Auditorium. According to the University of North Carolina (UNC) at Chapel Hill professor, overweight and obese women, as well as women who gain too much weight during their pregnancies, may be endangering their own health and the health of their children.

In her talk, "Maternal Obesity—The Number One Problem Facing Prenatal Care Providers in the New Millennium," Siega-Riz presented a great amount of evidence that these women have a significantly greater risk of suffering from metabolic syndrome-related diseases, of bearing children with birth defects (such as spina bifida), and of giving birth to babies who will experience problems with their own health.

Women are overweight and obese, and more of them are gaining excessive weight during pregnancy. Compounding the problem, Siega-Riz added, is the complacency of many pregnant women and, even more disturbing, their healthcare providers.

"Maternal obesity is not unique to the United States," Siega-Riz said as she began her lecture. "It is occurring globally." Many developing countries are facing the same problems as the United States, with obesity rates between 20 and 30 percent. Not only are rates increasing, Siega-Riz noted, but obesity is also emerging as a health-disparity issue due to its greater prevalence among minority women.

According to Siega-Riz, in the United States, about a third of women are overweight and 10 to 15 percent are obese. The majority of pregnant women are gaining 21 to 40 pounds during pregnancy, and since the 1990s, there has been a 30 percent increase in the number of women who gain 40 or more pounds. "Only about a third of women are gaining weight within the targeted weight gain recommendations," she said. In addition to the significant health problems that obesity contributes to on its own, such as diabetes and cardiovascular disease, Siega-Riz pointed to studies suggesting that about 25 percent of problems with fecundity and fertility are due to obesity.

Maternal overweight and obesity have been associated with a dramatic increase in risk for gestational diabetes, gestational hypertension, preeclampsia, caesarian delivery, fetal death, and birth defects. The effects of overweight and obesity persist beyond childbirth and include postpartum weight retention, postpartum anemia related to the higher rate of caesarian sections, shorter duration of breastfeeding, and persistent glucose intolerance. Moreover, with excessive weight gain, a woman is also more likely to find herself in a higher weight classification at twelve months postpartum than she was at conception, putting her at even greater risk for complications in a subsequent pregnancy.

Because of these trends, physicians are seeing a growing number of pregnant women weighing as much as 300 pounds. "Quite frankly, they don't know how to manage them," Siega-Riz observed. One study found that 33 percent of subjects reported receiving no advice on gestational weight gain from their providers. The few intervention studies thus far have failed to show promising results and have found poor rates of compliance with interventions on the part of physicians and pregnant women.

As she and her colleagues strive to close the gaps in research on gestational weight gain, Siega-Riz continues to push for translation of this research through education and policy change. She currently serves a member of the Institute of Medicine's (IOM) Committee to Reexamine IOM Pregnancy Weight Guidelines. In 2004, she served on the IOM's Committee to Review the WIC Food Packages. As a result of the recommendations from this committee, the United States Department of Agriculture (USDA) made the first major changes to the food packages since women, infants, and children's (WIC) inception 30 years ago. In November 2007, the March of Dimes recognized her distinguished achievements in research, education and clinical services in the field of maternal-fetal nutrition with the Agnes Higgins Award.

Chapter 22

Risk Factors for Sleep Apnea during Pregnancy

Snoring, older age, and obesity may increase a pregnant woman's risk for sleep apnea—interrupted breathing during sleep—according to researchers funded by the National Institutes of Health (NIH). The study, which appears in the *American Journal of Obstetrics and Gynecology* (AJOG), was supported by NIH's *Eunice Kennedy Shriver* National Institute of Child Health and Human Development (NICHD) and the National Heart, Lung, and Blood Institute (NHLBI).

"Our study found an easy, inexpensive way to screen large numbers of women at higher risk of sleep apnea during pregnancy," said study co-author Uma Reddy, M.D., of NICHD's Pregnancy and Perinatology Branch (PPB). "Right now, this means we'll be able to rapidly identify women who may benefit from further testing. Depending on what we learn from future studies, our findings could also lead to improvements in pregnancy outcomes."

In an earlier study of first-time pregnancies, the researchers found that sleep apnea increases a woman's risk for hypertensive disorders and gestational diabetes. Currently, there are no medical guidelines or treatment recommendations for sleep apnea during pregnancy. NIH currently supports a study of potential treatments

This chapter includes text excerpted from "NIH-Funded Researchers Identify Risk Factors for Sleep Apnea during Pregnancy," National Institutes of Health (NIH), February 13, 2018.

for pregnancy-related sleep apnea, and is planning a larger one to be conducted by the NICHD-funded Maternal-Fetal Medicine Units (MFMU) Network.

In the current study, participants responded to questionnaires about their sleep habits, snoring, and daytime sleepiness in early pregnancy (6 to 15 weeks) and mid-pregnancy (22 to 29 weeks). The women also underwent sleep-apnea testing using an at-home monitoring device.

The researchers found that 3.6 percent of 3,264 women in early pregnancy and 8.3 percent of 2,512 women in mid-pregnancy had sleep apnea. Risk factors for having the condition included frequent snoring (three or more nights per week), older maternal age, and being overweight or obese as determined by body mass index (BMI).

Because each woman's risk varies according to individual characteristics, the authors developed a calculator using maternal age, BMI, and frequency of snoring to arrive at her probability of sleep apnea in early and mid-pregnancy. This tool may be used by obstetric providers to identify women at risk for the condition, so they can be referred for definitive testing.

A common treatment for sleep apnea is continuous positive airway pressure (CPAP) therapy, which involves wearing a mask that fits over the nose or the nose and mouth. Air is pumped through a tube attached to the mask, increasing pressure into the airways to keep them from collapsing. Dr. Reddy explained, however, that it is not currently known if using CPAP therapy during pregnancy will prevent hypertension, diabetes, or other complications of sleep apnea. She added that pregnant women who have or think they have sleep apnea should discuss their concerns with a physician.

Chapter 23

Sex during Pregnancy

Many parents-to-be find it difficult to discuss sex during pregnancy, perhaps because the subject feels culturally taboo to them, but they can count on experiencing changes in their sex life during pregnancy. Because of this reality, it is important to find a balanced way to feel happy as a couple in the midst of these changes.

Some of common questions about sex during pregnancy are addressed below.

Is Sex Safe during Pregnancy?

Yes, sexual activity is considered safe during all stages of a healthy pregnancy. During a healthy, normal pregnancy, the risk of complications, such as preterm labor or miscarriage, are low for couples who enjoy sex during pregnancy. In fact, unless your healthcare provider advises you not to, it is absolutely safe for you to have sex up until your water breaks.

Is Pregnant Sex Different from Regular Sex?

Some women may feel discomfort during pregnant sex because of tender heavy breasts, hormonal fluctuations, exhaustion, increased self-consciousness about weight gain, increased influx of blood in the lower parts of the body (which causes heightened sensitivity and engorgement of the genitals), vaginal fluid changes, and so on, while others experience little discomfort.

Will Sex Harm the Fetus?

Penetration during intercourse will not harm the developing fetus, as it is cushioned by the amniotic fluid (watery yellow fluid within the amniotic sac) and encircled by the muscles of the uterus. The mucus plug seal in the cervix guards against infection.

Can Intercourse or Orgasm Cause a Miscarriage or Contractions?

In a healthy pregnancy, the answer is no. It will not provoke a miscarriage. The contractions during and after orgasm are totally different from labor. As a safety precaution, some providers may advise not to have sex during the final week of pregnancy as it is suspected that prostaglandins (hormones in semen) may stimulate labor contractions in past-due or full-term pregnancies.

Which Sex Positions Are Most Comfortable during Pregnancy?

As the pregnancy progresses, the missionary position (man on top) may not be comfortable for some couples. Alternative sex positions to try during pregnancy, which keep the weight off of the stomach, are:

- Straddling while the partner sits in a chair, table, or on a counter to control pace and penetration
- Women on top or doggy position in order to balance the weight between hands and knees
- Lying side-by-side (spooning position) to avoid deep penetration
- Open communication is the secret to determining what works best for the individual and the couple for pregnancy sex.

Are Condoms Necessary?

If the relationship is not mutually monogamous or if one partner chooses to have sex with a new partner, then condom use is the safest way to avoid sexually transmitted infections (STIs).

When Should You Not Have Sex during Pregnancy?

Healthcare providers will say "no sex" if they determine the pregnancy to be high risk with:

- A history or threat of preterm labor (premature uterine contractions/birth/delivery before 37 weeks of pregnancy)

- A history or threat of miscarriage

- Vaginal bleeding or cramps with no known cause

- Incompetent cervix—a condition in which the cervix becomes weak, which could lead to a premature/early opening of the cervix. This would raise the risk of a premature birth/ delivery.

- Placenta previa—a condition in which the placenta (a blood-rich structure that nourishes the fetus) lies too low

- Leakage of the amniotic fluid (the fluid that surrounds the fetus). This is also called "ruptured membrane" or "waters broken."

- Multiple fetuses—if the couple is expecting twins, triplets, or multiples

- Either parent is found to have a sexually transmitted disease (STD)

What Should You Not Do during Pregnancy Sex?

- Avoid deep penetration.

- Avoid holding your breath during penetration.

- Avoid direct nipple stimulation.

- Avoid lying flat on your back after the first trimester—always use a pillow under one side.

- Avoid anal sex (as suggested by some of the healthcare providers).

- Avoid blowing air into the partner's vagina during oral sex, as this can cause an air embolism (blockage of a blood vessel by an air bubble), which can be fatal to both mother and fetus.

- Avoid new sexual partners whose sexual history is unknown.

- Avoid all forms of sex (oral, anal, or vaginal) if the partner has an active STI since having an STI during pregnancy is potentially dangerous for both the parents-to-be and the unborn baby.

When Do You Have to Call the Doctor?

Orgasm in late pregnancy may cause mild contractions (called "Braxton Hicks contractions"), which are common near the end of the third trimester, but will resolve after a few minutes of rest. If the contractions continue, or you unusual symptoms such as developing pain, bleeding or leaking fluid, then contact your doctor right away. Always remember that "normal" is a relative term when discussing "sex during pregnancy," and make sure to discuss what feels right for both you and your partner.

References

1. Johnson, Traci C. MD, "Sex during and after Pregnancy," WebMD, January 21, 2017.

2. Hirsch, Larissa. MD, "Sex during Pregnancy," KidsHealth®/The Nemours Foundation, October 2016.

3. "Sex during Pregnancy: What's Ok, What's Not," Mayoclinic, July 10, 2018.

Chapter 24

Working and Traveling during Pregnancy

Chapter Contents

Section 24.1

Pregnancy and Your Job

This section contains text excerpted from the following sources: Text in this section begins with excerpts from "Reproductive Health and the Workplace," Centers for Disease Control and Prevention (CDC), April 20, 2017; Text under the heading "Know Your Pregnancy Rights" is excerpted from "Know Your Pregnancy Rights," Office on Women's Health (OWH), U.S. Department of Health and Human Services (HHS), January 30, 2019.

Pregnancy can affect your safety as a worker. If you are pregnant, discuss possible job hazards with your employer, health and safety office at work (if there is one), and doctor as soon as possible. Many pregnant women are able to adjust their job duties temporarily, or take extra steps to protect themselves.

Current occupational exposure limits were set based on studies of nonpregnant adults. What is considered safe for you, may not be safe for a fetus. Although most employees are able to safely do their job throughout pregnancy, pregnancy can sometimes affect worker safety.

If you are pregnant and working, you may have to consider that:

- Changes in your metabolism increase how quickly you absorb some chemicals (e.g., some metals)

- Because of physical changes, the personal protective equipment that you could wear correctly before pregnancy may not fit properly, such as lab coats or respirators

- When pregnant, changes in your immune system, lung capacity, and ligaments can alter your risk of injury or illness due to some workplace hazards

- A fetus might be more vulnerable to some chemicals because of its rapid growth and development, particularly early in pregnancy when organs are developing

Know Your Pregnancy Rights

When sharing your good news with coworkers, discrimination might be the last thing on your mind. But the truth is that many women are treated unfairly—or even fired—after revealing the news of their pregnancy.

As long as a pregnant woman is able to perform the major functions of her job, not hiring or firing her because she is pregnant is against the law. It is against the law to dock her pay or demote her to a lesser position because of pregnancy. It is also against the law to hold back benefits for pregnancy because a woman is not married. All are forms of pregnancy discrimination, and all are illegal.

Women are protected under the Pregnancy Discrimination Act (PDA). This act states that businesses with at least 15 employees must treat women who are pregnant in the same manner as other job applicants or employees with similar abilities or limitations.

The Family and Medical Leave Act (FMLA) also protects the jobs of workers who are employed by companies with 50 employees or more and who have worked for the company for at least 12 months. These companies must allow employees to take 12 weeks of unpaid leave for medical reasons, including pregnancy and childbirth. Your job cannot be given away during this 12-week period.

Many state laws also protect pregnant women's rights. These laws appear clear cut. But issues that arise on the job seldom are. Visit the U.S. Equal Employment Opportunity Commission (EEOC) website to learn more about your rights during pregnancy and what to do if you think your rights have been violated.

Section 24.2

Travel and Pregnancy

This section includes text excerpted from "Staying Healthy and Safe," Office on Women's Health (OWH), U.S. Department of Health and Human Services (HHS), January 30, 2019.

Everyday life does not stop once you are pregnant. Most healthy pregnant women are able to continue with their usual routine and activity level. That means going to work, running errands, and for some, traveling away from home. To take care of yourself and the fetus, consider these points before taking a long trip or traveling far from home:

- Talk to your doctor before making any travel decisions that will take you far from home. Ask if any of your health conditions may make travel during pregnancy unsafe. Also consider the destination. Is the food and water safe? Will you need immunizations before you go? Is there good medical care available in the event of an emergency? Will your health insurance cover medical care at your destination?

- Avoid sitting for long periods of time during car or air travel. Prolonged sitting can affect blood flow in your legs. Try to limit driving to no more than five or six hours each day. Take frequent breaks to stretch your legs. Stand up, and move your legs often during air travel. Wearing support pantyhose can also help blood flow.

- Occasional air travel is safe for most pregnant women, and most airlines will allow women to fly up to 36 weeks of pregnancy. Make sure to wear your seatbelt during the flight, and take steps to ease the discomforts of prolonged travel and sitting. Frequent air travel during pregnancy increases the risk of fetal exposure to cosmic radiation. If you are a pregnant pilot, aircrew member, or other frequent flier, check with your employer about flying restrictions.

- Bring a copy of your medical record and find out about the medical care available at your destination so you will be prepared in the event of an emergency.

- If you suspect a problem with your pregnancy during your trip, do not wait until you come home to see your doctor. Seek medical care right away.

Buckle Up.

Wearing a seatbelt during car and air travel is safe while pregnant. The lap strap should go under your stomach and across your hips. The shoulder strap should go between your breasts and to the side of your stomach. Make sure it fits snugly.

Section 24.3

International Travel during Pregnancy

This section includes text excerpted from "Pregnant Travelers,"
Centers for Disease Control and Prevention (CDC), October 31, 2017.

Pregnant women can generally travel safely with a little preparation. But they should avoid some destinations, including those with Zika and malaria risk. Learn about the steps you can take if you are pregnant and planning an international trip, especially to a developing country. Follow these tips to keep you and the fetus safe and healthy.

Zika and Malaria

The Zika virus is spread through mosquito bites and sex. Because Zika infection in a pregnant woman can cause severe birth defects, pregnant women should not travel to any area with risk of Zika. If you must travel to an area with Zika risk, take strict precautions to prevent mosquito bites and avoid sexual transmission. If you have a sex partner who lives in or has traveled to an area with Zika, you should use condoms for the rest of your pregnancy.

Pregnant women should also avoid travelling to areas with malaria, which can be more severe for women who are pregnant. Malaria can increase the risk for serious pregnancy problems, including premature birth, miscarriage, and stillbirth. If you must go to an area with malaria while you are pregnant, talk to your doctor about taking a drug to prevent malaria. Malaria is spread by mosquitoes, so you also should wear effective insect repellent and take other precautions to avoid mosquito bites.

Pretravel Care and Travel Health Insurance

The first thing you should do when planning an international trip is to make an appointment with a healthcare provider who specializes in travel medicine. You should ideally visit the travel clinic at least four to six weeks before you leave. A travel-medicine specialist can review your itinerary, make recommendations based on the health risks at your destination, and give you any vaccines you may need. You should also talk to your obstetrician (OB/GYN) about your trip for advice on whether it is safe for you to travel. Your travel-medicine doctor and your obstetrician may need to talk to each other about your care.

Next, consider how you are going to get care overseas if you need it. Your health insurance in the United States may not pay for medical care in another country, so check with your insurance company. Consider getting supplemental-travel health insurance, and make sure the policy will also cover the baby if you give birth during your trip. If you are traveling to a remote area, an insurance policy that covers medical evacuation will pay for your transportation to a high-quality hospital in case of emergency.

Transportation Issues

Before you book a flight, check how late in your pregnancy the airline will let you fly. Most will let you fly until 36 weeks, but some have an earlier cutoff. Your feet may become swollen on a long flight, so wear comfortable shoes and loose clothing and try to walk around every hour or so. Pregnancy makes blood clots during travel much more likely. To reduce your risk of a blood clot, your doctor may recommend compression stockings or leg exercises that you can do in your seat.

If you are going on a cruise, check with the cruise line to find out if it has specific guidance for pregnant women. Most will not allow you to travel after 24 to 28 weeks of pregnancy, and you may need to have a note from your doctor stating you are fit to travel.

Car crashes are a leading cause of injury for healthy U.S. travelers abroad. At your destination, always wear a seatbelt on a car or bus. A lap belt with a shoulder strap is best, and the straps should be placed carefully above and below your stomach.

Food and Water Safety

Travelers' diarrhea is caused by eating or drinking contaminated food or water. The dehydration caused by diarrhea can be more of a problem for pregnant women than for others. In addition, other bacteria and viruses spread by food or water can lead to more severe illnesses that can cause problems for a pregnant woman and the fetus. Therefore, if you are traveling in a developing country, you should carefully follow food and water safety measures:

- Eat only food that is cooked and served piping hot

- Do not eat cold food or food that has been sitting at room temperature (such as a buffet)

- Do not eat raw or undercooked meat or fish

- Eat fresh fruits and vegetables only if you can peel them or wash them in clean water

- Do not eat unpasteurized dairy products

- Drink only water, sodas, or sports drinks that are canned or bottled and sealed (carbonated is safer because the bubbles indicate that it was sealed at the factory)

- Do not drink anything with ice in it, as the ice may be made with contaminated water

If you get travelers' diarrhea, the best thing to do is drink plenty of safe liquids while you wait for it to go away on its own. However, your doctor may give you an antibiotic you can take in case diarrhea is moderate or severe. Diarrhea is considered "moderate" when it is distressing or interferes with planned activities, and "severe" when it is disabling or completely prevents planned activities. Do not take products containing bismuth, such as Pepto-Bismol or Kaopectate. These medicines are not recommended for pregnant women.

Chapter 25

Nicotine, Alcohol, and Substance Use during Pregnancy

Chapter Contents

Section 25.1

Smoking and Pregnancy

This section includes text excerpted from "Tobacco
Use and Pregnancy," Centers for Disease Control
and Prevention (CDC), September 29, 2017.

How Does Smoking during Pregnancy Harm My Health and the Fetus?

Most people know that smoking causes cancer, heart disease, and
other major health problems. Smoking during pregnancy causes additional health problems, including premature birth (being born too
early), certain birth defects, and infant death.

- Smoking makes it harder for a woman to get pregnant.

- Women who smoke during pregnancy are more likely to have a
  miscarriage than other women.

- Smoking can cause problems with the placenta—the source
  of the baby's food and oxygen during pregnancy. For example,
  the placenta can separate from the womb too early, causing
  bleeding, which is dangerous to the mother and the fetus.

- Smoking during pregnancy can cause a baby to be born too early
  or to have low birth weight, making it more likely the baby will
  be sick and have to stay in the hospital longer. A few babies may
  even die.

- Smoking during and after pregnancy is a risk factor of sudden
  infant death syndrome (SIDS). SIDS is an infant death for which
  a cause of the death cannot be found.

- Babies born to women who smoke are more likely to have certain
  birth defects, such as a cleft lip or cleft palate.

What Are E-Cigarettes? Are They Safer Than Regular Cigarettes in Pregnancy?

Electronic cigarettes (also called "electronic nicotine delivery systems or e-cigarettes") come in different sizes and shapes, including
"pens," "mods," (which are modified by the user) and "tanks." Most
e-cigarettes contain a battery, a heating device, and a cartridge to hold

liquid. The liquid typically contains nicotine, flavorings, and other chemicals. The battery-powered device heats the liquid in the cartridge into an aerosol that the user inhales.

Although the aerosol of e-cigarettes generally has fewer harmful substances than cigarette smoke, e-cigarettes and other products containing nicotine are not safe to use during pregnancy. Nicotine is a health danger for pregnant women and fetuses and can damage the developing brain and lungs. Also, some of the flavorings used in e-cigarettes may be harmful to a fetus.

How Many Women Smoke during Pregnancy?

According to the 2011 Pregnancy Risk Assessment and Monitoring System (PRAMS) data collected from 24 states:

- Approximately 10 percent of women reported smoking during the last 3 months of pregnancy.

- Of women who smoked 3 months before pregnancy, 55 percent quit during pregnancy. Among women who quit smoking during pregnancy, 40 percent started smoking again within 6 months after delivery.

What Are the Benefits of Quitting?

Quitting smoking will help you feel better and provide a healthier environment for the fetus.

When you stop smoking:

- The fetus will get more oxygen, even after just one day of not smoking.

- There is less risk that your baby will be born too early.

- There is a better chance that your baby will come home from the hospital with you.

- You will be less likely to develop heart disease, strokes, lung cancer, chronic lung disease, and other smoke-related diseases.

- You will be more likely to live to know your grandchildren.

- You will have more energy and breathe more easily.

- Your clothes, hair, and home will smell better.

- Your food will taste better.

- You will have more money that you can spend on other things.

- You will feel good about what you have done for yourself and your child.

How Does Other People's Smoke (Secondhand Smoke) Harm My Health and My Child's Health?

Breathing other people's smoke make children and adults who do not smoke sick. There is no safe level of breathing other people's smoke.

- Pregnant women who breathe other people's cigarette smoke are more likely to have a baby with a low birth weight.

- Babies who breathe in other people's cigarette smoke are more likely to have ear infections and more frequent asthma attacks.

- Babies who breathe in other people's cigarette smoke are more likely to die from Sudden Infant Death Syndrome (SIDS). SIDS is an infant death for which a cause of the death cannot be found.

In the United States, 58 million children and adults who do not smoke are exposed to secondhand smoke. Almost 25 million children and adolescents aged 3 to 19 years, or about 4 out of 10 children in this age group, are exposed to other people's cigarette smoke. Home and vehicles are the places where children are most exposed to cigarette smoke, and a major location of smoke exposure for adults too. Individuals can also be exposed to cigarette smoke in public places, restaurants, and at work.

What Can You Do to Avoid Other People's Smoke?

There is no safe level of exposure to cigarette smoke. Even breathing a little smoke can be harmful. The only way to fully protect yourself and your loved ones from the dangers of other people's smoke is through 100 percent smoke-free environments.

You can protect yourself and your family by:

- Making your home and car smoke-free.

- Asking people not to smoke around you and your children.

- Making sure that your children's day care center or school is smoke-free.

- Choosing restaurants and other businesses that are smoke-free. Thanking businesses for being smoke-free.

- Teaching children to stay away from other people's smoke.

- Avoiding all smoke. If you or your children have respiratory conditions, if you have heart disease, or if you are pregnant, the dangers are greater for you.

- Learn as much as you can by talking to your doctor, nurse, or healthcare provider about the dangers of secondhand smoke.

Section 25.2

Alcohol Use and Pregnancy

This section includes text excerpted from "Alcohol Use in Pregnancy," Centers for Disease Control and Prevention (CDC), March 27, 2018.

There is no known safe amount of alcohol use during pregnancy or while trying to get pregnant. There is also no safe time during pregnancy to drink. All types of alcohol are equally harmful, including all wines and beer. When a pregnant woman drinks alcohol, so does the fetus.

Women also should not drink alcohol if they are sexually active, and do not use effective contraception (birth control). This is because a woman might get pregnant and expose her baby to alcohol before she knows she is pregnant. Nearly half of all pregnancies in the United States are unplanned. Most women will not know they are pregnant for up to four to six weeks.

Fetal alcohol spectrum disorders (FASDs) are completely preventable if a woman does not drink alcohol during pregnancy. Why take the risk?

Why Alcohol Is Dangerous

Alcohol in the mother's blood passes to the fetus through the umbilical cord. Drinking alcohol during pregnancy can cause miscarriage, stillbirth, and a range of lifelong physical, behavioral, and intellectual disabilities. These disabilities are known as fetal alcohol spectrum disorders. Children with FASDs might have the following character-istics and behaviors:

- Abnormal facial features, such as a smooth ridge between the nose and upper lip (this ridge is called the "philtrum")
- Small head size
- Shorter-than-average height
- Low body weight
- Poor coordination
- Hyperactive behavior
- Difficulty with attention
- Poor memory
- Difficulty in school (especially with math)
- Learning disabilities
- Speech and language delays
- Intellectual disability or low IQ
- Poor reasoning and judgment skills
- Sleep and sucking problems as a baby
- Vision or hearing problems
- Problems with the heart, kidney, or bones

How Much Alcohol Is Dangerous

There is no known safe amount of alcohol to drink while pregnant.

When Alcohol Is Dangerous

There is no safe time to drink alcohol during pregnancy. Alcohol can cause problems for the developing fetus throughout pregnancy, including before a woman knows she is pregnant. Drinking alcohol in the first three months of pregnancy can cause the baby to have abnormal facial features. Growth and central nervous system prob-lems (such as low birth weight and behavioral problems) can occur from drinking alcohol anytime during pregnancy. The fetus's brain is developing throughout pregnancy and can be affected by exposure to alcohol at any time.

If a woman is drinking alcohol during pregnancy, it is never too late to stop. The sooner a woman stops drinking, the better it will be for both the fetus and herself.

Get Help.

If you are pregnant or trying to get pregnant and cannot stop drinking, get help. Contact your healthcare provider, local Alcoholics Anonymous, or local alcohol treatment center.

Section 25.3

Fetal Alcohol Spectrum Disorders

This section includes text excerpted from "Basics about FASDs,"
Centers for Disease Control and Prevention (CDC), May 10, 2018.

Fetal alcohol spectrum disorders (FASDs) are a group of conditions that can occur in a person whose mother drank alcohol during pregnancy. These effects can include physical problems and problems with behavior and learning. Often, a person with a FASD has a mix of these problems.

Cause and Prevention

FASDs are caused by a woman drinking alcohol during pregnancy. Alcohol in the mother's blood passes to the fetus through the umbilical cord. When a woman drinks alcohol, so does the fetus.

There is no known safe amount of alcohol during pregnancy or when trying to get pregnant. There is also no safe time to drink during pregnancy. Alcohol can cause problems for a developing fetus throughout pregnancy, including before a woman knows she is pregnant. All types of alcohol are equally harmful, including all wines and beer.

To prevent FASDs, a woman should not drink alcohol while she is pregnant, or when she might get pregnant. This is because a woman could get pregnant and not know for up to four to six weeks. In the United States, nearly half of pregnancies are unplanned.

If a woman is drinking alcohol during pregnancy, it is never too late to stop drinking. Because brain growth takes place throughout pregnancy, the sooner a woman stops drinking the safer it will be for her and the fetus.

FASDs are completely preventable if a woman does not drink alcohol during pregnancy—so why take the risk?

Signs and Symptoms

FASDs refer to the whole range of effects that can happen to a person whose mother drank alcohol during pregnancy. These conditions can affect each person in different ways, and can range from mild to severe.

A person with a FASD might have:

- Abnormal facial features, such as a smooth ridge between the nose and upper lip (this ridge is called the "philtrum")

- Small head size

- Shorter-than-average height

- Low body weight

- Poor coordination

- Hyperactive behavior

- Difficulty with attention

- Poor memory

- Difficulty in school (especially with math)

- Learning disabilities

- Speech and language delays

- Intellectual disability or low IQ

- Poor reasoning and judgment skills

- Sleep and sucking problems as a baby

- Vision or hearing problems

- Problems with the heart, kidneys, or bones

Types of Fetal Alcohol Spectrum Disorders

Different terms are used to describe FASDs, depending on the type of symptoms.

- **Fetal alcohol syndrome (FAS):** FAS represents the most involved end of the FASD spectrum. Fetal death is the most extreme outcome from drinking alcohol during pregnancy. People with FAS might have abnormal facial features, growth problems, and central nervous system (CNS) problems. People with FAS can have problems with learning, memory, attention, communication, vision, or hearing. They might have a mix of these problems. People with FAS often have a hard time in school and trouble getting along with others.

- **Alcohol-related neurodevelopmental disorder (ARND):** People with ARND might have intellectual disabilities and problems with behavior and learning. They might do poorly in school and have difficulties with math, memory, attention, judgment, and poor impulse control.

- **Alcohol-related birth defects (ARBD):** People with ARBD might have problems with the heart, kidneys, or bones or with hearing. They might have a mix of these.

- **Neurobehavioral disorder associated with prenatal alcohol exposure (ND-PAE):** ND-PAE was first included as a recognized condition in the Diagnostic and Statistical Manual 5 (DSM 5) of the American Psychiatric Association (APA) in 2013. A child or youth with ND-PAE will have problems in three areas: thinking and memory, where the child may have trouble planning or may forget material she or he has already learned; behavior problems, such as severe tantrums, mood issues (for example, irritability), and difficulty shifting attention from one task to another; and trouble with day-to-day living, which can include problems with bathing, dressing for the weather, and playing with other children. In addition, to be diagnosed with ND-PAE, the mother of the child must have consumed more than minimal levels of alcohol before the child's birth, which APA defines as more than 13 alcoholic drinks per month of pregnancy (that is, any 30-day period of pregnancy) or more than 2 alcoholic drinks in one sitting.

Diagnosis

The term FASDs is not meant for use as a clinical diagnosis. The Centers for Disease Control and Prevention (CDC) worked with a group of experts and organizations to review the research and develop guidelines for diagnosing fetal alcohol syndrome (FAS). The guidelines were developed for FAS only. The CDC and its partners are working to put together diagnostic criteria for other FASDs, such as alcohol-related neurodevelopmental disorder.

Diagnosing FAS can be hard because there is no medical test, such as a blood test, for it. And other disorders, such as attention deficit hyperactivity disorder (ADHD) and Williams syndrome, have some symptoms much like those associated with FAS.

To diagnose FAS, doctors look for:

- Abnormal facial features (such as a smooth ridge between the nose and upper lip)

- Lower-than-average height, weight, or both

- Central nervous system (CNS) problems (such as small head size, problems with attention and hyperactivity, and poor coordination)

- Prenatal alcohol exposure; although confirmation is not required to make a diagnosis.

Treatment

FASDs last a lifetime. There is no cure for FASDs, but research shows that early intervention treatment services can improve a child's development.

There are many types of treatment options, including medication to help with some symptoms, behavior and education therapy, parent training, and other alternative approaches. No one treatment is right for every child. Good treatment plans will include close monitoring, followups, and changes as needed along the way.

Also, "protective factors" can help reduce the effects of FASDs and help people with these conditions reach their full potential.

Protective factors include:

- Diagnosis before six years of age

- Loving, nurturing, and stable home environment during the school years

- Absence of violence

- Involvement in special education and social services

Get Help

If you or the doctor thinks there could be a problem, ask the doctor for a referral to a specialist (someone who knows about FASDs), such as a developmental pediatrician, child psychologist, or clinical geneticist. In some cities, there are clinics with staffs that have special training in diagnosing and treating children with FASDs. To find doctors and clinics in your area visit the National and State Resource Directory from the National Organization on Fetal Alcohol Syndrome (NOFAS).

At the same time, as you ask the doctor for a referral to a specialist, call your state or territory's early-intervention program to request a free evaluation to find out if your child can get services to help. This is sometimes called a "child find evaluation." You do not need to wait for a doctor's referral or a medical diagnosis to make this call.

Where to call for a free evaluation from the state depends on your child's age:

If your child is younger than three years old, Call your state or area's early intervention program and say: "I have concerns about my child's development, and I would like to have my child evaluated to find out if she/he is eligible for early intervention services."

If your child is three years old or older, contact your local public school system.

Even if your child is not old enough for kindergarten or enrolled in a public school, call your local elementary school or board of education and ask to speak with someone who can help you have your child evaluated.

Section 25.4

Substance Use during Pregnancy

This section includes text excerpted from "Substance Use in Women,"
National Institute on Drug Abuse (NIDA), July 2018.

Regular use of some drugs can cause neonatal abstinence syndrome
(NAS), in which the baby goes through withdrawal upon birth. Most
research in this area has focused on the effects of opioids (prescription pain relievers or heroin). However, data has shown that use of
alcohol, barbiturates, benzodiazepines, and caffeine during pregnancy
may also cause the infant to show withdrawal symptoms at birth. The
type and severity of an infant's withdrawal symptoms depend on the
drug(s) used, how long and how often the drugs were used, how her
body breaks the drug down, and whether the infant was born full term
or prematurely.

Symptoms of drug withdrawal in a newborn can develop immediately or up to 14 days after birth and can include:

- Blotchy skin coloring

- Diarrhea

- Excessive or high-pitched crying

- Abnormal sucking reflex

- Fever

- Hyperactive reflexes

- Increased muscle tone

- Irritability

- Poor feeding

- Rapid breathing

- Seizures

- Sleep problems

- Slow weight gain

- Stuffy nose and sneezing

- Sweating

- Trembling
- Vomiting

Effects of using some drugs could be long-term and possibly fatal to the baby:

- Birth defects
- Low birth weight
- Premature birth
- Small head circumference
- Sudden infant death syndrome (SIDS)

Chapter 26

Prenatal Radiation Exposures and Home Monitoring

Chapter Contents

Section 26.1

X-Rays, Pregnancy, and You

This section includes text excerpted from "X-Rays, Pregnancy and You," U.S. Food and Drug Administration (FDA), December 9, 2017.

Pregnancy is a time to take good care of yourself and the fetus. Many things are especially important during pregnancy, such as eating right, cutting out cigarettes and alcohol, and being careful about the prescription and over-the-counter (OTC) drugs you take. Diagnostic X-rays and other medical radiation procedures of the abdominal area also deserve extra attention during pregnancy.

Diagnostic X-rays can give the doctor important and even life-saving information about a person's medical condition. But like many things, diagnostic X-rays have risks as well as benefits. They should be used only when they will give the doctor information needed to treat you.

You will probably never need an abdominal X-ray during pregnancy. But sometimes, because of a particular medical condition, your physician may feel that a diagnostic X-ray of your abdomen or lower torso is needed. If this should happen, do not worry. The risk to you and the fetus is very small, and the benefit of finding out about your medical condition is far greater. In fact, the risk of not having a needed X-ray could be much greater than the risk from the radiation. But even small risks should not be taken if they are unnecessary.

You can reduce those risks by telling your doctor if you are, or think you might be, pregnant whenever an abdominal X-ray is prescribed. If you are pregnant, the doctor may decide that it would be best to cancel the X-ray examination, to postpone it, or to modify it to reduce the amount of radiation. Or, depending on your medical needs, and realizing that the risk is very small, the doctor may feel that it is best to proceed with the X-ray as planned. In any case, you should feel free to discuss the decision with your doctor.

What Kind of X-rays Can Affect the Fetus?

During most X-ray examinations—like those of the arms, legs, head, teeth, or chest—your reproductive organs are not exposed to the direct X-ray beam. So these kinds of procedures, when properly done, do not involve any risk to the fetus. However, X-rays of the mother's lower torso—abdomen, stomach, pelvis, lower back, or kidneys—may expose the fetus to the direct X-ray beam. They are of more concern.

What Are the Possible Effects of X-rays?

There is scientific disagreement about whether the small amounts of radiation used in diagnostic radiology can actually harm a fetus, but it is known that a fetus is very sensitive to the effects of things such as radiation, certain drugs, excess alcohol, and infection. This is true, in part, because the cells are rapidly dividing and growing into specialized cells and tissues. If radiation or other agents were to cause changes in these cells, there could be a slightly increased chance of birth defects or certain illnesses, such as leukemia, later in life.

It should be pointed out, however, that the majority of birth defects and childhood diseases occur even if the mother is not exposed to any known harmful agent during pregnancy. Scientists believe that heredity and random errors in the developmental process are responsible for most of these problems.

What If I'm X-Rayed before I Know I'm Pregnant?

Do not be alarmed. Remember that the possibility of any harm to you and the fetus from an X-ray is very small. There are, however, rare situations in which a woman who is unaware of her pregnancy may receive a very large number of abdominal X-rays over a short period, or she may receive radiation treatment of the lower torso. Under these circumstances, the woman should discuss the possible risks with her doctor.

How You Can Help Minimize the Risks

- Most important, tell your physician if you are pregnant or think you might be. This is important for many medical decisions, such as drug prescriptions and nuclear medicine procedures, as well as X-rays. And remember, this is true even in the very early weeks of pregnancy.

- Occasionally, a woman may mistake the symptoms of pregnancy for the symptoms of a disease. If you have any of the symptoms of pregnancy—nausea, vomiting, breast tenderness, fatigue— consider whether you might be pregnant, and tell your doctor or X-ray technologist (the person doing the examination) before having an X-ray of the lower torso. A pregnancy test may be called for.

- If you are pregnant, or think you might be, do not hold a child who is being X-rayed. If you are not pregnant, and you are asked to hold a child during an X-ray, be sure to ask for a lead apron to protect your reproductive organs. This is to prevent damage to your genes that could be passed on and cause harmful effects in your future descendants.

- Whenever an X-ray is requested, tell your doctor about any similar X-rays you have had recently. It may not be necessary to do another. It is a good idea to keep a record of the X-ray examinations you and your family have had taken so you can provide this kind of information accurately.

- Feel free to talk with your doctor about the need for an X-ray examination. You should understand the reason X-rays are requested in your particular case.

Section 26.2

Ultrasound Imaging and Pregnancy

This section includes text excerpted from "Ultrasound Imaging," U.S. Food and Drug Administration (FDA), August 29, 2018.

Ultrasound imaging (sonography) uses high-frequency sound waves to view inside the body. Because ultrasound images are captured in real-time, they can also show movement of the body's internal organs as well as blood flowing through the blood vessels. Unlike X-ray imaging, there is no ionizing radiation exposure associated with ultrasound imaging.

In an ultrasound exam, a transducer (probe) is placed directly on the skin or inside a body opening. A thin layer of gel is applied to the skin so that the ultrasound waves are transmitted from the transducer through the gel into the body.

The ultrasound image is produced based on the reflection of the waves off of the body structures. The strength (amplitude) of the sound signal and the time it takes for the wave to travel through the body provide the information necessary to produce an image.

Uses

Ultrasound imaging is a medical tool that can help a physician evaluate, diagnose, and treat medical conditions. Common ultrasound imaging procedures include:

- Abdominal ultrasound (to visualize abdominal tissues and organs)
- Bone sonometry (to assess bone fragility)
- Breast ultrasound (to visualize breast tissue)
- Doppler fetal heart rate monitors (to listen to the fetal heartbeat)
- Doppler ultrasound (to visualize blood flow through a blood vessel, organs, or other structures)
- Echocardiogram (to view the heart)
- Fetal ultrasound (to view the fetus in pregnancy)
- Ultrasound-guided biopsies (to collect a sample of tissue)
- Ophthalmic ultrasound (to visualize ocular structures
- Ultrasound-guided needle placement (in blood vessels or other tissues of interest)

Benefits/Risks

Ultrasound imaging has been used for over 20 years and has an excellent safety record. It is based on nonionizing radiation, so it does not have the same risks as X-rays or other types of imaging systems that use ionizing radiation.

Although ultrasound imaging is generally considered safe when used prudently by appropriately trained healthcare providers, ultrasound energy has the potential to produce biological effects on the body. Ultrasound waves can heat the tissues slightly. In some cases, it can also produce small pockets of gas in body fluids or tissues (cavitation). The long-term consequences of these effects are still unknown. Because of the particular concern for effects on the fetus, organizations such as the American Institute of Ultrasound in Medicine (AIUM) have advocated prudent use of ultrasound imaging in pregnancy. Furthermore, the use of ultrasound solely for nonmedical purposes, such as obtaining fetal keepsake videos, has been discouraged. Keepsake images or videos are reasonable if they are produced during a medically-indicated exam, and if no additional exposure is required.

Information for Patients Including Expectant Mothers

For all medical-imaging procedures, the U.S. Food and Drug Administration (FDA) recommends that patients talk to their healthcare provider to understand the reason for the examination, the medical information that will be obtained, the potential risks, and how the results will be used to manage the medical condition or pregnancy. Because ultrasound is not based on ionizing radiation, it is particularly useful for women of childbearing age when computed tomography (CT) or other imaging methods would otherwise result in exposure to radiation.

Expectant Mothers

Ultrasound is the most widely used medical-imaging method for viewing the fetus during pregnancy. Routine examinations are performed to assess and monitor the health status of the fetus and mother. Ultrasound examinations provide parents with a valuable opportunity to view and hear the heartbeat of the fetus, bond, and capture images to share with family and friends.

In fetal ultrasound, three-dimensional (3D) ultrasound allows the visualization of some facial features and possibly other parts, such as fingers and toes of the fetus. Four-dimensional (4D) ultrasound is 3D ultrasound in motion. While ultrasound is generally considered to be safe with very low risks, the risks may increase with unnecessary prolonged exposure to ultrasound energy, or when untrained users operate the device.

Expectant mothers should also be aware of purchasing over-the-counter (OTC) fetal heartbeat monitoring systems (also called "doptones"). These devices should only be used by trained healthcare providers when medically necessary. Use of these devices by untrained persons could expose the fetus to prolonged and unsafe energy levels, or could provide information that is interpreted incorrectly by the user.

Section 26.3

Pregnant Women Should Avoid Fetal Keepsake Images and Heartbeat Monitors

This section includes text excerpted from "Avoid Fetal "Keepsake" Images, Heartbeat Monitors," U.S. Food and Drug Administration (FDA), September 10, 2018.

Ultrasound imaging is the most widely used medical-imaging method during pregnancy.

Fetal ultrasound imaging provides real-time images of the fetus. Doppler fetal ultrasound heartbeat monitors are hand-held ultrasound devices that let you listen to the heartbeat of the fetus. Both are prescription devices designed to be used by trained healthcare professionals. They are not intended for over-the-counter (OTC) sale or use, and the U.S. Food and Drug Administration (FDA) strongly discourages their use for creating fetal keepsake images and videos.

"Although there is a lack of evidence of any harm due to ultrasound imaging and heartbeat monitors, prudent use of these devices by trained healthcare providers is important," says Shahram Vaezy, Ph.D., an FDA biomedical engineer. "Ultrasound can heat tissues slightly, and in some cases, it can also produce very small bubbles (cavitation) in some tissues."

The long-term effects of tissue heating and cavitation are not known. Therefore, ultrasound scans should be done only when there is a medical need, based on a prescription, and performed by appropriately-trained operators.

Fetal keepsake videos are controversial because there is no medical benefit gained from exposing the fetus to ultrasound. The FDA is aware of several enterprises in the United States that are commercializing ultrasonic imaging by making fetal keepsake videos. In some cases, the ultrasound machine may be used for as long as an hour to get a video of the fetus.

While the FDA recognizes that fetal imaging can promote bonding between the parents and the developing fetus, such opportunities are routinely provided during prenatal care. In creating fetal keepsake videos, there is no control on how long a single imaging session will last, how many sessions will take place, or whether the ultrasound systems will be operated properly. By contrast, Veazy says, "Proper use of ultrasound equipment pursuant to a prescription ensures that a woman will receive professional care that contributes to her health and to the health of her fetus."

Doppler Ultrasound Heartbeat Monitors

Similar concerns surround the OTC sale and use of Doppler ultrasound heartbeat monitors. These devices, which are used for listening to the heartbeat of a fetus, are legally marketed as "prescription devices," and should only be used by, or under the supervision of, a healthcare professional.

"When the product is purchased over the counter and used without consultation with a healthcare professional taking care of the pregnant woman, there is no oversight of how the device is used. Also, there is little or no medical benefit expected from the exposure," Vaezy says. "Furthermore, the number of sessions or the length of a session in scanning a fetus is uncontrolled, and that increases the potential for harm to the fetus and eventually the mother."

Section 26.4

Home Uterine Monitors Are Not Useful for Predicting Premature Birth

This section includes text excerpted from "Common Tests for Preterm Birth Not Useful for Routine Screening of First-Time Pregnancies," National Institutes of Health (NIH), March 14, 2017.

Two methods thought to hold promise in predicting preterm delivery in first-time pregnancies identified only a small proportion of cases, and do not appear suitable for widespread screening, according to a large study by a National Institutes of Health (NIH) research network.

The study focused on spontaneous preterm delivery—labor that occurs naturally—rather than delivery initiated for medical need, such as cesarean surgery or induced labor.

The study's authors evaluated routine ultrasound examination of the uterine cervix, the lower part of the uterus that shortens and opens during labor. Previous studies have indicated that a short cervix early in pregnancy could be a warning sign of impending preterm birth. The researchers also evaluated testing for fetal fibronectin, a glue-like protein that secures the amniotic sac to the inside of the uterus. Some studies have suggested that the presence of fetal fibronectin in the vagina early in pregnancy could signal early labor.

However, after screening more than 9,000 women throughout pregnancy, each test identified only a small proportion of the women who would eventually deliver preterm.

"These methods of assessing women in their first pregnancy do not identify most of those who will later go on to have a spontaneous preterm delivery," said the study's senior author, Uma Reddy, M.D., of the Pregnancy and Perinatology Branch at NIH's *Eunice Kennedy Shriver* National Institute of Child Health and Human Development (NICHD). "There is a need to develop better screening tests that can be performed early in pregnancy."

The article appears in the *Journal of the American Medical Association (JAMA)*.

The study included 9,410 women pregnant with a single fetus at 8 research centers in the United States. It was conducted as part of the Nulliparous Pregnancy Outcomes Study: Monitoring Mothers-to-Be (nuMoM2b), which aims to improve the care of women during their first pregnancy and to find new ways to identify impending preterm birth and other adverse pregnancy conditions.

The women underwent ultrasound testing to measure cervical length at 16 to 22 weeks of pregnancy, and again from 22 to 31 weeks of pregnancy. Fetal fibronectin tests were conducted at 6 to 14 weeks, 16 to 22 weeks, and 22 to 30 weeks. A short cervix was defined as less than 25 mm.

Of the women tested at 16 to 22 weeks, 35 of 439 women (8 percent) who delivered spontaneously before the 37th week of pregnancy had a short cervix. At 22 to 31 weeks, 94 of 403 women (23.3 percent) who delivered prematurely had a short cervix.

For the fibronectin test at 16 to 22 weeks, 30 of 410 women (7.3 percent) who delivered spontaneously before the 37th week had high fibronectin levels. At 22 to 30 weeks, 31 of 384 women (8.1 percent) who delivered prematurely had high fibronectin levels. The authors defined a high fibronectin level as 50 ng/mL or greater.

The researchers found no benefit to combining the results of the two tests. They concluded that, alone and together, the methods did not identify enough preterm births to support routine screening of first-time pregnancies.

Chapter 27

Common Safety Concerns during Pregnancy

Chapter Contents

Section 27.1

Hot Tubs, High Temperatures, and Pregnancy Risks

This section includes text excerpted from "Operating Public Hot Tubs," Centers for Disease Control and Prevention (CDC), May 10, 2014. Reviewed February 2019.

Low water volumes combined with high temperatures and heavy bather loads make operating a public hot tub challenging. The result can be low disinfectant levels that allow the growth and spread of a variety of germs (e.g., *Pseudomonas* and *Legionella*) that can cause skin and respiratory recreational water illnesses (RWIs). Operators that focus on hot tub maintenance and operation to ensure continuous, high water quality are the first line of defense in preventing the spread of RWIs.

- Obtain state or local authority-recommended operator and chemical-handling training.

- Ensure availability of trained operation staff during weekends when hot tubs are used most.

- Maintain free chlorine (2 to 4 parts per million or ppm) or bromine (4 to 6 ppm) levels continuously.

- Maintain the pH level of the water at 7.2 to 7.8.

- Test pH and disinfectant levels at least twice per day (hourly when in heavy use).

- Maintain accurate records of disinfectant/pH measurements and maintenance activities.

- Maintain filtration and recirculation systems according to manufacturer recommendations.

- Inspect accessible recirculation-system components for a slime layer and clean as needed.

- Scrub hot tub surfaces to remove any slime layer.

- Enforce bather-load limits.

- Drain and replace all or portions of the water on a weekly to monthly basis, depending on usage and water quality. Depending on filter type, clean filter or replace filter media before refilling the hot tub.

- Treat the hot tub with a biocidal shock treatment on a daily to weekly basis, depending on water quality and frequency of water replacement.

- Institute a preventive maintenance program to replace equipment or parts before they fail (e.g., feed pump tubing and sensor probes).

- Provide disinfection guidelines for fecal accidents and body fluid spills.

- Develop a clear communication chain for reporting operation problems.

- Cover hot tubs, if possible, to minimize loss of disinfectant and reduce the levels of environmental contamination (e.g., debris and dirt).

- Educate hot tub users about appropriate hot tub use.

Additional Hot Tub Safety Measures

- Prevent the water temperature from exceeding 104°F (40°C).

- Exclude children less than five years old from using hot tubs.

- Maintain a locked safety cover for the hot tub when possible.

- Recommend that all pregnant women consult a physician before hot tub use, particularly in the first trimester.

- Prevent entrapment injuries with appropriate drain design and configuration.

Section 27.2

Cosmetics and Pregnancy

This section includes text excerpted from "Cosmetics and Pregnancy,"
U.S. Food and Drug Administration (FDA), March 6, 2018.

The U.S. Food and Drug Administration (FDA) sometimes receives questions about the safe use of cosmetics during pregnancy. If you are pregnant and have concerns about cosmetic products or ingredients, contact your healthcare provider. While the FDA cannot give medical advice, some general safety information can be provided.

What the Law Says about Cosmetic Safety

It is important to know that the law does not require cosmetic products or ingredients to have FDA approval before they go on the market. However, cosmetics must be safe when consumers use them according to product labeling, or as the products are customarily used.

Companies and individuals who manufacture or market cosmetics are legally responsible for making sure their products are safe. The FDA can take action against an unsafe cosmetic that does not comply with the law, but first, they need reliable information showing that it is unsafe when people use it as intended.

The law treats color additives differently. Color additives must be approved by the FDA before they are used in cosmetics or other FDA-regulated products. Some must even be from batches certified in the FDA's own labs.

The law also makes a special exception for coal-tar hair dyes, which include most permanent, semi-permanent, and temporary hair dyes on the market. The FDA cannot take action against a coal-tar hair dye if it has this statement on the label—along with instructions for doing a skin test.

"Caution—This product contains ingredients which may cause skin irritation on certain individuals and a preliminary test according to accompanying directions should first be made. This product must not be used for dyeing the eyelashes or eyebrows; to do so may cause blindness."

How U.S. Food and Drug Administration Monitors Cosmetic Safety

The FDA monitors the safety of cosmetics in several ways. For example, the FDA periodically buys cosmetics and analyzes them, especially if they are aware of a potential problem. The FDA scientists keep up with the latest research and the FDA conducts its own research as well. The FDA also evaluate reports of problems that are sent by consumers who have had bad reactions, to watch for trends that will tell if a particular product may require action on the FDA's part.

When the FDA into the safety of a cosmetic product or ingredient on the market, they consider factors such as how it is used and who is likely to use it. This includes whether there are likely to be safety concerns when women use the product during pregnancy. When the FDA identifies a safety problem, they let the public know and take action against the product.

Safety Information in Cosmetic Labeling

Cosmetics must be labeled properly. For example, they must have any directions for use and any warnings needed to make sure consumers use the product safely. Also, cosmetics marketed on a retail basis to consumers, such as in stores or person-to-person, must have a list of ingredients on the label. For cosmetics sold by mail order, including online, this list must be on the label, in a catalog, on a website, enclosed with the shipment, or sent separately when the consumer asks for it. This list lets consumers know if a product contains ingredients they want to avoid.

Some Personal Care Products That Are Not Cosmetics

Not all personal care products, including those you might use during and after pregnancy, are cosmetics. For example, a product that is intended to affect the structure or function of your body, or to treat or prevent disease, is regulated as a drug, or sometimes both a cosmetic and a drug. This is true even if it affects how you look. Stretch mark treatments, creams for treating irritated or cracked nipples, sunscreens, antiperspirants, and treatments for dandruff and acne are some common examples.

Generally, nonprescription drugs must conform to special regulations, called "monographs," for their product category or be approved by the FDA before they go on the market.

Part Four

High-Risk Pregnancies

Chapter 28

What Is a High-Risk Pregnancy?

A high-risk pregnancy is one that threatens the health or life of the mother or her fetus. It often requires specialized care from specially trained providers. Some pregnancies become high risk as they progress, while some women are at increased risk for complications even before they get pregnant for a variety of reasons. Early and regular prenatal care helps many women have healthy pregnancies and deliveries without complications.

What Are Some Factors That Make a Pregnancy High Risk?

Several factors can make a pregnancy high risk, including existing health conditions, the mother's age, lifestyle, and health issues that happen before or during pregnancy.

This chapter contains text excerpted from the following sources: Text in this chapter begins with excerpts from "What Is a High-Risk Pregnancy?" *Eunice Kennedy Shriver* National Institute of Child Health and Human Development (NICHD), January 31, 2017; Text under the heading "What Are Some Factors That Make a Pregnancy High Risk?" is excerpted from "What Are Some Factors That Make a Pregnancy High Risk?" *Eunice Kennedy Shriver* National Institute of Child Health and Human Development (NICHD), November 6, 2018.

Existing Health Conditions

- **High blood pressure.** Even though high blood pressure can be risky for the mother and fetus, most women with slightly high blood pressure and no other diseases have healthy pregnancies and healthy deliveries because they get their blood pressure under control before pregnancy. Uncontrolled high blood pressure, however, can damage the mother's kidneys and increase the risk for low birth weight or preeclampsia. It is very important for women to have their blood pressure checked at every prenatal visit so that healthcare providers can detect any changes and make decisions about treatment.

- **Polycystic ovary syndrome (PCOS).** Women with PCOS have higher rates of pregnancy loss before 20 weeks of pregnancy, diabetes during pregnancy (gestational diabetes), preeclampsia, and cesarean section.

- **Diabetes.** It is important for women with diabetes to manage their blood sugar levels both before getting pregnant and throughout pregnancy. During the first few weeks of pregnancy, often before a woman even knows she is pregnant, high blood sugar levels can cause birth defects. Even women whose diabetes is well under control may have changes in their metabolism during pregnancy that require extra care or treatment to promote a healthy birth. Babies of mothers with diabetes tend to be large and are likely to have low blood sugar soon after birth, which is yet another reason for women with diabetes to keep tight control of their blood sugar.

- **Kidney disease.** Women with mild kidney disease often have healthy pregnancies. But kidney disease can cause difficulties getting and staying pregnant, as well as problems during pregnancy, including preterm delivery, low birth weight, and preeclampsia. Pregnant women with kidney disease require additional treatments, changes in diet and medication, and frequent visits to their healthcare provider.

- **Autoimmune disease.** Conditions such as lupus and multiple sclerosis can increase the risk of problems during pregnancy and delivery. Women with lupus are at an increased risk for preterm birth and stillbirth. Some women may find that their symptoms improve during pregnancy, while others have flare-ups and other challenges. Certain medicines to treat autoimmune diseases may be harmful to the fetus, meaning a woman with an autoimmune disease will need to work closely with a healthcare provider throughout pregnancy.

- **Thyroid disease.** The thyroid is a small gland in the neck that makes hormones that help control heart rate and blood pressure. Uncontrolled thyroid disease, such as an overactive or underactive thyroid, can cause problems for the fetus, such as heart failure, poor weight gain, and brain development problems. Thyroid problems are usually treatable with medicine or surgery.

- **Obesity.** Being obese before pregnancy is associated with a number of risks for poor pregnancy outcomes. Obesity before pregnancy is associated with an increased risk of structural problems with the fetus's heart. There can also be problems if overweight or obese women gain too much weight during pregnancy. Obesity increases the chance of developing diabetes during pregnancy, which can contribute to difficult births. Obesity can also cause a fetus to be larger than normal, making the birth process more difficult. It increases the risk of sleep apnea and disordered sleep breathing during pregnancy.

- **Human immunodeficiency virus (HIV)/acquired immunodeficiency syndrome (AIDS).** HIV can pass to a fetus during pregnancy, labor and delivery, and breastfeeding. Fortunately, there are effective treatments that can reduce and prevent the spread of HIV from mother to fetus or child. Medications for the mother and for the infant, as well as surgical delivery of the baby before the "water breaks" and feeding formula instead of breastfeeding, can prevent mother-to-child transmission and has led to a dramatic decrease in transmission—to less than one percent in the United States and other developed countries.

- **Zika infection.** Although scientists and healthcare providers have known about Zika for decades, the link between Zika infection during pregnancy, risks, and birth defects has only recently come to light. Research supported by the *Eunice Kennedy Shriver* National Institute of Child Health and Human Development (NICHD) has shown that infants born to mothers who were infected with Zika just before and during pregnancy were at higher risk for different problems with the brain and nervous system. The most noticeable is microcephaly, a condition in which the head is smaller than normal. Zika infection during pregnancy can also increase the woman's risk of pregnancy loss and stillbirth. Researchers are still just learning the possible mechanisms of Zika's effects on pregnancy.

Age

- **Young age.** Pregnant teens are more likely to develop pregnancy-related high blood pressure and anemia (lack of healthy red blood cells) and to go through preterm (early) labor and delivery than women who are older. Teens are also more likely to not know they have a sexually transmitted infection (STI). Some STIs can cause problems with the pregnancy or for the fetus. Teens may be less likely to get prenatal care or to keep prenatal appointments. Prenatal care is important because it allows a healthcare provider to evaluate, identify, and treat risks, such as counseling teens not to take certain medications during pregnancy, sometimes before these risks become problems.

- **First-time pregnancy after age 35.** Most older first-time mothers have normal pregnancies, but research shows that older women are at higher risk for certain problems than younger women, including:

  - Pregnancy-related high blood pressure (called "gestational hypertension") and diabetes (called "gestational diabetes").

  - Pregnancy loss

  - Ectopic pregnancy (when the embryo attaches itself outside the uterus), a condition that can be life-threatening

  - Cesarean (surgical) delivery

  - Delivery complications, such as excessive bleeding

  - Prolonged labor (lasting more than 20 hours)

  - Labor that does not advance

  - Genetic disorders, such as Down syndrome, in the baby

Lifestyle Factors

- **Alcohol use.** Drinking alcohol during pregnancy can increase the fetus's risk for fetal alcohol spectrum disorders (FASDs), sudden infant death syndrome (SIDS), and other problems.

FASDs have a variety of effects on the fetus that results from a pregnant woman drinking alcohol during pregnancy. The effects range from mild to severe, and they include intellectual and developmental disabilities; behavior problems; abnormal facial features; and disorders of the heart, kidneys, bones, and hearing difficulties. FASDs are completely preventable; if a woman does not drink alcohol while she is pregnant, her child will not have an FASD. Women who drink also are more likely to have a miscarriage or stillbirth. Currently, research shows that there is no safe amount of alcohol to drink while pregnant.

- **Tobacco use.** Smoking during pregnancy puts the fetus at risk for preterm birth, certain birth defects, and SIDS. One study showed that smoking doubled or even tripled the risk of stillbirth, or a fetal death after 20 weeks of pregnancy. Research has also found that smoking during pregnancy leads to changes in an infant's immune system. Secondhand smoke also puts a woman and her developing fetus at increased risk for health problems.

- **Drug use.** Research shows that smoking marijuana and taking drugs during pregnancy can also harm the fetus and affect infant health. One study showed that smoking marijuana and using illegal drugs doubled the risk of stillbirth. Research also shows that smoking marijuana during pregnancy can interfere with normal brain development in the fetus, possibly causing long-term problems.

Conditions of Pregnancy

- **Multiple gestation.** Pregnancy with twins, triplets, or more fetuses is called "multiple gestation," which increases the risk of infants being born prematurely (before 37 weeks of pregnancy). Both giving birth after age 30 and taking fertility drugs have been linked with multiple births. Having three or more fetuses increases the chance that a woman will need to deliver through cesarean section. Twins and triplets are more likely to be smaller for their size than single infants. If infants are born prematurely, they are more likely to have difficulty breathing.

- **Gestational diabetes.** Gestational diabetes occurs when a woman who did not have diabetes before develops diabetes when she is pregnant. Gestational diabetes can cause problems for both the mother and fetus, including preterm labor and delivery, and high blood pressure. It also increases the risk that a woman and her baby will develop type 2 diabetes later in life. Many women with gestational diabetes have healthy pregnancies because they work with a healthcare provider to manage their condition.

- **Preeclampsia and eclampsia.** Preeclampsia is a sudden increase in a pregnant woman's blood pressure after the 20th week of pregnancy. It can affect the mother's kidneys, liver, and brain. The condition can be fatal for both the mother and the fetus or cause long-term health problems. Eclampsia is a more severe form of preeclampsia that includes seizures and can lead to a coma.

- **Previous preterm birth.** Women who went into labor or who had their baby early (before 37 weeks of pregnancy) with a previous pregnancy are at higher risk for preterm labor and birth with their current pregnancy. Healthcare providers will want to monitor women at high risk for preterm labor and birth in case treatment is needed. Women who become pregnant within 12 months after their latest delivery may be at an increased risk for preterm birth. Women who have recently given birth may want to talk with a healthcare provider about contraception to help delay the next pregnancy.

- **Birth defects or genetic conditions in the fetus.** In some cases, healthcare providers can detect health problems in the fetus during pregnancy. Depending on the nature of the problems, the pregnancy may be considered high risk because treatments are needed while the fetus is still in the womb or immediately after birth. If certain forms of spina bifida are detected in the fetus, the problems can be repaired before birth. Certain heart problems that are common among infants with Down syndrome need to be corrected with surgery immediately after birth. Knowing a fetus has Down syndrome before birth can help healthcare providers and parents be prepared to give treatment right away.

Chapter 29

Common Risky Pregnancies

Chapter Contents

Section 29.1

Teen Pregnancy

This section contains text excerpted from the following
sources: Text in this section begins with excerpts from "Teenage
Pregnancy," MedlinePlus, National Institutes of Health (NIH),
November 2, 2018; Text under the heading "Adverse Effects
of Teen Pregnancy" is excerpted from "Adverse Effects,"
Youth.gov, October 17, 2012. Reviewed February 2019.

Most teenage girls do not plan to get pregnant, but many do. Teen
pregnancies carry extra health risks to both the mother and the fetus.
Often, teens do not get prenatal care soon enough, which can lead
to problems later on. They have a higher risk for pregnancy-related
high blood pressure and its complications. Risks for the fetus include
premature birth and a low birth weight.

If you are a pregnant teen, you can help yourself and the fetus
by:

- Getting regular prenatal care

- Taking your prenatal vitamins for your health and to prevent
  some birth defects

- Avoiding smoking, alcohol, and drugs

- Using a condom if you are having sex, to prevent sexually
  transmitted diseases (STDs) that could hurt your fetus

Adverse Effects of Teen Pregnancy

The high social and economic costs of teen pregnancy and childbearing can have short- and long-term negative consequences for teen
parents, their children, and their community. Through recent research,
it has been recognized that pregnancy and childbirth have a significant
impact on the educational outcomes of teen parents.

- By age 22, only around 50 percent of teen mothers have received
  a high school diploma and only 30 percent have earned a
  General Education Development (GED) certificate, whereas 90
  percent of women who did not give birth during adolescence
  receive a high school diploma.

- Only about 10 percent of teen mothers complete a 2- or 4-year
  college program

- Teen fathers have a 25 to 30 percent lower probability of graduating from high school than teenage boys who are not fathers

Children who are born to teen mothers also experience a wide range of problems. For example, they are more likely to:

- Have a higher risk for low birth weight and infant mortality

- Have lower levels of emotional support and cognitive stimulation

- Have fewer skills and are less prepared to learn when they enter kindergarten

- Have behavioral problems and chronic medical conditions

- Rely more heavily on publicly funded healthcare

- Have higher rates of foster care placement

- Be incarcerated at some time during adolescence

- Have lower school achievement and dropout of high school

- Give birth as a teen

- Be unemployed or underemployed as a young adult

These immediate and long-lasting effects continue for teen parents and their children even after adjusting for the factors that increased the teen's risk for pregnancy, such as growing up in poverty, having parents with low levels of education, growing up in a single-parent family, and having low attachment to and performance in school.

Teen pregnancy costs U.S. taxpayers about $11 billion per year due to increased healthcare and foster care, increased incarceration rates among children of teen parents, and lost tax revenue because of lower educational attainment and income among teen mothers. Some recent cost studies estimate that the cost may be as high as $28 billion per year or an average of $5,500 for each teen parent. The majority of this cost is associated with teens who give birth before age 18.

Section 29.2

Multiple Pregnancy: Twins, Triplets, and Beyond

This section includes text excerpted from "Twins, Triplets, and Other Multiples," Office on Women's Health (OWH), U.S. Department of Health and Human Services (HHS), January 30, 2019.

Information about Multiples

In 2005, 133,122 twins and 6,208 triplets were born in the United States. In 1980, there were only 69,339 twin and 1,337 triplet births.

Why the increase? For one, more women are having babies after age 30. Women in their 30s are more likely than younger women to conceive more than one fetus naturally. Another reason is that more women are using fertility treatments to help them conceive.

How Twins Are Formed

Twins form in one of two ways:

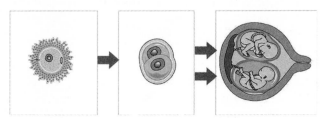

Figure 29.1. *Identical Twins*

Identical twins occur when a single fertilized egg splits into two. Identical twins look almost exactly alike and share the exact same genes. Most identical twins happen by chance.

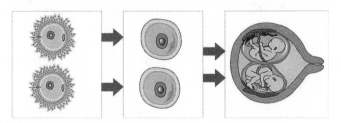

Figure 29.2. *Fraternal Twins*

Fraternal twins occur when two, separate eggs are fertilized by two, separate sperm. Fraternal twins do not share the exact same genes—they are no more alike than they are to their siblings from different pregnancies. Fraternal twins tend to run in some families.

Multiple births can be fraternal, identical, or a combination. Multiples associated with fertility treatments are mainly fraternal.

Pregnancy with Multiples

Years ago, most twins came as a surprise. Now, thanks to advances in prenatal care, most women learn about a multiple pregnancy early. You might suspect you are pregnant with multiples if you have more severe body changes, including:

- Rapid weight gain in the first trimester

- Intense nausea and vomiting

- Extreme breast tenderness

Your doctor can confirm whether you are carrying more than one fetus through ultrasound. If you are pregnant with twins or other multiples, you will need to see your doctor more often than women who are carrying only one fetus because your risk of complications is greater. Women carrying more than one fetus are at higher risk of:

- Preterm birth

- Low birth weight

- Preeclampsia

- Gestational diabetes

- Cesarean birth

More frequent prenatal visits help your doctor to monitor your and your fetuses' health. Your doctor will also tell you how much weight to gain, if you need to take extra vitamins, and how much activity is safe. With close monitoring, your babies will have the best chance of being born near term and at a healthy weight.

After delivery and once your babies come home, you may feel overwhelmed and exhausted. Ask for help from your partner, family, and friends. Volunteer help and support groups for parents of multiples also can ease the transition.

Chapter 30

Asthma and Pregnancy

What Is Asthma?

Asthma is a chronic lung disease that affects the bronchial tubes. Your bronchial tubes carry air into and out of your lungs. When you breathe, your lungs take in oxygen. The oxygen travels through your bloodstream to all parts of your body.

In people who have asthma, the lungs and walls of the bronchial tubes become inflamed and oversensitive. When people with asthma breathe in "asthma triggers," such as smoke, air pollution, cold air, mold, or chemicals, the bronchial tubes tighten in response. This limits airflow and makes it difficult to breathe. Asthma triggers may be different for each person and may change over time.

What Are the Symptoms of Asthma?

Asthma symptoms include:

- Wheezing

- Coughing

- Shortness of breath

- Chest tightness

This chapter includes text excerpted from "Asthma," Office on Women's Health (OWH), U.S. Department of Health and Human Services (HHS), December 27, 2018.

267

You may have only one or two of these symptoms, or you may get all of them. You may also get asthma symptoms only at night or in cold weather. Or you may get asthma symptoms after exposure to an allergen or another trigger, or when you have a cold or are exercising.

What Are Common Asthma Triggers?

Many different things can trigger an asthma attack. And what triggers one person's asthma may not trigger another person's asthma. Common asthma triggers include:

- Tobacco smoke
- Animal urine, saliva, and dander (dead skin that comes from pets, such as cats and dogs)
- Dust mites
- Cockroaches
- Air pollution
- Mold
- Pollens and other allergens in the air (such as from trees and grass)
- Fragrances (including personal care products, such as lotions, or household products, such as candles that have fragrance added)
- Physical activity (called "exercise-induced asthma")
- Cold air
- Wood smoke
- Preservatives in alcohol called "sulfites"
- Certain chemicals in cleaning products or other types of chemicals you might use at work or at home

How Does Asthma Affect Pregnancy?

Many women who have asthma do not have any problems during pregnancy. But asthma can cause problems for you and the fetus during pregnancy because of changing hormone levels. A fetus depends on the air you breathe in for oxygen. Asthma attacks during pregnancy can prevent the fetus from getting enough oxygen.

Pregnant women with asthma have a higher risk of:

- Preeclampsia

- Gestational diabetes

- Problems with the placenta, including placental abruption

- Premature birth (babies born before 37 weeks of pregnancy)

- Low birth weight baby (less than 5 and a half pounds)

- Cesarean section (C-section)

- Serious bleeding after childbirth (called "postpartum hemorrhage")

Pregnancy may also make asthma symptoms seem worse due to acid reflux or heartburn. If you have asthma and are thinking about becoming pregnant, talk to your doctor or nurse. Having your asthma under control before you get pregnant can help prevent problems during pregnancy.

How Is Asthma Diagnosed?

Many people develop asthma during childhood, but asthma can happen at any age. Asthma can be difficult to diagnose. Asthma symptoms can be similar to those of other conditions, such as chronic obstructive pulmonary disease (COPD), pneumonia, bronchitis, anxiety disorders, and heart disease.

To diagnose asthma, your doctor or nurse may:

- Ask about your symptoms and what seems to trigger them.

- Ask about your health history.

- Do a physical exam.

- Ask about your daily habits.

- Ask what types of allergens or irritants might be in your workplace or home that could trigger your asthma symptoms.

Your doctor or nurse may also do tests including:

- **Spirometry.** A machine called a spirometer measures how much air you can breathe. It also measures how fast you can blow air out. Your doctor or nurse may give you medicines and then retest you to see if the results are better after you take the medicines.

- **Bronchoprovocation.** Your doctor or nurse tests your lung function using spirometry. During the test, you will put stress on your lungs by exercising or breathing in increasing doses of a special chemical or cold air.

Your doctor or nurse may want to test for other problems that might be causing your symptoms. These include sleep apnea, vocal cord problems, or stomach acid backing up into the throat.

How Is Asthma Treated?

Asthma is a chronic disease. This means that it can be treated but not cured. However, some people are able to manage asthma so that symptoms do not happen again or happen rarely.

You can take steps to control asthma and prevent problems by:

- Working with your doctor or nurse to set up and follow a personal asthma action plan

- Taking medicines as your doctor or nurse prescribes them for you. Asthma medicines fall into two groups: long-term control medicines and quick relief or "rescue" medicines. Asthma medicines work by opening the lung airways or by reducing the inflammation in the lungs. Some asthma medicines are pills, but most come from an inhaler (you breathe the medicine in).

- Staying away from your asthma triggers

- Getting a flu shot. The flu can be very dangerous for women with asthma.

Is Asthma Medicine Safe to Take during Pregnancy?

Some asthma medicines may be safe to take during pregnancy. Talk to your doctor or nurse about whether it is safe to continue taking your medicine during pregnancy.

Your doctor or nurse may suggest a different medicine to take. Do not stop taking your medicine or change your medicine without talking to your doctor or nurse first. Not using medicine that you need may be more harmful to you and the fetus than using medicine. Untreated asthma can cause serious problems during pregnancy.

Also, talk with your doctor or nurse about getting a flu shot. The flu can be very dangerous for women with asthma, especially during pregnancy when your immune system is different from normal.

Chapter 31

Cancer and Pregnancy

Chapter Contents

Section 31.1

Breast Cancer and Pregnancy

This section includes text excerpted from "Breast Cancer
Treatment during Pregnancy (PDQ®)—Patient Version,"
National Cancer Institute (NCI), December 28, 2018.

Breast cancer is a disease in which malignant (cancer) cells form in the tissues of the breast.

The breast is made up of lobes and ducts. Each breast has 15 to 20 sections called "lobes." Each lobe has many smaller sections called "lobules." Lobules end in dozens of tiny bulbs that can make milk. The lobes, lobules, and bulbs are linked by thin tubes called "ducts."

Each breast also has blood vessels and lymph vessels. The lymph vessels carry an almost colorless, watery fluid called "lymph." Lymph vessels carry lymph between lymph nodes. Lymph nodes are small, bean-shaped structures found throughout the body. They filter lymph and store white blood cells that help fight infection and disease. Groups of lymph nodes are found near the breast in the axilla (under the arm), above the collarbone, and in the chest.

Sometimes breast cancer occurs in women who are pregnant or have just given birth. Breast cancer occurs about once in every 3,000 pregnancies. It occurs most often in women aged 32 to 38 years. Because many women are choosing to delay having children, it is likely that the number of new cases of breast cancer during pregnancy will increase.

Signs of Breast Cancer

These and other signs may be caused by breast cancer or by other conditions. Check with your doctor if you have any of the following:

- A lump or thickening in or near the breast or in the underarm area

- A change in the size or shape of the breast

- A dimple or puckering in the skin of the breast

- A nipple turned inward into the breast

- Fluid, other than breast milk, from the nipple, especially if it is bloody

- Scaly, red, or swollen skin on the breast, nipple, or areola (the dark area of skin around the nipple)

- Dimples in the breast that look like the skin of an orange, called "peau d'orange"

Tests for Breast Cancer

It may be difficult to detect (find) breast cancer early in pregnant or nursing women. The breasts usually get larger, tender, or lumpy in women who are pregnant, nursing, or have just given birth. This occurs because of normal hormone changes that take place during pregnancy. These changes can make small lumps difficult to detect. The breasts may also become denser. It is more difficult to detect breast cancer in women with dense breasts using mammography. Because these breast changes can delay diagnosis, breast cancer is often found at a later stage in these women.

Breast exams should be part of prenatal and postnatal care. To detect breast cancer, pregnant and nursing women should examine their breasts themselves. Women should also receive clinical breast exams during their regular prenatal and postnatal check-ups. Talk to your doctor if you notice any changes in your breasts that you did not expect or that worry you.

The following tests and procedures may be used:

- Physical exam and history

- Clinical breast exam (CBE)

- Ultrasound exam

- Mammogram

- Biopsy

If cancer is found, tests are done to study the cancer cells.

Decisions about the best treatment are based on the results of these tests and the age of the fetus. The tests give information about:

- How quickly the cancer may grow

- How likely it is that the cancer will spread to other parts of the body

- How well certain treatments might work

- How likely the cancer is to recur (come back)

Tests may include the following:

- Estrogen and progesterone receptor test

273

- Human epidermal growth factor type 2 receptor (HER2/neu) test
- Multigene tests
  - Oncotype DX
  - MammaPrint

Certain factors affect prognosis (chance of recovery) and treatment options.

The chance of recovery and treatment options depend on the following:

- The stage of the cancer (the size of the tumor and whether it is in the breast only or has spread to other parts of the body)
- The type of breast cancer
- The age of the fetus
- Whether there are signs or symptoms
- The patient's general health

After breast cancer has been diagnosed, tests are done to find out if cancer cells have spread within the breast or to other parts of the body. The process used to find out if the cancer has spread within the breast or to other parts of the body is called "staging." The information gathered from the staging process determines the stage of the disease. It is important to know the stage in order to plan treatment.

Some procedures may expose the fetus to harmful radiation or dyes. These procedures are done only if absolutely necessary. Certain actions can be taken to expose the fetus to as little radiation as possible, such as the use of a lead-lined shield to cover the abdomen.

The following tests and procedures may be used to stage breast cancer during pregnancy:

- Chest X-ray
- Bone scan
- Ultrasound exam
- Magnetic resonance imaging (MRI)

Treatment Options

Treatment options for pregnant women depend on the stage of the disease and the age of the fetus.

Three types of standard treatment are used:

Surgery

Most pregnant women with breast cancer have surgery to remove the breast. Some of the lymph nodes under the arm may be removed so they can be checked under a microscope by a pathologist for signs of cancer.

Types of surgery to remove the cancer include:

- Modified-radical mastectomy
- Breast-conserving surgery

After the doctor removes all of the cancer that can be seen at the time of surgery, some patients may be given chemotherapy or radiation therapy after surgery to kill any cancer cells that are left. For pregnant women with early-stage breast cancer, radiation therapy and hormone therapy are given after the baby is born. Treatment given after surgery, to lower the risk that the cancer will come back, is called "adjuvant therapy."

Radiation Therapy

Radiation therapy is a cancer treatment that uses high-energy X-rays or other types of radiation to kill cancer cells or keep them from growing. There are two types of radiation therapy:

- External radiation therapy uses a machine outside the body to send radiation to the cancer.
- Internal radiation therapy uses a radioactive substance sealed in needles, seeds, wires, or catheters that are placed directly into or near the cancer.

The way the radiation therapy is given depends on the type and stage of the cancer being treated.

External radiation therapy may be given to pregnant women with early stage (stage I or II) breast cancer after the baby is born. Women with late stage (stage III or IV) breast cancer may be given external radiation therapy after the first 3 months of pregnancy or, if possible, radiation therapy is delayed until after the baby is born.

Chemotherapy

Chemotherapy is a cancer treatment that uses drugs to stop the growth of cancer cells, either by killing the cells or by stopping the cells from dividing. When chemotherapy is taken by mouth or injected into a vein or muscle, the drugs enter the bloodstream and can reach cancer cells throughout the body (systemic chemotherapy). When chemotherapy is placed directly into the cerebrospinal fluid, an organ, or a body cavity such as the abdomen, the drugs mainly affect cancer cells in those areas (regional chemotherapy).

The way the chemotherapy is given depends on the type and stage of the cancer being treated. Systemic chemotherapy is used to treat breast cancer during pregnancy.

Chemotherapy is usually not given during the first three months of pregnancy. Chemotherapy given after this time does not usually harm the fetus, but may cause early labor or low birth weight.

Ending the pregnancy does not seem to improve the mother's chance of survival. Because ending the pregnancy is not likely to improve the mother's chance of survival, it is not usually a treatment option. Treatment for breast cancer may cause side effects.

Treatment Options for Breast Cancer during Pregnancy
Early Stage Breast Cancer

Pregnant women with early-stage breast cancer (stage I and stage II) are usually treated in the same way as patients who are not pregnant, with some changes to protect the fetus. Treatment may include the following:

- Modified radical mastectomy, if the breast cancer was diagnosed early in pregnancy

- Breast-conserving surgery, if the breast cancer is diagnosed later in pregnancy. Radiation therapy may be given after the baby is born.

- Modified radical mastectomy or breast-conserving surgery during pregnancy. After the first three months of pregnancy, certain types of chemotherapy may be given before or after surgery.

Hormone therapy and trastuzumab should not be given during pregnancy.

Late-Stage Breast Cancer

There is no standard treatment for patients with late-stage breast cancer (stage III or stage IV) during pregnancy. Treatment may include the following:

- Radiation therapy

- Chemotherapy

Radiation therapy and chemotherapy should not be given during the first 3 months of pregnancy.

Special Issues about Breast Cancer during Pregnancy

Lactation (breast milk production) and breastfeeding should be stopped if surgery or chemotherapy is planned. If surgery is planned, breastfeeding should be stopped to reduce blood flow in the breasts and make them smaller. Many chemotherapy drugs, especially cyclophosphamide and methotrexate, may occur in high levels in breast milk and may harm the nursing baby. Women receiving chemotherapy should not breastfeed. Stopping lactation does not improve the mother's prognosis. Breast cancer does not appear to harm the fetus. Breast cancer cells do not seem to pass from the mother to the fetus. Pregnancy does not seem to affect the survival of women who have had breast cancer in the past. For women who have had breast cancer, pregnancy does not seem to affect their survival.

However, some doctors recommend that a woman should wait two years after treatment for breast cancer before trying to have a baby, so that any early return of the cancer would be detected. This may affect a woman's decision to become pregnant. The fetus does not seem to be affected if the mother has had breast cancer.

Section 31.2

Gestational Trophoblastic Tumors

This section includes text excerpted from "Gestational
Trophoblastic Disease Treatment (PDQ®)—Patient Version,"
National Cancer Institute (NCI), May 3, 2018.

Gestational trophoblastic disease (GTD) is a group of rare diseases
in which abnormal trophoblast cells grow inside the uterus after conception. In a GTD, a tumor develops inside the uterus from tissue that
forms after conception (the joining of sperm and egg). This tissue is
made of trophoblast cells and normally surrounds the fertilized egg
in the uterus. Trophoblast cells help connect the fertilized egg to the
wall of the uterus and form part of the placenta (the organ that passes
nutrients from the mother to the fetus).

Sometimes there is a problem with the fertilized egg and trophoblast cells. Instead of a healthy fetus developing, a tumor forms. Until
there are signs or symptoms of the tumor, the pregnancy will seem
like a normal pregnancy.

Most GTD is benign (not cancer) and does not spread, but some
types become malignant (cancer) and spread to nearby tissues or distant parts of the body.

Gestational trophoblastic disease (GTD) is a general term that
includes different types of disease:

- Hydatidiform moles (HM)

  - Complete HM

  - Partial HM

- Gestational trophoblastic neoplasia (GTN)

  - Invasive moles

  - Choriocarcinomas

  - Placental-site trophoblastic tumors (PSTT; very rare)

  - Epithelioid trophoblastic tumors (ETT; even more rare)

Hydatidiform mole (HM) is the most common type of GTD. HMs
are slow-growing tumors that look like sacs of fluid. An HM is also
called a "molar pregnancy." The cause of hydatidiform moles is not
known.

HMs may be complete or partial:

- A complete HM forms when sperm fertilizes an egg that does not contain the mother's Deoxyribonucleic acid (DNA). The egg has DNA from the father, and the cells that were meant to become the placenta are abnormal.

- A partial HM forms when sperm fertilizes a normal egg and there are two sets of DNA from the father in the fertilized egg. Only part of the fetus forms, and the cells that were meant to become the placenta are abnormal.

Most hydatidiform moles are benign, but they sometimes become cancer. Having one or more of the following risk factors increases the risk that a hydatidiform mole will become cancer:

- A pregnancy before 20 or after 35 years of age

- A very high level of beta-human chorionic gonadotropin (β-hCG), a hormone made by the body during pregnancy

- A large tumor in the uterus

- An ovarian cyst larger than six centimeters

- High blood pressure during pregnancy

- An overactive thyroid gland (extra thyroid hormone is made)

- Severe nausea and vomiting during pregnancy

- Trophoblastic cells in the blood, which may block small blood vessels

- Serious blood clotting problems caused by the HM

Gestational trophoblastic neoplasia (GTN) is a type of GTD that is almost always malignant.

GTN includes the following:

- **Invasive moles:** Invasive moles are made up of trophoblast cells that grow into the muscle layer of the uterus. Invasive moles are more likely to grow and spread than a hydatidiform mole. Rarely, a complete or partial HM may become an invasive mole. Sometimes an invasive mole will disappear without treatment.

- **Choriocarcinomas:** A choriocarcinoma is a malignant tumor that forms from trophoblast cells and spreads to the muscle

279

layer of the uterus and nearby blood vessels. It may also spread to other parts of the body, such as the brain, lungs, liver, kidney, spleen, intestines, pelvis, or vagina. A choriocarcinoma is more likely to form in women who have had any of the following:

• Molar pregnancy, especially with a complete hydatidiform mole

• Normal pregnancy

• Tubal pregnancy (the fertilized egg implants in the fallopian tube rather than the uterus)

• Miscarriage

• **Placental-site trophoblastic tumors:** A placental-site trophoblastic tumor (PSTT) is a rare type of GTN that forms where the placenta attaches to the uterus. The tumor forms from trophoblast cells and spreads into the muscle of the uterus and into blood vessels. It may also spread to the lungs, pelvis, or lymph nodes. A PSTT grows very slowly and signs or symptoms may appear months or years after a normal pregnancy.

• **Epithelioid trophoblastic tumors:** An epithelioid trophoblastic tumor (ETT) is a very rare type of GTN that may be benign or malignant. When the tumor is malignant, it may spread to the lungs.

Age and a previous molar pregnancy affect the risk of GTD. Anything that increases your risk of getting a disease is called a "risk factor." Having a risk factor does not mean that you will get cancer; not having risk factors does not mean that you will not get cancer. Talk to your doctor if you think you may be at risk. Risk factors for GTD include the following:

• Being pregnant when you are younger than 20 or older than 35 years of age

• Having a personal history of hydatidiform mole

Signs of Gestational Trophoblastic Disease

Signs of GTD include abnormal vaginal bleeding and a uterus that is larger than normal. These and other signs and symptoms may be caused by GTD or by other conditions. Check with your doctor if you have any of the following:

• Vaginal bleeding not related to menstruation

- A uterus that is larger than expected during pregnancy
- Pain or pressure in the pelvis
- Severe nausea and vomiting during pregnancy
- High blood pressure with headache and swelling of feet and hands early in the pregnancy
- Vaginal bleeding that continues for longer than normal after delivery
- Fatigue, shortness of breath, dizziness, and a fast or irregular heartbeat caused by anemia

GTD sometimes causes an overactive thyroid. Signs and symptoms of an overactive thyroid include the following:

- Fast or irregular heartbeat
- Shakiness
- Sweating
- Frequent bowel movements
- Trouble sleeping
- Feeling anxious or irritable
- Weight loss

Tests for Gestational Trophoblastic Disease

The following tests and procedures may be used:

- Physical exam and history
- Pelvic exam
- Ultrasound exam of the pelvis
- Blood chemistry studies
- Serum tumor marker test
- Urinalysis

Prognosis and Treatment Options

Gestational trophoblastic disease usually can be cured. Treatment and prognosis depend on the following:

- The type of GTD
- Whether the tumor has spread to the uterus, lymph nodes, or distant parts of the body

- The number of tumors and where they are in the body

- The size of the largest tumor

- The level of β-hCG in the blood

- How soon the tumor was diagnosed after the pregnancy began

- Whether GTD occurred after a molar pregnancy, miscarriage, or normal pregnancy

- Previous treatment for gestational trophoblastic neoplasia

Treatment options also depend on whether the woman wishes to become pregnant in the future.

After GTN has been diagnosed, tests are done to find out if cancer has spread from where it started to other parts of the body.

The process used to find out the extent or spread of cancer is called "staging." The information gathered from the staging process helps determine the stage of disease. For GTN, the stage is one of the factors used to plan treatment.

The following tests and procedures may be done to help find out the stage of the disease:

- Chest X-ray

- Computed tomography (CT) scan (CAT scan)

- Magnetic resonance imaging (MRI) with gadolinium

- Lumbar puncture

Treatment for Gestational Trophoblastic Neoplasia

Invasive moles and choriocarcinomas are treated based on risk groups. The stage of the invasive mole or choriocarcinoma is one factor used to determine risk group. Other factors include the following:

- The age of the patient when the diagnosis is made

- Whether the GTN occurred after a molar pregnancy, miscarriage, or normal pregnancy

- How soon the tumor was diagnosed after the pregnancy began

- The level of beta-human chorionic gonadotropin (β-hCG) in the blood

- The size of the largest tumor

- Where the tumor has spread to and the number of tumors in the body

- How many chemotherapy drugs the tumor has been treated with (for recurrent or resistant tumors)

There are two risk groups for invasive moles and choriocarcinomas: low risk and high risk. Patients with low-risk disease usually receive less aggressive treatment than patients with high-risk disease.

Placental-site trophoblastic tumor (PSTT) and epithelioid trophoblastic tumor (ETT) treatments depend on the stage of disease.

Recurrent and Resistant Gestational Trophoblastic Neoplasia

Recurrent GTN is cancer that has recurred (come back) after it has been treated. Cancer may come back in the uterus or in other parts of the body. GTN that does not respond to treatment is called "resistant GTN."

There are different types of treatment for patients with GTD.

Different types of treatment are available for patients with GTD. Some treatments are standard (the currently-used treatment), and some are being tested in clinical trials. Before starting treatment, patients may want to think about taking part in a clinical trial. A treatment clinical trial is a research study meant to help improve current treatments or obtain information on new treatments for patients with cancer. When clinical trials show that a new treatment is better than the standard treatment, the new treatment may become the standard treatment.

Clinical trials are taking place in many parts of the country. Choosing the most appropriate cancer treatment is a decision that ideally involves the patient, family, and healthcare team.

Three types of standard treatment are used:

Surgery

The doctor may remove the cancer using one of the following operations:

- **Dilatation and curettage (D and C) with suction evacuation:** A surgical procedure to remove abnormal tissue and parts of the inner lining of the uterus. The cervix is dilated, and the material inside the uterus is removed with a small vacuum-like device. The walls of the uterus are then gently scraped with a curette (spoon-shaped instrument) to remove any material that may remain in the uterus. This procedure may be used for molar pregnancies.

- **Hysterectomy:** Surgery to remove the uterus, and sometimes the cervix. If the uterus and cervix are taken out through the vagina, the operation is called a "vaginal hysterectomy." If the uterus and cervix are taken out through a large incision (cut) in the abdomen, the operation is called a "total abdominal hysterectomy." If the uterus and cervix are taken out through a small incision in the abdomen using a laparoscope, the operation is called a "total laparoscopic hysterectomy."

After the doctor removes all the cancer that can be seen at the time of the surgery, some patients may be given chemotherapy to kill any cancer cells that are left. Treatment given after the surgery, to lower the risk that the cancer will come back, is called "adjuvant therapy."

Chemotherapy

Chemotherapy is a cancer treatment that uses drugs to stop the growth of cancer cells, either by killing the cells or by stopping them from dividing. When chemotherapy is taken by mouth or injected into a vein or muscle, the drugs enter the bloodstream and can reach cancer cells throughout the body (systemic chemotherapy). When chemotherapy is placed directly into the cerebrospinal fluid, an organ, or a body cavity such as the abdomen, the drugs mainly affect cancer cells in those areas (regional chemotherapy). The way the chemotherapy is given depends on the type and stage of the cancer being treated, or whether the tumor is low-risk or high-risk. Combination chemotherapy is treatment using more than one anti-cancer drug.

Radiation Therapy

Radiation therapy is a cancer treatment that uses high-energy X-rays or other types of radiation to kill cancer cells or keep them from growing. There are two types of radiation therapy:

- External radiation therapy uses a machine outside the body to send radiation toward the cancer.

- Internal radiation therapy uses a radioactive substance sealed in needles, seeds, wires, or catheters that are placed directly into or near the cancer.

The way the radiation therapy is given depends on the type of GTD being treated. External radiation therapy is used to treat GTD. New types of treatment are being tested in clinical trials.

Treatment for GTD may cause side effects. Patients may want to think about taking part in a clinical trial. For some patients, taking part in a clinical trial may be the best treatment choice. Clinical trials are part of the cancer research process. Clinical trials are done to find out if new cancer treatments are safe and effective or better than the standard treatment.

Many of today's standard treatments for cancer are based on earlier clinical trials. Patients who take part in a clinical trial may receive the standard treatment or be among the first to receive a new treatment. Patients who take part in clinical trials also help improve the way cancer will be treated in the future. Even when clinical trials do not lead to effective new treatments, they often answer important questions and help move research forward.

Patients can enter clinical trials before, during, or after starting their cancer treatment.

Some clinical trials only include patients who have not yet received treatment. Other trials test treatments for patients whose cancer has not gotten better. There are also clinical trials that test new ways to stop cancer from recurring (coming back) or reduce the side effects of cancer treatment.

Clinical trials are taking place in many parts of the country. Follow-up tests may be needed. Some of the tests that were done to diagnose the cancer or to find out the stage of the cancer may be repeated. Some tests will be repeated in order to see how well the treatment is working. Decisions about whether to continue, change, or stop treatment may be based on the results of these tests.

Some of the tests will continue to be done from time to time after treatment has ended. The results of these tests can show if your condition has changed or if the cancer has recurred. These tests are sometimes called "follow-up tests" or "check-ups."

Blood levels of β-hCG will be checked for up to six months after treatment has ended. This is because a β-hCG level that is higher than normal may mean that the tumor has not responded to treatment or it has become cancer.

Treatment for Gestational Trophoblastic Disease
Hydatidiform Moles

Treatment of a hydatidiform mole may include the following:

• Surgery (Dilatation and curettage with suction evacuation) to remove the tumor

After surgery, β-hCG blood tests are done every week until the β-hCG level returns to normal. Patients also have follow-up doctor visits monthly for up to six months. If the level of β-hCG does not return to normal or increases, it may mean the hydatidiform mole was not completely removed, and it has become cancer. Pregnancy causes β-hCG levels to increase, so your doctor will ask you not to become pregnant until follow-up is finished.

For disease that remains after surgery, treatment is usually chemotherapy. You can search for trials based on the type of cancer, the age of the patient, and where the trials are being done.

Gestational Trophoblastic Neoplasia
Low-Risk Gestational Trophoblastic Neoplasia

Treatment of low-risk gestational trophoblastic neoplasia (GTN) (invasive mole or choriocarcinoma) may include the following:

• Chemotherapy with one or more anticancer drugs. Treatment is given until the β-hCG level is normal for at least three weeks after treatment ends.

If the level of β-hCG in the blood does not return to normal or the tumor spreads to distant parts of the body, chemotherapy regimens used for high-risk metastatic GTN are given.

You can use the National Cancer Institute (NCI) clinical trial search to find NCI-supported cancer clinical trials that are accepting patients. You can search for trials based on the type of cancer, the age of the patient, and where the trials are being done. General information about clinical trials is also available.

High-Risk Metastatic Gestational Trophoblastic Neoplasia

Treatment of high-risk metastatic gestational trophoblastic neoplasia (invasive mole or choriocarcinoma) may include the following:

• Combination chemotherapy

- Intrathecal chemotherapy and radiation therapy to the brain (for cancer that has spread to the lung, to keep it from spreading to the brain)
- High-dose chemotherapy or intrathecal chemotherapy and/or radiation therapy to the brain (for cancer that has spread to the brain)

Placental-Site Gestational Trophoblastic Tumors and Epithelioid Trophoblastic Tumors

Treatment of stage I placental-site gestational trophoblastic tumors and epithelioid trophoblastic tumors may include the following:

- Surgery to remove the uterus

Treatment of stage II placental-site gestational trophoblastic tumors and epithelioid trophoblastic tumors may include the following:

- Surgery to remove the tumor, which may be followed by combination chemotherapy

Treatment of stage III and IV placental-site gestational trophoblastic tumors and epithelioid trophoblastic tumors may include the following:

- Combination chemotherapy
- Surgery to remove cancer that has spread to other places, such as the lung or abdomen

Recurrent or Resistant Gestational Trophoblastic Neoplasia

Treatment of recurrent or resistant gestational trophoblastic tumor may include the following:

- Chemotherapy with one or more anticancer drugs for tumors previously treated with surgery
- Combination chemotherapy for tumors previously treated with chemotherapy
- Surgery for tumors that do not respond to chemotherapy

Chapter 32

For Women with Diabetes: Your Guide to Pregnancy

If you have diabetes and plan to have a baby, you should try to get your blood glucose levels close to your target range before you get pregnant.

Staying in your target range during pregnancy, which may be different than when you are not pregnant, is also important. High blood glucose, also called "blood sugar," can harm the fetus during the first weeks of pregnancy, even before you know you are pregnant. If you have diabetes and are already pregnant, see your doctor as soon as possible to make a plan to manage your diabetes. Working with your healthcare team and following your diabetes management plan can help you have a healthy pregnancy and a healthy baby.

If you develop diabetes for the first time while you are pregnant, you have gestational diabetes.

How Can Diabetes Affect the Fetus?

A fetus's organs, such as the brain, heart, kidneys, and lungs, start forming during the first eight weeks of pregnancy. High blood-glucose levels can be harmful during this early stage and can increase the

This chapter includes text excerpted from "Pregnancy If You Have Diabetes," National Institute of Diabetes and Digestive and Kidney Diseases (NIDDK), January 2017.

chance that the fetus will have birth defects, such as heart defects or defects of the brain or spine.

High blood-glucose levels during pregnancy can also increase the chance that your baby will be born too early, weigh too much, or have breathing problems or low blood-glucose right after birth.

High blood glucose also can increase the chance that you will experience a miscarriage or a stillbirth. A stillborn means the fetus dies in the womb during the second half of pregnancy.

How Can My Diabetes Affect Me during Pregnancy?

Hormonal and other changes in your body during pregnancy affect your blood glucose levels, so you might need to change how you manage your diabetes. Even if you have had diabetes for years, you may need to change your meal plan, physical activity routine, and medicines. If you have been taking an oral diabetes medicine, you may need to switch to insulin. As you get closer to your due date, your management plan might change again.

What Health Problems Could I Develop during Pregnancy Because of My Diabetes?

Pregnancy can worsen certain long-term diabetes problems, such as eye problems and kidney disease, especially if your blood glucose levels are too high.

You also have a greater chance of developing preeclampsia, sometimes called "toxemia," which is when you develop high blood pressure and too much protein in your urine during the second half of pregnancy. Preeclampsia can cause serious or life-threatening problems for you and the fetus. The only cure for preeclampsia is to give birth. If you have preeclampsia and have reached 37 weeks of pregnancy, your doctor may want to deliver your baby early. Before 37 weeks, you and your doctor may consider other options to help the fetus develop as much as possible before birth.

How Can I Prepare for Pregnancy If I Have Diabetes?

If you have diabetes, keeping your blood glucose as close to normal as possible before and during your pregnancy is important to stay healthy and have a healthy baby. Getting checkups before and during pregnancy, following your diabetes meal plan, being physically active as your healthcare team advises, and taking diabetes medicines if you need to will help you manage your diabetes. Stopping smoking and taking vitamins as your doctor advises also can help you and the fetus stay healthy.

Work with Your Healthcare Team

Regular visits with members of a healthcare team who are experts in diabetes and pregnancy will ensure that you and the fetus get the best care. Your healthcare team may include:

- A medical doctor who specializes in diabetes care, such as an endocrinologist or a diabetologist

- An obstetrician with experience treating women with diabetes

- A diabetes educator who can help you manage your diabetes

- A nurse practitioner who provides prenatal care during your pregnancy

- A registered dietitian to help with meal planning

- Specialists who diagnose and treat diabetes-related problems, such as vision problems, kidney disease, and heart disease

- A social worker or psychologist to help you cope with stress, worry, and the extra demands of pregnancy

You are the most important member of the team. Your healthcare team can give you expert advice, but you are the one who must manage your diabetes every day.

Get a Checkup

Have a complete checkup before you get pregnant or as soon as you know you are pregnant. Your doctor should check for:

- High blood pressure

- Eye disease

- Heart and blood vessel disease

- Nerve damage

291

- Kidney disease

- Thyroid disease

Pregnancy can make some diabetes health problems worse. To help prevent this, your healthcare team may recommend adjusting your treatment before you get pregnant.

Do Not Smoke

Smoking can increase your chance of a stillbirth or premature birth. Smoking is especially harmful for people with diabetes. Smoking can increase diabetes-related health problems such as eye disease, heart disease, and kidney disease.

If you smoke or use other tobacco products, stop. Ask for help so you do not have to do it alone. You can start by calling the national quitline at 800-QUIT-NOW (800-784-8669). For tips on quitting, go to Smokefree.gov.

See a Registered Dietitian Nutritionist

If you do not already see a dietitian, you should start seeing one before you get pregnant. Your dietitian can help you learn what to eat, how much to eat, and when to eat to reach or stay at a healthy weight before you get pregnant. Together, you and your dietitian will create a meal plan to fit your needs, schedule, food preferences, medical conditions, medicines, and physical activity routine.

During pregnancy, some women need to make changes in their meal plan, such as adding extra calories, protein, and other nutrients. You will need to see your dietitian every few months during pregnancy as your dietary needs change.

Be Physically Active

Physical activity can help you reach your target blood-glucose numbers. Being physically active can also help keep your blood pressure and cholesterol levels in a healthy range, relieve stress, strengthen your heart and bones, improve muscle strength, and keep your joints flexible.

Before getting pregnant, make physical activity a regular part of your life. Aim for 30 minutes of activity five days of the week.

Talk with your healthcare team about what activities are best for you during your pregnancy.

How to Eat Better and Be More Active While You Are Pregnant
Avoid Alcohol

You should avoid drinking alcoholic beverages while you are trying to get pregnant and throughout pregnancy. When you drink, the alcohol also affects the fetus. Alcohol can lead to serious, lifelong health problems for your baby.

Adjust Your Medicines

Some medicines are not safe during pregnancy, and you should stop taking them before you get pregnant. Tell your doctor about all the medicines you take, such as those for high cholesterol and high blood pressure. Your doctor can tell you which medicines to stop taking, and may prescribe a different medicine that is safe to use during pregnancy.

Doctors most often prescribe insulin for both type 1 and type 2 diabetes during pregnancy. If you are already taking insulin, you might need to change the kind, the amount, or how and when you take it. You may need less insulin during your first trimester but probably will need more as you go through pregnancy. Your insulin needs may double or even triple as you get closer to your due date. Your health-care team will work with you to create an insulin routine to meet your changing needs.

Take Vitamin and Mineral Supplements

Folic acid is an important vitamin for you to take before and during pregnancy to protect the fetus's health. You will need to start taking folic acid at least one month before you get pregnant. You should take a multivitamin or supplement that contains at least 400 micrograms (mcg) of folic acid. Once you become pregnant, you should take 600 mcg daily. Ask your doctor if you should take other vitamins or minerals, such as iron or calcium supplements, or a multivitamin.

What Do I Need to Know about Blood-Glucose Testing before and during Pregnancy?

How often you check your blood glucose levels may change during pregnancy. You may need to check them more often than you do now. If you did not need to check your blood glucose before pregnancy, you will probably need to start. Ask your healthcare team how often and at what times you should check your blood glucose levels. Your blood glucose targets will change during pregnancy. Your healthcare team also may want you to check your ketone levels if your blood glucose is too high.

Target Blood-Glucose Levels before Pregnancy

When you are planning to become pregnant, your daily blood-glucose targets may be different than your previous targets. Ask your healthcare team which targets are right for you.

You can also use an electronic blood-glucose tracking system on your computer or mobile device. Record the results every time you check your blood glucose. Your blood-glucose records can help you and your healthcare team decide whether your diabetes care plan is working. You also can make notes about your insulin and ketones. Take your tracker with you when you visit your healthcare team.

Target Blood-Glucose Levels during Pregnancy

Recommended daily target blood-glucose numbers for most pregnant women with diabetes are:

- Before meals, at bedtime, and overnight: 90 or less

- One hour after eating: 130 to 140 or less

- Two hours after eating: 120 or less

Ask your doctor what targets are right for you. If you have type 1 diabetes, your targets may be higher so you do not develop low blood glucose, also called "hypoglycemia."

A1C Numbers

Another way to see whether you are meeting your targets is to have an A1C blood test. Results of the A1C test reflect your average blood-glucose levels during the past three months. Most women with diabetes should aim for an A1C as close to normal as possible—ideally below 6.5 percent—before getting pregnant. After the first three months of pregnancy, your target may be as low as six percent. These targets may be different than A1C goals you have had in the past. Your doctor can help you set A1C targets that are best for you.

Ketone Levels

When your blood glucose is too high or if you are not eating enough, your body might make ketones. Ketones in your urine or blood mean your body is using fat for energy instead of glucose. Burning large amounts of fat instead of glucose can be harmful to your health and the fetus's health.

You can prevent serious health problems by checking for ketones. Your doctor might recommend you test your urine or blood daily for ketones or when your blood glucose is above a certain level, such as 200. If you use an insulin pump, your doctor might advise you to test for ketones when your blood-glucose level is higher than expected. Your healthcare team can teach you how and when to test your urine or blood for ketones.

Talk with your doctor about what to do if you have ketones. Your doctor might suggest making changes in the amount of insulin you take or when you take it. Your doctor also may recommend a change in meals or snacks if you need to consume more carbohydrates.

What Tests Will Check the Fetus's Health during Pregnancy?

You will have tests throughout your pregnancy, such as blood tests and ultrasounds, to check the fetus's health. Talk with your healthcare team about what prenatal tests you will have and when you might have them.

Chapter 33

Epilepsy and Pregnancy

What Are Epilepsies

The epilepsies are chronic neurological disorders in which clusters of nerve cells, or neurons, in the brain sometimes signal abnormally and cause seizures. Neurons normally generate electrical and chemical signals that act on other neurons, glands, and muscles to produce human thoughts, feelings, and actions. During a seizure, many neurons fire (signal) at the same time—as many as 500 times a second, which is much faster than normal. This surge of excessive electrical activity happening at the same time causes involuntary movements, sensations, emotions, and behaviors and the temporary disturbance of normal neuronal activity may cause a loss of awareness.

In general, a person is not considered to have epilepsy until she or he has had 2 or more unprovoked seizures separated by at least 24 hours. In contrast, a provoked seizure is caused by a known precipitating factor such as a high fever, nervous system infections, acute traumatic brain injury, or fluctuations in blood sugar or electrolyte levels.

Anyone can develop epilepsy. About 2.3 million adults and more than 450,000 children and adolescents in the United States currently live with epilepsy. Each year, an estimated 150,000 people are diagnosed with epilepsy. Epilepsy affects both males and females of all races, ethnic backgrounds, and ages.

This chapter includes text excerpted from "The Epilepsies and Seizures: Hope through Research," National Institute of Neurological Disorders and Stroke (NINDS), August 8, 2018.

The majority of those diagnosed with epilepsy have seizures that can be controlled with drug therapies and surgery. However, as much as 30 to 40 percent of people with epilepsy continue to have seizures because available treatments do not completely control their seizures (called "intractable" or "medication-resistant epilepsy").

What Causes Epilepsies

The epilepsies have many possible causes, but for up to half of people with epilepsy a cause is not known. In other cases, the epilepsies are clearly linked to genetic factors, developmental brain abnormalities, infection, traumatic brain injury, stroke, brain tumors, or other identifiable problems. Anything that disturbs the normal pattern of neuronal activity, from illness to brain damage to abnormal brain development, can lead to seizures.

The epilepsies may develop because of an abnormality in brain wiring, an imbalance of nerve signaling in the brain, or some combination of these factors. In some pediatric conditions, abnormal brain wiring causes other problems, such as intellectual impairment.

In other persons, the brain's attempt to repair itself after a head injury, stroke, or other problem may inadvertently generate abnormal nerve connections that lead to epilepsy. Brain malformations and abnormalities in brain wiring that occur during brain development also may disturb neuronal activity and lead to epilepsy.

Examples of conditions that can lead to epilepsy include:

- Brain tumors, including those associated with neurofibromatosis or tuberous sclerosis complex, two inherited conditions that cause benign tumors, called "hamartomas," to grow in the brain

- Head trauma

- Alcoholism or alcohol withdrawal

- Alzheimer disease

- Strokes, heart attacks, and other conditions that deprive the brain of oxygen (a significant portion of new-onset epilepsy in elderly people is due to stroke or other cerebrovascular disease (CeVD)).

- Abnormal blood vessel formation (arteriovenous malformations) or bleeding in the brain (hemorrhage)

- Inflammation of the brain

- Infections such as meningitis, human immunodeficiency virus (HIV), and viral encephalitis

Cerebral palsy or other developmental neurological abnormalities may also be associated with epilepsy. Epilepsies often co-occur in people with abnormalities of brain development or other neurodevelopmental disorders. Seizures are more common among individuals with an autism spectrum disorder (ASD) or intellectual impairment.

What Triggers a Seizure

Seizure triggers include alcohol consumption or alcohol withdrawal, dehydration or missing meals, stress, and hormonal changes associated with the menstrual cycle. In surveys of people with epilepsy, stress is the most commonly reported seizure trigger. Exposure to toxins or poisons such as lead or carbon monoxide, street drugs, or even excessively large doses of antidepressants or other prescribed medications also can trigger seizures.

Sleep deprivation is a powerful trigger of seizures. Sleep disorders are common among people with the epilepsies and appropriate treatment of coexisting sleep disorders can often lead to improved control of seizures. Certain types of seizures tend to occur during sleep, while others are more common during times of wakefulness, suggesting to physicians how to best adjust a person's medication.

For some people, visual stimulation can trigger seizures in a condition known as "photosensitive epilepsy." Stimulation can include such things as flashing lights or moving patterns.

Is Epilepsy Dangerous in Pregnancy?

Women with epilepsy are often concerned about whether they can become pregnant and have a healthy child. Epilepsy itself does not interfere with the ability to become pregnant. Children of parents with epilepsy have about a five percent risk of developing the condition at some point during life, in comparison to about a one percent risk in a child in the general population. However, the risk of developing epilepsy increases if a parent has a clearly hereditary form of the disorder. Parents who are worried that their epilepsy may be hereditary may wish to consult a genetic counselor to determine their risk of passing on the disorder.

Other potential risks to the fetus of a woman with epilepsy or on antiseizure medication include increased risk for major congenital malformations (also known as "birth defects") and adverse effects on the developing brain. The types of birth defects that have been most commonly reported with antiseizure medications include cleft lip or cleft palate, heart problems, abnormal spinal-cord development (spina bifida), urogenital defects, and limb skeletal defects. Some antiseizure medications, particularly valproate, are known to increase the risk of having a child with birth defects and/or neurodevelopmental problems, including learning disabilities, general intellectual disabilities, and ASD. It is important that a woman work with a team of providers that includes her neurologist and her obstetrician to learn about any special risks associated with her epilepsy and the medications she may be taking.

Prior to a planned pregnancy, a woman with epilepsy should meet with her healthcare team to reassess the current need for antiseizure medications and to determine the optimal medication to balance seizure control and avoid birth defects and the lowest dose for going into a planned pregnancy. Any transitions to either a new medication or dosage should be phased in prior to the pregnancy, if possible. If a woman's seizures are controlled for the nine months prior to pregnancy, she is more likely to continue to have seizure control during pregnancy. For all women with epilepsy during pregnancy, approximately 15 to 25 percent will have seizure worsening, but another 15 to 25 percent will have seizure improvement. As a woman's body changes during pregnancy, the dose of seizure medication may need to be increased. For most medicines, monthly monitoring of blood levels of the antiseizure medicines can help to assure continued seizure control. Many of the birth defects seen with antiseizure medications occur in the first six weeks of pregnancy, often before a woman is aware she is pregnant. Pregnant women with epilepsy should get plenty of sleep and avoid other triggers or missed medications to avoid worsening of seizures.

Most pregnant women with epilepsy can deliver with the same choices as women without any medical complications. During the labor and delivery, it is important that the woman be allowed to take her same formulations and doses of antiseizure drugs at her usual times; it is often helpful for her to bring her medications from home. If a seizure does occur during labor and delivery, intravenous short-acting medications can be given if necessary. It is unusual for the newborns of women with epilepsy to experience symptoms of withdrawal from the mother's antiseizure medication (unless she is on phenobarbital or a standing dose of benzodiazepines), but the symptoms resolve quickly, and there are usually no serious or long-term effects.

The use of antiseizure medications is considered safe for women who choose to breastfeed their child. On very rare occasions, the baby may become excessively drowsy or feed poorly, and these problems should be closely monitored. However, experts believe the benefits of breastfeeding outweigh the risks except in rare circumstances. One large study showed that the children who were breastfed by mothers with epilepsy on antiseizure medications performed better on learning and developmental scales than the babies who were not breastfed. It is common for the antiseizure medication dosing to be adjusted again in the postpartum setting, especially if the dose was altered during pregnancy.

With the appropriate selection of safe antiseizure medicines during pregnancy, use of supplemental folic acid, and ideally, with prepregnancy planning, most women with epilepsy can have a healthy pregnancy with good outcomes for themselves and their child.

Chapter 34

Lupus and Pregnancy

Lupus is a chronic (lifelong) autoimmune disease that can damage any part of the body, including the skin, joints, and organs. About 9 out of 10 adults with lupus are women. Some women have only mild symptoms. But, for others, lupus can cause severe problems. Women with lupus need to be especially careful to manage their symptoms when planning a pregnancy.

What Are the Different Types of Lupus?

There are several different types of lupus:

- **Systemic lupus erythematosus** (SLE) is the most common and most serious type of lupus, which affects all parts of the body.

- **Cutaneous lupus erythematosus** (CLE), which affects only the skin

- **Drug-induced lupus**, a short-term type of lupus caused by certain medicines

- **Neonatal lupus**, a rare type of lupus that affects newborn babies

---

This chapter contains text excerpted from the following sources: Text in this chapter begins with excerpts from "Lupus and Women," Office on Women's Health (OWH), U.S. Department of Health and Human Services (HHS), July 12, 2018; Text beginning with the heading "How Does Pregnancy Affect Lupus?" is excerpted from "Pregnancy and Lupus," Office on Women's Health (OWH), U.S. Department of Health and Human Services (HHS), July 12, 2018.

How Does Pregnancy Affect Lupus?

Pregnant women with lupus have a higher risk for certain pregnancy complications than women who do not have lupus.

- **You may get flares during pregnancy.** The flares happen most often in the first or second trimester. Most flares are mild. But some flares require medicine right away or may cause you to deliver early. Always call your doctor right away if you get the warning signs of a lupus flare.

- **About 2 in 10 pregnant women with lupus get preeclampsia, a serious condition that must be treated right away.** The risk of preeclampsia is higher in women with lupus who have a history of kidney disease. If you get preeclampsia, you might notice sudden weight gain, swelling of the hands and face, blurred vision, dizziness, or stomach pain. You might have to deliver your baby early.

- **Pregnancy can raise your risk for other problems, especially if you take corticosteroids.** These problems include high blood pressure, diabetes, and kidney problems. Good nutrition during pregnancy can help prevent these problems during pregnancy. Regular doctor visits can help find problems, such as these, early so they can be treated to keep you and the fetus as healthy as possible.

Is It Safe for Women to Get Pregnant with Lupus?

Yes. Women with lupus can safely become pregnant. If your disease is under control, pregnancy is unlikely to cause flares. However, you will need to start planning for pregnancy well before you get pregnant.

- **Your disease should be under control or in remission for six months before you get pregnant.** Getting pregnant when your lupus is active could result in miscarriage, stillbirth, or other serious health problems for you or your baby.

- **Pregnancy is very risky for certain groups of women with lupus.** These include women with high blood pressure, lung disease, heart failure, chronic kidney failure, kidney disease, or a history of preeclampsia. It also may include women who have had a stroke or a lupus flare within the past six months.

You will need to find an obstetrician (a doctor who is specially trained to care for women during pregnancy) who manages high-risk pregnancies and who can work closely with your regular doctor.

How Can I Tell If the Changes in My Body Are Normal during Pregnancy or a Sign of a Flare?

You may not be able to tell the difference between changes in your body due to pregnancy and warning signs of a lupus flare. Tell your doctor about any new symptoms. You and your doctor can figure out whether your symptoms are because of your pregnancy or your lupus. This way, you can help prevent or control any flares that do happen.

I Have Lupus and Am Pregnant. Will My Baby Be Healthy?

Most likely, yes. Most babies born to mothers with lupus are healthy.

Rarely, infants are born with a condition called "neonatal lupus." Certain antibodies found in the mother can cause neonatal lupus. At birth, an infant with neonatal lupus may have a skin rash, liver problems, or low blood-cell levels.

Infants with neonatal lupus can develop a serious heart defect called "congenital heart block." But, in most babies, neonatal lupus goes away after three to six months and does not come back.

Your doctor will test for neonatal lupus during your pregnancy. Treatment can also begin at or before birth.

Can I Breastfeed If I Have Lupus?

Yes. Breastfeeding is possible for mothers with lupus. However, some medicines can pass through your breastmilk to your infant. Talk to your doctor or nurse about whether breastfeeding is safe with the medicines you use to control your lupus.

Chapter 35

Sickle Cell Disease and Pregnancy

Sickle cell disease (SCD) is a group of inherited red blood cells disorders. People who have sickle cell disease have an abnormal protein in their red blood cells. In the United States, most people who have sickle cell disease are of African ancestry, but the condition is also common in people with a Hispanic background. Because the disease runs in families, couples planning to have children can have genetic testing.

Early signs and symptoms of sickle cell disease include swelling of the hands and feet; symptoms of anemia, including fatigue, or extreme tiredness; and jaundice. Over time, sickle cell disease can lead to complications such as infections, delayed growth, and episodes of pain, called "pain crises." Most children who have sickle cell disease are pain-free between crises, but adolescents and adults may also suffer with chronic, ongoing pain. Over a lifetime, sickle cell disease can harm a patient's spleen, brain, eyes, lungs, liver, heart, kidneys, penis, joints, bones, or skin.

A blood and bone marrow transplant is currently the only cure for sickle cell disease, and only a small number of people who have sickle disease are able to have the transplant. There are effective

This chapter contains text excerpted from the following sources: Text in this chapter begins with excerpts from "Sickle Cell Disease," National Heart, Lung, and Blood Institute (NHLBI), December 3, 2018; Text beginning with the heading "Pregnant Women with Sickle Cell Disease" is excerpted from "Sickle Cell Disease and Pregnancy," Centers for Disease Control and Prevention (CDC), August 9, 2017.

307

treatments that can reduce symptoms and prolong life. Early diagnosis and regular medical care to prevent complications also contribute to an improved well-being. Sickle cell disease is a life-long illness. The severity of the disease varies widely from person to person.

Signs and Symptoms

If a person has sickle cell disease, it is present at birth. But most infants do not have any problems from the disease until they are about five or six months of age. Every state in the United States, the District of Columbia, and the U.S. territories require that all newborn babies receive screening for sickle cell disease. When a child has sickle cell disease, parents are notified before the child has symptoms.

Some children with sickle cell disease will start to have problems early on, and some later. Early symptoms of sickle cell disease may include:

- A yellowish color of the skin, known as "jaundice," or whites of the eyes, known as "icterus," that occurs when a large number of red cells undergo hemolysis

- Fatigue or fussiness from anemia

- Painful swelling of the hands and feet, known as "dactylitis"

The signs and symptoms of sickle cell disease will vary from person to person and can change over time. Most of the signs and symptoms of sickle cell disease are related to complications of the disease.

Diagnosis

Your doctor may diagnose sickle cell disease based on the results from tests to confirm the results from various screening tests.

Screening Tests

People who do not know whether they make sickle hemoglobin or another abnormal hemoglobin, such as SC, Sβ thalassemia, and SE, can find out by having their blood tested. This way, they can learn whether they carry a gene—or have the trait—for an abnormal hemoglobin that they could pass on to a child.

When each parent has this information, he or she can be better informed about the chances of having a child with some type of sickle cell disease, such as hemoglobin SS, SC, Sβ thalassemia, or others.

Newborn Screening

When a child has sickle cell disease, early diagnosis is important to better prevent complications.

Every state in the United States, the District of Columbia, and the U.S. territories require that every baby is tested for sickle cell disease as part of a newborn screening program. In newborn screening programs, blood from a heel prick is collected in "spots" on a special paper. The hemoglobin from this blood is then analyzed in special labs. Newborn screening results are sent to the doctor who ordered the test and to the child's primary doctor.

If a baby is found to have sickle cell disease, health providers from a special follow-up newborn screening group contact the family directly to make sure that the parents know the results. The child is always retested to be sure that the diagnosis is correct.

Newborn screening programs also find out whether the baby has an abnormal hemoglobin trait. If so, the parents are informed, and counseling is offered. Remember that when a child has sickle cell trait or sickle cell disease, a future sibling or the child's own future child may be at risk. These possibilities should be discussed with the primary care doctor, a blood specialist called a "hematologist," or a genetic counselor.

Prenatal Screening

Doctors can also diagnose sickle cell disease before a baby is born. This is done using a sample of amniotic fluid, the liquid in the sac surrounding a growing embryo, or of tissue taken from the placenta, the organ that attaches the umbilical cord to the mother's womb.

Testing before birth can be done as early as 8 to 10 weeks into the pregnancy. This testing looks for the sickle hemoglobin gene rather than the abnormal hemoglobin.

Treatment

A blood and bone marrow transplant is currently the only cure for some patients who have sickle cell disease. After early diagnosis, the goal is health maintenance to prevent complications and medicines and treatments to manage complications, including chronic pain.

Health Maintenance to Prevent Complications

Babies with sickle cell disease may see a hematologist, a doctor with special training in blood diseases such as sickle cell disease. For infants, the first sickle cell disease visit should take place before 8 weeks of age.

If someone was born in a country that does not perform newborn screening, he or she might be diagnosed with sickle cell disease later in childhood. These people should also be referred as soon as possible for special care.

All people who have sickle cell disease should see their healthcare providers every 3 to 12 months, depending on the person's age. Your doctor or medical team can help to prevent problems by taking certain steps:

- Educating families about the disease and what to watch out for

- Examining the person

- Giving medicines and immunizations

- Performing tests

Pregnant Women with Sickle Cell Disease

A woman with SCD is more likely to have problems during pregnancy that can affect her health and the health of the fetus than a woman without SCD. During pregnancy, the disease can become more severe, and pain episodes can occur more often. A pregnant woman with SCD is at a higher risk of preterm labor, having a low-birth-weight baby or other complications. However, with early prenatal care and careful monitoring throughout pregnancy, a woman with SCD can have a healthy pregnancy.

SCD is recessive, which means that both parents must pass on the sickle cell gene for a child to be born with SCD. During pregnancy there is a test to find out if the baby will have SCD, sickle cell trait (SCT), or neither one. The test usually is done after the second month of pregnancy.

Women who have SCT also can have a healthy pregnancy. Women with SCD or SCT might want to see a genetic counselor for information about the disease and the chances that SCD or SCT will be passed to their child.

Pregnancy Complications

Pregnancies in women who have sickle cell disease can be risky for both the mother and the fetus.

Mothers may have medical complications that include:

- Blood clots
- High blood pressure
- Increased pain episodes
- Infections

They also are at higher risk for:

- Miscarriages
- Premature births
- Small-for-date or underweight babies

Chapter 36

Thyroid Disease and Pregnancy

Thyroid disease is a group of disorders that affects the thyroid gland. The thyroid is a small, butterfly-shaped gland in the front of your neck that makes thyroid hormones. Thyroid hormones control how your body uses energy, so they affect the way nearly every organ in your body works—even the way your heart beats.

Sometimes the thyroid makes too much or too little of these hormones. Too much thyroid hormone is called "hyperthyroidism" and can cause many of your body's functions to speed up. "Hyper" means the thyroid is overactive. Too little thyroid hormone is called "hypothyroidism" and can cause many of your body's functions to slow down. "Hypo" means the thyroid is underactive.

If you have thyroid problems, you can still have a healthy pregnancy and protect the fetus's health by having regular thyroid-function tests and taking any medicines that your doctor prescribes.

What Role Do Thyroid Hormones Play in Pregnancy?

Thyroid hormones are crucial for normal development of the fetus's brain and nervous system. During the first trimester—the first three

This chapter includes text excerpted from "Thyroid Disease and Pregnancy," National Institute of Diabetes and Digestive and Kidney Diseases (NIDDK), December 2017.

months of pregnancy—the fetus depends on your supply of thyroid hormone, which comes through the placenta. At around 12 weeks, a fetus's thyroid starts to work on its own, but it does not make enough thyroid hormone until 18 to 20 weeks of pregnancy.

Two pregnancy-related hormones—human chorionic gonadotropin (hCG) and estrogen—cause higher measured thyroid hormone levels in your blood. The thyroid enlarges slightly in healthy women during pregnancy, but usually not enough for a healthcare professional to feel during a physical exam.

Thyroid problems can be hard to diagnose in pregnancy due to higher levels of thyroid hormones and other symptoms that occur in both pregnancy and thyroid disorders. Some symptoms of hyperthyroidism or hypothyroidism are easier to spot and may prompt your doctor to test you for these thyroid diseases.

Another type of thyroid disease, postpartum thyroiditis, can occur after your baby is born.

Hyperthyroidism in Pregnancy
What Are the Symptoms of Hyperthyroidism in Pregnancy?

Some signs and symptoms of hyperthyroidism often occur in normal pregnancies, including faster heart rate, trouble dealing with heat, and tiredness.

Other signs and symptoms can suggest hyperthyroidism:

- Fast and irregular heartbeat

- Shaky hands

- Unexplained weight loss or failure to have normal pregnancy weight gain

What Causes Hyperthyroidism in Pregnancy?

Hyperthyroidism in pregnancy is usually caused by Graves disease and occurs in 1 to 4 of every 1,000 pregnancies in the United States. Graves disease is an autoimmune disorder. With this disease, your immune system makes antibodies that cause the thyroid to make too much thyroid hormone. This antibody is called "thyroid stimulating immunoglobulin," or TSI.

Graves disease may first appear during pregnancy. However, if you already have Graves disease, your symptoms could improve in your second and third trimesters. Some parts of your immune system are less active later in pregnancy, so your immune system makes less TSI. This may be why symptoms improve. Graves disease often gets worse again in the first few months after your baby is born, when TSI levels go up again. If you have Graves disease, your doctor will most likely test your thyroid function monthly throughout your pregnancy and may need to treat your hyperthyroidism. Thyroid hormone levels that are too high can harm your health and the fetus's.

How Can Hyperthyroidism Affect Me and the Fetus?

Untreated hyperthyroidism during pregnancy can lead to:

- Miscarriage
- Premature birth
- Low birth weight
- Preeclampsia—a dangerous rise in blood pressure in late pregnancy
- Thyroid storm—a sudden, severe worsening of symptoms
- Congestive heart failure

Rarely, Graves disease may also affect a fetus's thyroid, causing it to make too much thyroid hormone. Even if your hyperthyroidism was cured by radioactive iodine treatment to destroy thyroid cells or surgery to remove your thyroid, your body still makes the TSI antibody. When levels of this antibody are high, TSI may travel to the fetus's bloodstream. Just as TSI caused your own thyroid to make too much thyroid hormone, it can also cause the fetus's thyroid to make too much.

Tell your doctor if you have had surgery or radioactive iodine treatment for Graves disease so she or he can check your TSI levels. If they are very high, your doctor will monitor the fetus for thyroid-related problems later in your pregnancy.

An overactive thyroid in a newborn can lead to:

- A fast heart rate, which can lead to heart failure
- Early closing of the soft spot in the baby's skull
- Poor weight gain
- Irritability

Sometimes an enlarged thyroid can press against your baby's windpipe and make it hard for your baby to breathe. If you have Graves disease, your healthcare team should closely monitor you and your newborn.

How Do Doctors Diagnose Hyperthyroidism in Pregnancy?

Your doctor will review your symptoms and do some blood tests to measure your thyroid hormone levels. Your doctor may also look for antibodies in your blood to see if Graves disease is causing your hyperthyroidism.

How Do Doctors Treat Hyperthyroidism during Pregnancy?

If you have mild hyperthyroidism during pregnancy, you probably won't need treatment. If your hyperthyroidism is linked to hyperemesis gravidarum, you only need treatment for vomiting and dehydration.

If your hyperthyroidism is more severe, your doctor may prescribe antithyroid medicines, which cause your thyroid to make less thyroid hormone. This treatment prevents too much of your thyroid hormone from getting into the fetus's bloodstream. You may want to see a specialist, such as an endocrinologist or expert in maternal-fetal medicine, who can carefully monitor the fetus to make sure you are getting the right dose.

Doctors most often treat pregnant women with the antithyroid medicine propylthiouracil (PTU) during the first three months of pregnancy. Another type of antithyroid medicine, methimazole, is easier to take and has fewer side effects, but is slightly more likely to cause serious birth defects than PTU. Birth defects with either type of medicine are rare. Sometimes doctors switch to methimazole after the first trimester of pregnancy. Some women no longer need antithyroid medicine in the third trimester.

Small amounts of antithyroid medicine move into the fetus's bloodstream and lower the amount of thyroid hormone the fetus makes. If you take antithyroid medicine, your doctor will prescribe the lowest possible dose to avoid hypothyroidism in the fetus, but enough to treat the high thyroid hormone levels that can also affect the fetus.

Antithyroid medicines can cause side effects in some people, including:

- Allergic reactions, such as rashes and itching

- A decrease in the number of white blood cells in the body, which can make it harder for your body to fight infection, in rare cases

- Liver failure, in rare cases

Stop your antithyroid medicine and call your doctor right away if you develop any of these symptoms while taking antithyroid medicines:

- Yellowing of your skin or the whites of your eyes, called "jaundice"

- Dull pain in your abdomen

- Constant sore throat

- Fever

If you do not hear back from your doctor the same day, you should go to the nearest emergency room.

You should also contact your doctor if any of these symptoms develop for the first time while you are taking antithyroid medicines:

- Increased tiredness or weakness

- Loss of appetite

- Skin rash or itching

- Easy bruising

If you are allergic to or have severe side effects from antithyroid medicines, your doctor may consider surgery to remove part or most of your thyroid gland. The best time for thyroid surgery during pregnancy is in the second trimester.

Radioactive iodine treatment is not an option for pregnant women because it can damage the fetus's thyroid gland.

Hypothyroidism in Pregnancy
What Are the Symptoms of Hypothyroidism in Pregnancy?

Symptoms of an underactive thyroid are often the same for pregnant women as for other people with hypothyroidism. Symptoms include:

- Extreme tiredness

- Trouble dealing with cold

- Muscle cramps

- Severe constipation

- Problems with memory or concentration

Most cases of hypothyroidism in pregnancy are mild and may not have symptoms.

What Causes Hypothyroidism in Pregnancy?

Hypothyroidism in pregnancy is usually caused by Hashimoto disease and occurs in 2 to 3 out of every 100 pregnancies. Hashimoto disease is an autoimmune disorder. In Hashimoto disease, the immune system makes antibodies that attack the thyroid, causing inflammation and damage that make it less able to make thyroid hormones.

How Can Hypothyroidism Affect Me and the Fetus?

Untreated hypothyroidism during pregnancy can lead to:

- Preeclampsia—a dangerous rise in blood pressure in late pregnancy
- Anemia
- Miscarriage
- Low birth weight
- Stillbirth
- Congestive heart failure, in rare cases

These problems occur most often with severe hypothyroidism.

Because thyroid hormones are so important to a fetus's brain and nervous system development, untreated hypothyroidism—especially during the first trimester—can cause low IQ (intelligence quotient) and problems with normal development.

How Do Doctors Diagnose Hypothyroidism in Pregnancy?

Your doctor will review your symptoms and do some blood tests to measure your thyroid hormone levels. Your doctor may also look for certain antibodies in your blood to see if Hashimoto disease is causing your hypothyroidism.

How Do Doctors Treat Hypothyroidism during Pregnancy?

Treatment for hypothyroidism involves replacing the hormone that your own thyroid can no longer make. Your doctor will most likely prescribe levothyroxine, a thyroid hormone medicine that is the same as T4, one of the hormones the thyroid normally makes. Levothyroxine is safe for the fetus and especially important until the fetus can make its own thyroid hormone.

Your thyroid makes a second type of hormone, T3. Early in pregnancy, T3 cannot enter the fetus's brain like T4 can. Instead, any T3 that the fetus's brain needs is made from T4. T3 is included in a lot of thyroid medicines made with animal thyroid, such as Armour Thyroid, but is not useful for a fetus's brain development. These medicines contain too much T3 and not enough T4, and should not be used during pregnancy. Experts recommend only using levothyroxine (T4) while you are pregnant.

Some women with subclinical hypothyroidism—a mild form of the disease with no clear symptoms—may not need treatment.

If you had hypothyroidism before you became pregnant and are taking levothyroxine, you will probably need to increase your dose. Most thyroid specialists recommend taking two extra doses of thyroid medicine per week, starting right away. Contact your doctor as soon as you know you are pregnant.

Your doctor will most likely test your thyroid hormone levels every 4 to 6 weeks for the first half of your pregnancy, and at least once after 30 weeks. You may need to adjust your dose a few times.

Postpartum Thyroiditis
What Is Postpartum Thyroiditis?

Postpartum thyroiditis is an inflammation of the thyroid that affects about 1 in 20 women during the first year after giving birth and is more common in women with type 1 diabetes. The inflammation causes stored thyroid hormone to leak out of your thyroid gland. At first, the leakage raises the hormone levels in your blood, leading to hyperthyroidism. The hyperthyroidism may last up to three months. After that, some damage to your thyroid may cause it to become underactive. Your hypothyroidism may last up to a year after your baby is born. However, in some women, hypothyroidism does not go away.

Not all women who have postpartum thyroiditis go through both phases. Some only go through the hyperthyroid phase, and some only the hypothyroid phase.

What Are the Symptoms of Postpartum Thyroiditis?

The hyperthyroid phase often has no symptoms, or only mild ones. Symptoms may include irritability, trouble dealing with heat, tiredness, trouble sleeping, and a fast heartbeat.

Symptoms of the hypothyroid phase may be mistaken for the "baby blues"—the tiredness and moodiness that sometimes occur after the baby is born. Symptoms of hypothyroidism may also include trouble dealing with cold; dry skin; trouble concentrating; and tingling in your hands, arms, feet, or legs. If these symptoms occur in the first few months after your baby is born or you develop postpartum depression, talk with your doctor as soon as possible.

What Causes Postpartum Thyroiditis?

Postpartum thyroiditis is an autoimmune condition similar to Hashimoto disease. If you have postpartum thyroiditis, you may have already had a mild form of autoimmune thyroiditis that flares up after you give birth.

How Do Doctors Diagnose Postpartum Thyroiditis?

If you have symptoms of postpartum thyroiditis, your doctor will order blood tests to check your thyroid hormone levels.

How Do Doctors Treat Postpartum Thyroiditis?

The hyperthyroid stage of postpartum thyroiditis rarely needs treatment. If your symptoms are bothering you, your doctor may prescribe a beta-blocker, a medicine that slows your heart rate. Antithyroid medicines are not useful in postpartum thyroiditis, but if you have Graves disease, it may worsen after your baby is born and you may need antithyroid medicines.

You are more likely to have symptoms during the hypothyroid stage. Your doctor may prescribe thyroid hormone medicine to help with your symptoms. If your hypothyroidism does not go away, you will need to take thyroid hormone medicine for the rest of your life.

Is It Safe to Breastfeed While I Am Taking Beta-Blockers, Thyroid Hormone, or Antithyroid Medicines?

Certain beta-blockers are safe to use while you are breastfeeding because only a small amount shows up in breast milk. The lowest possible dose to relieve your symptoms is best. Only a small amount of thyroid hormone medicine reaches your baby through breast milk, so it is safe to take while you are breastfeeding. However, in the case of antithyroid drugs, your doctor will most likely limit your dose to no more than 20 milligrams (mg) of methimazole, or less commonly, 400 mg of PTU.

Thyroid Disease and Eating during Pregnancy

Because the thyroid uses iodine to make thyroid hormone, iodine is an important mineral for you while you are pregnant. During pregnancy, your baby gets iodine from your diet. You will need more iodine when you are pregnant—about 250 micrograms a day. Good sources of iodine are dairy foods, seafood, eggs, meat, poultry, and iodized salt—salt with added iodine. Experts recommend taking a prenatal vitamin with 150 micrograms of iodine to make sure you are getting enough, especially if you do not use iodized salt. You also need more iodine while you are breastfeeding, since your baby gets iodine from breast milk. However, too much iodine from supplements, such as seaweed, can cause thyroid problems. Talk with your doctor about an eating plan that is right for you and what supplements you should take.

Chapter 37

Eating Disorders during Pregnancy

Adequate nutrition is vital during pregnancy to ensure the health and well-being of both the mother and the fetus. As a result, pregnancy may present challenges for women who are struggling with or recovering from eating disorders. Pregnancy creates physical and emotional changes that can be stressful for anyone, but especially for women who have preexisting mental health conditions. Even women who believe they have put their disordered eating behaviors in the past may be vulnerable to relapse due to the bodily changes associated with pregnancy. The normal weight gain during pregnancy can trigger symptoms of anorexia, for instance, while the feelings of fullness as the fetus grows can create an urge to purge among people with bulimia. The food cravings that often occur during pregnancy can also be problematic for people with binge-eating disorder.

If left untreated during pregnancy, active eating disorders can cause serious complications that jeopardize the health of both the mother and the fetus. Mothers with eating disorders are more likely to deliver by cesarean section and experience postpartum depression. Meanwhile, babies born to mothers with eating disorders have a high risk of premature delivery, low birth weight, and small head circumference. On the other hand, some women find it easier to avoid disordered eating

"Eating Disorders during Pregnancy," © 2016 Omnigraphics. Reviewed February 2019.

behavior during pregnancy as their focus shifts to protecting the health and welfare of the fetus. Given the importance of nutrition throughout pregnancy, however, women with eating disorders should seek professional advice and treatment to ensure that the condition does not interfere with the normal growth and development of the fetus.

Recognizing the Signs of Eating Disorders

Eating disorders may impact a woman's reproductive health even before she becomes pregnant. Women with anorexia or bulimia often experience irregularity or cessation of menstrual cycles, for instance, which can affect fertility and reduce the likelihood of conception. Therefore, doctors recommend that women bring eating disorders under control and maintain a healthy weight for several months before trying to get pregnant. Even in such cases, however, some women find that the bodily changes associated with pregnancy may trigger or exacerbate the symptoms of eating disorders. Some of the common signs that a woman is struggling with an eating disorder during pregnancy include:

- Weight loss or very limited weight gain throughout the pregnancy

- Anxiety about being overweight

- Restricting food intake, skipping meals, or eliminating major food groups

- Vomiting or purging to get rid of calories consumed

- Extreme (to the point of exhaustion) or excessive exercising to stay thin

- Chronic fatigue, dizziness, or fainting

- Depression, lack of interest in socializing, or avoidance of family and friends

If these signs appear during pregnancy, it is important to seek treatment to ensure a healthy outcome for both the mother and the fetus.

Understanding the Risks of Eating Disorders

Left untreated, eating disorders can have debilitating effects on the health of both the pregnant woman and the fetus. Understanding the risks posed by eating disorders may encourage expectant mothers to get the help they need to have a healthy pregnancy. Some of the potential health risks for a pregnant woman with an eating disorder include:

- Severe dehydration or malnutrition
- High blood pressure (preeclampsia), gestational diabetes, or anemia
- Cardiac irregularities
- Miscarriage, stillbirth, or premature labor
- Complications during delivery and increased risk of cesarean section
- Extended time required to heal from childbirth
- Postpartum depression
- Difficulties in breastfeeding
- Low self-esteem and poor body image
- Social withdrawal, isolation, and marital or family conflicts

Eating disorders also carry a number of serious risks for the developing fetus, including:

- Malnutrition, abnormal fetal growth, or poor development
- Premature birth
- Respiratory distress
- Small head circumference
- Low birth weight (with anorexia or bulimia)
- High birth weight (with binge-eating disorder)
- Feeding difficulties

The seriousness of these risks, along with the natural maternal instinct to protect the developing fetus, enables some women to effectively manage their eating disorders during pregnancy.

Managing Eating Disorders in Pregnancy

For some women, on the other hand, the physical and emotional changes that occur during pregnancy may trigger or worsen eating disorder symptoms. Those with anorexia, for instance, may struggle with their inability to fully control their eating and weight gain while pregnant.

Pregnant women who are struggling with eating disorders should see a counselor or therapist to help guide them through pregnancy-related changes, fears about weight gain, and concerns about body image. In addition, they should work with a nutritionist or dietitian to learn about nutritional requirements during pregnancy, ensure that caloric intake is sufficient to support fetal development, and create appropriate meal plans. Finally, they should inform their obstetrician about their eating disorder and make regular visits to track prenatal growth. The pregnancy may be classified as "high risk" so that the healthcare provider can carefully monitor the health of both the mother and the fetus. Additional tips to help alleviate concerns and manage eating disorders during pregnancy include:

- Remember that the source of weight gain is a growing fetus

- Avoid the scale, and ask the healthcare provider not to share your weight during checkups

- Try to ignore, or at least not dwell on, comments others make about your pregnant body

- Avoid looking at magazines that feature unrealistic postnatal weight-loss stories

Maintaining Health after Childbirth

Even when women with eating disorders manage to keep them under control during pregnancy, many tend to suffer relapses following childbirth. Women face extreme social pressure to lose pregnancy weight as quickly as possible. As a result, many women feel that they must begin a weight-loss diet or exercise regimen immediately after their baby has been born. This pressure to shed pounds can trigger disordered eating behaviors. Experts recommend focusing instead on the remarkable physical accomplishment of growing and delivering a healthy baby. This focus can help women accept the changes in body shape and appearance that may have resulted from pregnancy and childbirth.

Experts also stress that it is important for women to take care of their own health following childbirth. Women with eating disorders are particularly susceptible to postnatal depression, so they should watch out for symptoms and seek professional help if they appear.

Many women with eating disorders also express concerns about their ability to breastfeed. As long as the eating disorder is under control, it should not affect breastfeeding. But it is important to remember that restricting caloric intake during breastfeeding can reduce both the quantity and quality of breastmilk. Adequate nutrition is also important to ensure that new mothers have the energy, health, and well-being necessary to love, care for, and enjoy their infant.

References

1. "Eating Disorders and Pregnancy," Eating Disorder Hope, May 25, 2013.

2. "Eating Disorders and Pregnancy," Eating Disorders Victoria, June 24, 2015.

3. "Pregnancy and Eating Disorders," American Pregnancy Association, July 2015.

Chapter 38

Do Obesity and Overweight Affect Pregnancy?

How much a woman weighs when she gets pregnant and how much weight she gains during pregnancy can affect her health and that of the fetus. Entering pregnancy with a normal body mass index (BMI) and gaining weight within the recommended levels during pregnancy are important ways to protect a mother's and a child's health.

The Institute of Medicine (IOM) recommends the following ranges of weight gain during pregnancy for American women:

- Pregnant women who are underweight (BMI of less than 18.5) should gain 28 to 40 pounds.

- Pregnant women at a normal weight (BMI of 18.5 to 24.9) should gain 25 to 35 pounds.

- Overweight pregnant women (BMI of 25 to 29.9) should gain 15 to 25 pounds.

- Obese pregnant women (BMI greater than 30) should limit weight gain to 11 to 20 pounds.

This chapter includes text excerpted from "Do Obesity and Overweight Affect Pregnancy?" *Eunice Kennedy Shriver* National Institute of Child Health and Human Development (NICHD), December 1, 2016.

Obesity-Related Health Risks for Mothers

Women who are overweight or obese during pregnancy face several possible health risks, including high blood pressure, gestational diabetes, and an increased chance of needing a cesarean delivery.

Gestational diabetes is diabetes that begins during pregnancy. Women who have had gestational diabetes are at a higher lifetime risk for obesity and type 2 diabetes.

Obesity-Related Health Risks for Fetuses

The developing fetuses of obese women also are at an increased risk for health problems. For example, researchers found a connection between maternal obesity and neural-tube defects, in which the brain or spinal column does not form properly in early development. Also, research suggests that obesity increases a woman's chance of giving birth to a child with a heart defect by around 15 percent.

Gestational diabetes also can cause problems for a newborn, including dangerously low blood sugar, large body size that may cause injuries at birth, and high bilirubin levels, which can cause other health problems.

Children whose mothers had gestational diabetes also are at a higher lifetime risk for obesity and type 2 diabetes.

Preventing Obesity and Overweight in Pregnancy

In light of the rise in rates of obesity in the United States, the American Congress of Obstetricians and Gynecologists (ACOG) encourages women to seek guidance about nutrition and weight reduction from a healthcare provider if they are overweight and considering getting pregnant.

Good nutrition, staying active, and gaining the right amount of weight are important ways to promote a healthy pregnancy.

Part Five

Pregnancy Complications

Chapter 39

Understanding Pregnancy Complications

Chapter Contents

333

Section 39.1

What Are Some Common Complications of Pregnancy?

This section includes text excerpted from "Pregnancy Complications," Office on Women's Health (OWH), U.S. Department of Health and Human Services (HHS), January 30, 2019.

Sometimes pregnancy problems arise even in healthy women. Some prenatal tests done during pregnancy can help prevent these problems or spot them early. Following the doctor's advice will boost the chances of having a safe delivery and a strong, healthy baby.

Health Problems during Pregnancy
Anemia

Lower than normal number of healthy red blood cells. Symptoms may include:

• Feel tired or weak

• Look pale

• Feel faint

• Shortness of breath

Treating the underlying cause of the anemia will help restore the number of healthy red blood cells. Women with pregnancy-related anemia are helped by taking iron and folic acid supplements. Your doctor will check your iron levels throughout pregnancy to be sure anemia does not happen again.

Depression

Extreme sadness during pregnancy or after birth (postpartum) Symptoms may include:

• Intense sadness

• Helplessness and irritability

• Appetite changes

• Thoughts of harming self or baby

Women who are pregnant might be helped with one or a combination of treatment options, including:

- Therapy

- Support groups

- Medicines

A mother's depression can affect the fetus's development, so getting treatment is important for both mother and the fetus.

Ectopic Pregnancy

When a fertilized egg implants outside of the uterus, usually in the fallopian tube
Symptoms may include:

- Abdominal pain

- Shoulder pain

- Vaginal bleeding

- Feeling dizzy or faint

With ectopic pregnancy, the egg cannot develop. Drugs or surgery is used to remove the ectopic tissue so your organs are not damaged.

Fetal Problems

The fetus has a health issue, such as poor growth or heart problems

- The fetus is moving less than normal

- The fetus is smaller than normal for gestational age

- Some problems have no symptoms, but are found with prenatal tests

Treatment depends on results of tests to monitor the fetus's health. If a test suggests a problem, this does not always mean the fetus is in trouble. It may only mean that the mother needs special care until the baby is delivered. This can include a wide variety of things, such as bed rest, depending on the mother's condition. Sometimes, the baby has to be delivered early.

Gestational Diabetes

Too high blood sugar levels during pregnancy

- Usually, there are no symptoms. Sometimes, extreme thirst, hunger, or fatigue

- Screening test shows high blood sugar levels

Most women with pregnancy-related diabetes can control their blood sugar levels by a following a healthy meal plan from their doctor. Some women also need insulin to keep blood sugar levels under control. Doing so is important because poorly controlled diabetes increases the risk of:

- Preeclampsia

- Early delivery

- Cesarean birth

- Having a big baby, which can complicate delivery

- Baby born with low blood sugar, breathing problems, and jaundice

High Blood Pressure (Pregnancy Related)

High blood pressure that starts after 20 weeks of pregnancy and goes away after birth

High blood pressure without other signs and symptoms of preeclampsia

The health of the mother and fetus are closely watched to make sure high blood pressure is not preeclampsia.

Hyperemesis Gravidarum

Severe, persistent nausea and vomiting during pregnancy—more extreme than "morning sickness"

- Nausea that does not go away

- Vomiting several times every day

- Weight loss

- Reduced appetite

- Dehydration

- Feeling faint or fainting

Dry, bland foods and fluids together is the first line of treatment. Sometimes, medicines are prescribed to help nausea. Many women with hyperemesis gravidarum (HG) have to be hospitalized so they can be fed fluids and nutrients through a tube in their veins. Usually, women with HG begin to feel better by the 20th week of pregnancy. But some women vomit and feel nauseated throughout all three trimesters.

Miscarriage

Pregnancy loss from natural causes before 20 weeks. As many as 20 percent of pregnancies end in miscarriage. Often, miscarriage occurs before a woman even knows she is pregnant.

Signs of a miscarriage can include:

- Vaginal spotting or bleeding*

- Cramping or abdominal pain

- Fluid or tissue passing from the vagina

Spotting early in pregnancy doesn't mean miscarriage is certain. Still, contact your doctor right away if you have any bleeding.

Placenta Previa

Placenta covers part or entire opening of cervix inside of the uterus

- Vaginal bleeding

- Cramping, abdominal pain, and uterine tenderness

When the separation is minor, bed rest for a few days usually stops the bleeding. Moderate cases may require complete bed rest. Severe cases (when more than half of the placenta separates) can require immediate medical attention and early delivery of the baby.

Preeclampsia

A condition starting after 20 weeks of pregnancy that causes high blood pressure and problems with the kidneys and other organs. Also called "toxemia."

- High blood pressure

- Swelling of hands and face

- Too much protein in urine

- Stomach pain
- Blurred vision
- Dizziness
- Headaches

The only cure is delivery, which may not be best for the baby. Labor will probably be induced if condition is mild and the woman is near term (37 to 40 weeks of pregnancy). If it is too early to deliver, the doctor will watch the health of the mother and the fetus very closely. She may need medicines and bed rest at home or in the hospital to lower her blood pressure. Medicines also might be used to prevent the mother from having seizures.

Preterm Labor

Going into labor before 37 weeks of pregnancy

- Increased vaginal discharge
- Pelvic pressure and cramping
- Back pain radiating to the abdomen
- Contractions

Medicines can stop labor from progressing. Bed rest is often advised. Sometimes, a woman must deliver early. Giving birth before 37 weeks is called "preterm birth." Preterm birth is a major risk factor for future preterm births.

Section 39.2

How Health Problems before Pregnancy Complicate Pregnancy

This section includes text excerpted from "Pregnancy Complications," Office on Women's Health (OWH), U.S. Department of Health and Human Services (HHS), January 30, 2019.

Before pregnancy, make sure to talk to your doctor about health problems you have now or have had in the past. If you are receiving treatment for a health problem, your doctor might want to change the way your health problem is managed. Some medicines used to treat health problems could be harmful if taken during pregnancy. At the same time, stopping medicines that you need could be more harmful than the risks posed should you become pregnant. Be assured that you are likely to have a normal, healthy baby when health problems are under control and you get good prenatal care.

Health Problems before Pregnancy
Asthma

Poorly controlled asthma may increase risk of preeclampsia, poor weight gain in the fetus, preterm birth, cesarean birth, and other complications. If pregnant women stop using asthma medicine, even mild asthma can become severe.

Depression

Depression that persists during pregnancy can make it hard for a woman to care for herself and the fetus. Having depression before pregnancy also is a risk factor for postpartum depression.

Diabetes

High blood-glucose (sugar) levels during pregnancy can harm the fetus and worsen a woman's long-term diabetes complications. Doctors advise getting diabetes under control at least three to six months before trying to conceive.

Eating Disorders

Body image changes during pregnancy can cause eating disorders to worsen. Eating disorders are linked to many pregnancy complications,

339

including birth defects and premature birth. Women with eating disorders also have higher rates of postpartum depression.

Epilepsy and Other Seizure Disorders

Seizures during pregnancy can harm the fetus, and increase the risk of miscarriage or stillbirth. But using medicine to control seizures might cause birth defects. For most pregnant women with epilepsy, using medicine poses less risk to their own health and the health of the fetus than stopping medicine.

High Blood Pressure

Having chronic high blood pressure puts a pregnant woman and the fetus at risk for problems. Women with high blood pressure have a higher risk of preeclampsia and placental abruption (when the placenta separates from the wall of the uterus). The likelihood of preterm birth and low birth weight also is higher.

Human Immunodeficiency Virus

Human immunodeficiency virus (HIV) can be passed from a woman to her baby during pregnancy or delivery. Yet this risk is less than 1 percent if a woman takes certain HIV medicines during pregnancy. Women who have HIV and want to become pregnant should talk to their doctors before trying to conceive. Good prenatal care will help protect the fetus from HIV and keep the mother healthy.

Migraine

Migraine symptoms tend to improve during pregnancy. Some women have no migraine attacks during pregnancy. Certain medicines commonly used to treat headaches should not be used during pregnancy. A woman who has severe headaches should speak to her doctor about ways to relieve symptoms safely.

Overweight and Obesity

Recent studies suggest that the heavier a woman is before she becomes pregnant, the greater her risk of a range of pregnancy complications, including preeclampsia and preterm delivery. Overweight and obese women who lose weight before pregnancy are likely to have healthier pregnancies.

Sexually Transmitted Infections

Some sexually transmitted infections (STIs) can cause early labor, a woman's water to break too early, and infection in the uterus after birth. Some STIs also can be passed from a woman to her baby during pregnancy or delivery. Some ways STIs can harm the baby include: low birth weight, dangerous infections, brain damage, blindness, deafness, liver problems, or stillbirth.

Thyroid Disease

Uncontrolled hyperthyroidism (overactive thyroid) can be dangerous to the mother and cause health problems such as heart failure and poor weight gain in the fetus. Uncontrolled hypothyroidism (underactive thyroid) also threatens the mother's health and can cause birth defects.

Uterine Fibroids

Uterine fibroids are not uncommon, but few cause symptoms that require treatment. Uterine fibroids rarely cause miscarriage. Sometimes, fibroids can cause preterm or breech birth. Cesarean delivery may be needed if a fibroid blocks the birth canal.

Section 39.3

Is Infection a Complicating Factor?

This section includes text excerpted from "Pregnancy Complications," Office on Women's Health (OWH), U.S. Department of Health and Human Services (HHS), January 30, 2019.

Yes. During pregnancy, the fetus is protected from many illnesses, such as the common cold or a passing stomach bug. But some infections can be harmful to your pregnancy, the fetus, or both. Easy steps, such as hand washing, practicing safe sex, and avoiding certain foods, can help protect you from some infections.

Infections during Pregnancy

Bacterial Vaginosis

A vaginal infection that is caused by an overgrowth of bacteria normally found in the vagina.

Bacterial vaginosis (BV) has been linked to preterm birth and low birth weight babies.

Symptoms may include:

- Grey or whitish discharge that has a foul, fishy odor

- Burning when passing urine or itching

- Some women have no symptoms

How to prevent BV is unclear. BV is not passed through sexual contact, although it is linked with having a new or more than one sex partner. Women with symptoms should be tested for BV. Antibiotics are used to treat BV.

Cytomegalovirus

A common virus that can cause disease in infants whose mothers are infected with cytomegalovirus (CMV) during pregnancy. CMV infection in infants can lead to hearing loss, vision loss, and other disabilities.

Symptoms may include:

- Mild illness that may include fever, sore throat, fatigue, and swollen glands

- Some women have no symptoms

Good hygiene is the best way to keep from getting CMV.

No treatment is currently available. But studies are looking at antiviral drugs for use in infants. Work to create a CMV vaccine also is underway.

Group B Strep

Group B strep (GBS) is a type of bacteria often found in the vagina and rectum of healthy women. One in four women has it. GBS usually is not harmful to you, but can be deadly to your baby if passed during childbirth.

There are no symptoms.

You can keep from passing GBS to your baby by getting tested at 35 to 37 weeks. This simply involves swabbing the vagina and rectum and does not hurt.

If you have GBS, an antibiotic given to you during labor will protect the fetus from infection. Make sure to tell the labor and delivery staff that you are a group B strep carrier when you check into the hospital.

Hepatitis B Virus

A viral infection that can be passed to baby during birth. Newborns that get infected have a 90 percent chance of developing life-long infection. This can lead to liver damage and liver cancer. A vaccine can keep newborns from getting HBV. But 1 in 5 newborns of mothers who are HBV positive do not get the vaccine at the hospital before leaving.

There may be no symptoms. Or symptoms can include:

- Nausea, vomiting, and diarrhea

- Dark urine and pale bowel movements

- Whites of eyes or skin looks yellow

Lab tests can find out if the mother is a carrier of hepatitis B.

You can protect your baby for life from HBV with the hepatitis B vaccine, which is a series of three shots:

- First dose of hepatitis B vaccine plus HBIG shot given to baby at birth

- Second dose of hepatitis B vaccine given to baby at 1 to 2 months old

- Third dose of hepatitis B vaccine given to baby at 6 months old (but not before 24 weeks old)

Influenza (Flu)

Flu is a common viral infection that is more likely to cause severe illness in pregnant women than in women who are not pregnant. Pregnant woman with flu also have a greater chance for serious problems for the fetus, including premature labor and delivery.

Symptoms may include:

- Fever (sometimes) or feeling feverish/chills

- Cough

- Sore throat
- Runny or stuffy nose
- Muscle or body aches
- Headaches
- Feeling tired
- Vomiting and diarrhea (sometimes)

Getting a flu shot is the first and most important step in protecting against flu. The flu shot given during pregnancy is safe and has been shown to protect both the mother and the fetus (up to 6 months old) from flu. (The nasal spray vaccine should not be given to women who are pregnant.)

If you get sick with flu-like symptoms call your doctor right away. If needed, the doctor will prescribe an antiviral medicine that treats the flu.

Listeriosis

An infection with the harmful bacteria called "listeria." It is found in some refrigerated and ready-to-eat foods. Infection can cause early delivery or miscarriage.

Symptoms may include:

- Fever, muscle aches, chills
- Sometimes diarrhea or nausea
- If progress, severe headache and stiff neck

Avoid foods that can harbor listeria. Antibiotics are used to treat listeriosis.

Parvovirus B19 (Fifth Disease)

Most pregnant women who are infected with this virus do not have serious problems. But there is a small chance the virus can infect the fetus. This raises the risk of miscarriage during the first 20 weeks of pregnancy. Fifth disease can cause severe anemia in women who have red blood cell disorders, such as sickle cell disease or immune system problems.

Symptoms may include:

- Low-grade fever
- Tiredness

- Rash on face, trunk, and limbs

- Painful and swollen joints

There is no specific treatment, except for blood transfusions that might be needed for people who have problems with their immune systems or with red blood cell disorders. There is no vaccine to help prevent infection with this virus.

Sexually Transmitted Infection

An infection that is passed through sexual contact. Many sexually transmitted infections (STIs) can be passed to the fetus or during birth. Some effects include stillbirth, low birth weight, and life-threatening infections. STIs also can cause a woman's water to break too early or preterm labor.

Symptoms may include:

- Symptoms depend on the STI. Often, a woman has no symptoms, which is why screening for STIs during pregnancy is so important.

- STIs can be prevented by practicing safe sex. A woman can keep from passing an STI to the fetus by being screened early in pregnancy.

Treatments vary depending on the STI. Many STIs are treated easily with antibiotics.

Toxoplasmosis

This infection is caused by a parasite, which is found in cat feces, soil, and raw or undercooked meat. If passed to a fetus, the infection can cause hearing loss, blindness, or intellectual disabilities.

Symptoms may include:

- Mild flu-like symptoms, or possibly no symptoms.

You can lower your risk by:

- Washing hands with soap after touching soil or raw meat

- Washing produce before eating

- Cooking meat completely

- Washing cooking utensils with hot, soapy water

- Not cleaning cats' litter boxes

Medicines are used to treat a pregnant woman and the fetus. Sometimes, the fetus is treated with medicine after birth.

Urinary Tract Infection

Bacterial infection in urinary tract. If untreated, it can spread to the kidneys, which can cause preterm labor.

Symptoms may include:

- Pain or burning when urinating

- Frequent urination

- Pelvis, back, stomach, or side pain

- Shaking, chills, fever, sweats

Urinary tract infections (UTIs) are treated with antibiotics.

Yeast Infection

An infection caused by an overgrowth of bacteria normally found in the vagina. Yeast infections are more common during pregnancy than in other times of a woman's life. They do not threaten the health of the fetus. But they can be uncomfortable and difficult to treat in pregnancy.

Symptoms may include:

- Extreme itchiness in and around the vagina

- Burning, redness, and swelling of the vagina and the vulva

- Pain when passing urine or during sex

- A thick, white vaginal discharge that looks like cottage cheese and does not have a bad smell

Vaginal creams and suppositories are used to treat yeast infection during pregnancy.

Chapter 40

Amniotic Fluid Abnormalities

In colloquial terms, amniotic fluid is referred to as a pregnant woman's "water." This watery fluid surrounds the fetus in the uterus. Both the fluid and fetus are contained in a membrane called the "amniotic sac," which develops 12 days after conception. The fluid is clear to pale yellow in color and is made up of combination of water, proteins, electrolytes, carbohydrates, lipids, phospholipids, and urea, with some fetal cells. The amount of fluid increases with gestational age and the normal volume varies from 800 to 1000 mL. The volume is measured using a method called "amniotic fluid index" (AFI).

Amniotic fluid acts as a life-support system to:

- Cushion and protect the fetus

- Allow room for the fetus to move and develop

- Maintain a relatively constant temperature

- Aid fetal lung development

- Develop the fetus's digestive system (as the fetus swallows the fluid)

- Act as a barrier to infections

- Protect against the squeezing and compression of the umbilical cord (the cord that carries food and oxygen from the mother to the fetus)

"Amniotic Fluid Abnormalities," © 2019 Omnigraphics. Reviewed February 2019.

Common Problems and Complications
Abnormal Odor

A foul-smelling odor may be a sign of infection and may present in conjunction with a fever. A woman whose water breaks at home and who notices a foul-smelling odor should contact her doctor immediately.

Abnormal Color

Color that differs from clear or pale yellow is an anomaly.

- Green or brown-colored fluid in near- or full-term pregnancies indicates "meconium," or the first fecal movement of the fetus, which contributes to the change in color. This is an indication that the baby is in distress or that the pregnancy has extended long enough for the fetus to pass the first stool in utero.

- Blood-tinged fluid during pregnancy may be an indication of cervix dilation or other placental problems.

- Dark-colored fluid may be an indication of the death of a fetus during pregnancy (intrauterine fetal demise (IUFD)).

"Water Breaks" Too Early

If the "water breaks" too early, this can affect both the mother and fetus. This occurrence is called "preterm premature rupture of membranes" (PPROM/PROM). Resulting complications include impaired fetal development, early labor and delivery, and possible infection. In such cases, bed rest, intravenous (IV) antibiotics, corticosteroid administration for facilitation of fetal lung maturity, and delaying labor to increase the survival chances of the fetus. If born early, the fetus will require neonatal care.

Too Little Amniotic Fluid—Oligohydramnios

Oligo means "less or scanty," and a decreased amount of amniotic fluid in the uterus is called "oligohydramnios."
The causes include:

- Urinary tract malformation—a birth defect in the urinary tract causing less fetal urine output

- Stunted growth of the fetus (not reaching expected growth)

- Chromosomal abnormality

- Placenta not functioning normally
- PROM
- Post-term pregnancy (pregnancy lasting longer than 40 weeks)
- Taking certain drugs, such as angiotensin-converting enzyme (ACE) inhibitors enalapril, captopril, nonsteroidal anti-inflammatory drugs (NSAIDs), aspirin, ibuprofin, and so on during the second or third trimester

If oligohydramnios is detected in the first half of the pregnancy, then the complications are serious and include:

- Potter syndrome—a combination of immature lungs and other deformities
- Fetal compression that may result in a flattened nose, recessed chin, limb deformities, and other developmental abnormalities
- Stillbirth or an increased chance of miscarriage

If oligohydramnios is detected in the second half of pregnancy, the complications include:

- Intrauterine growth restriction (IUGR)—slower growth of the fetus than expected
- Placental-cord compression and meconium-stained fluid (dark-colored amniotic fluid)
- Preterm birth—the fetus becomes unable to tolerate labor (making cesarean delivery necessary)

Too Much Amniotic Fluid—Polyhydramnios

A high accumulation of amniotic fluid is called "polyhydramnios." Most of the causes are unknown, but known causes include:

- Maternal diabetes—elevated blood-glucose levels in the mother either before getting pregnant (a personal history of diabetes) or during pregnancy (diabetes that developed during gestation)
- Multiple births or having more than one fetus. Twin–twin transfusion syndrome (TTTS)—in identical-twin pregnancies results in one twin receiving a high amount of blood and the other receiving too little.
- Rh incompatibility (Rhesus disease)—mismatched blood types in the mother and the fetus (Rh antibodies produced by the pregnant woman enter the fetus's blood)

- Fluid buildup in the baby (hydrops fetalis)

- Fetal birth defects, such as defects of the brain, spinal cord (spina bifida), heart (fetal arrhythmia), blocked esophagus, gut atresia, and others

- Infection during pregnancy

Woman with polyhydramnios may experience some of the following symptoms:

- Heartburn

- Constipation

- Swelling of feet and abdominal wall

- Breathlessness

- Heaviness of bump with uterine contractions and discomfort

- Fetal malposition such as breech presentation

The fluid accumulation stretches the uterus and puts more pressure on the pregnant woman's diaphragm, which leads to several other problems, including:

- Breathing issues

- Bleeding from the vagina post delivery due to a lack of uterine muscle tone

- Preterm labor

- PROM

- Prolapsed umbilical cord (the umbilical cord coming out of the vagina before the fetus)

- Placental abruption (early detachment of the placenta from the walls of the uterus)

Intra-Amniotic Infection

This infection develops when bacteria from the vagina enters the uterus and infects tissues around the fetus. Infection of these tissues (such as the amniotic fluid, placenta, the membranes around the fetus, or a combination of these) is collectively called as "intra-amniotic infection."

Intra-amniotic infection can cause:

- PPROM

- Less oxygen in the blood around the time of delivery

- Body-wide (systemic) infections, such as sepsis, pneumonia, or meningitis

- Seizures

- Cerebral palsy

- In certain cases, death

Amniotic Fluid Embolism

Amniotic fluid entering the woman's bloodstream causes a serious reaction and can damage the lungs and heart. A common complication is disseminated intravascular coagulation, in which small blood clots develop throughout the bloodstream. This results in widespread bleeding and a massive loss of blood and is a medical emergency. Immediate diagnosis and treatment are essential when a pregnant woman presents with the following symptoms:

- Sudden difficulty breathing

- Low blood pressure

- Widespread, uncontrolled bleeding

Blood transfusion and injection of a blood-clotting factor may be lifesaving. Women may require assistance with breathing or drugs to help contractions of the heart. In such cases, immediate delivery of the baby using forceps or a vacuum extractor, or even a cesarean delivery, may be done to save the fetus when it is old enough to survive outside the uterus.

Healthcare providers evaluate these abnormalities with the help of ultrasound and determine the best treatment plan based on the severity of the condition.

References

1. Carter, Brian S. "Polyhydramnios and Oligohydramnios," Medscape, September 20, 2017.

2. "Polyhydramnios," Mayoclinic, November 18, 2017.

3. Dulay, Antonette T. MD. "Problems with Amniotic Fluid," MSD Manual, March 2018.

Chapter 41

Bleeding and Blood Clots in Pregnancy

Chapter Contents

Section 41.1

Bleeding during Early Pregnancy

This section contains text excerpted from the following sources:
Text under the heading "What Is "Spotting" during Pregnancy, and
Does It Mean a Pregnancy Loss Is Occurring?" is excerpted from
"Other FAQs about Pregnancy Loss (Before 20 Weeks of Pregnancy),"
Eunice Kennedy Shriver National Institute of Child Health and
Human Development (NICHD), September 1, 2017; Text under the
heading "More than One Day of Early-Pregnancy Bleeding Linked
to Lower Birthweight" is excerpted from "More Than One Day of
Early-Pregnancy Bleeding Linked to Lower Birthweight," National
Institutes of Health (NIH), May 9, 2018.

What Is "Spotting" during Pregnancy, and Does It Mean a Pregnancy Loss Is Occurring?

"Spotting" is the term used to describe light bleeding from the vagina. Many pregnant women have spotting and mild cramping during early pregnancy, but it does not always indicate pregnancy loss or another problem.

According to the American College of Obstetricians and Gynecologists (ACOG), up to 20 percent of pregnant women experience light bleeding in the first trimester. In many cases, spotting at this stage of pregnancy does not indicate a problem.

Research also shows that spotting may occur during the second and third trimesters. It can result from factors such as infection, or it could be a signal of labor. Heavy vaginal bleeding at any point in pregnancy can mean there is a problem. Women who experience this type of bleeding should contact their healthcare provider immediately.

Likewise, pregnant women who have any of the symptoms of pregnancy loss—vaginal bleeding more than spotting, abdominal cramps, low back pain—should also contact their healthcare providers immediately.

More Than One Day of Early-Pregnancy Bleeding Linked to Lower Birthweight

Women who experience vaginal bleeding for more than one day during the first trimester of pregnancy may be more likely to have a smaller baby, compared to women who do not experience bleeding in the first trimester, suggest researchers at the National Institutes of Health (NIH). On average, full-term babies born to women with more than one day of bleeding in the first trimester were about three ounces lighter than those born to women with no bleeding during this time. Additionally, infants born to women with more than a day of first-trimester bleeding were roughly twice as likely to be small for gestational age, a category that includes infants who are healthy but small, as well as those whose growth has been restricted because of insufficient nutrition or oxygen or other causes.

The authors caution that the decrease in birthweight of infants born to women with vaginal bleeding was small. More studies are needed to determine if these infants are at risk for any additional health risks in infancy or later in life.

"The good news is that only one day of bleeding was not significantly associated with reduced growth," said the study's senior author, Katherine L. Grantz, M.D., an investigator in the *Eunice Kennedy Shriver* National Institute of Child Health and Human Development (NICHD) Epidemiology Branch. "But our results suggest that even if the bleeding stops before the second trimester, a pregnancy with more than one day of bleeding is at somewhat of a greater risk for a smaller baby."

According to the study authors, first trimester vaginal bleeding occurs in 16 to 25 percent of pregnancies. Earlier studies on whether bleeding is associated with adverse pregnancy outcomes have been inconclusive. The researchers analyzed data from the NICHD Fetal Growth Study, which enrolled women ages 18 to 40 at 12 hospitals in the United States. The study used ultrasound to track fetal growth throughout pregnancy. Of the roughly 2,300 women in the analysis, 410 (17.8%) had bleeding in the first trimester. Of these, 176 bled for one day and 234 bled for more.

The researchers also analyzed birthweight outcomes in a secondary analysis limited to 2,116 women with birthweight data available. Compared to women with no bleeding, fetuses of women with more than one day of bleeding were 68 to 107 grams (approximately 2 to 4 ounces) lighter in weeks 35 to 39 of pregnancy. The average birth weight of these babies who were full-term was about three ounces lighter than infants born to women who did not bleed at all. Infants who were small for gestational age were delivered to 148 women in the nonbleeding group (8.5%), nine women in the one-day group (5.7%), and 33 women (15.7%) in the group that had more than a day of bleeding.

Dr. Grantz added that when ultrasound exams indicate that the fetus is small for gestational age, physicians typically increase the number of exams to monitor the pregnancy more closely.

Section 41.2

Blood Clots during Pregnancy

This section includes text excerpted from "Venous
Thromboembolism (Blood Clots) and Pregnancy," Centers for
Disease Control and Prevention (CDC), August 29, 2018.

While everyone is at risk for developing a blood clot (also called
"venous thromboembolism" or VTE), pregnancy increases that risk
fivefold.

Why Do Pregnant Women Have a Higher Risk of Developing a Blood Clot?

Women are especially at risk for blood clots during pregnancy,
childbirth, and the three-month period after delivery. Here's why:

- During pregnancy, a woman's blood clots more easily to lessen
  blood loss during labor and delivery.

- Pregnant women may also experience less blood flow to the legs
  later in pregnancy because the blood vessels around the pelvis
  are pressed upon by the fetus.

Several other factors may also increase a pregnant woman's risk
for a blood clot:

- A family or personal history of blood clots or a blood clotting
  disorder

- Delivery by cesarean (C-section)

- Prolonged immobility (not moving a lot), such as during bed rest
  or recovery after delivery

- Complications of pregnancy and childbirth

- Certain long-term medical conditions, such as heart or lung
  conditions, or diabetes

Take Steps to Protect Yourself and Your Baby from Blood Clots during Pregnancy and after Delivery

- Know the signs and symptoms of blood clots

- A blood clot occurring in the legs or arms is called "deep vein thrombosis" (DVT). Signs and symptoms of a DVT include:

  - Swelling of the affected limb

  - Pain or tenderness not caused by injury

  - Skin that is warm to the touch, red, or discolored

If you have these signs or symptoms, alert your doctor as soon as possible.

- A blood clot in the legs or arms can break off and travel to the lungs. This is called a "pulmonary embolism" (PE) and can be life-threatening. Signs and symptoms of a PE include:

  - Difficulty breathing

  - Chest pain that worsens with a deep breath or cough

  - Coughing up blood

  - Faster than a normal or irregular heartbeat

Seek immediate medical attention if you experience any of these signs or symptoms.

- Talk with your healthcare provider about factors that might increase your risk for a blood clot. Let your provider know if you or anyone else in your family has ever had a blood clot.

- Follow your healthcare provider's instructions closely during pregnancy and after delivery.

  - In general, if a pregnant woman is at high risk for a blood clot or experiences a blood clot during pregnancy or after delivery, she may be prescribed a medicine called "low-molecular-weight heparin." This medicine, injected under the skin, is used to prevent or treat blood clots during and after pregnancy. Be sure to talk with your healthcare provider to understand the best course of management for you.

Chapter 42

Cholestasis of Pregnancy

Intrahepatic cholestasis of pregnancy (ICP) is a disorder of the liver that occurs in women during pregnancy. Cholestasis is a condition that impairs the release of bile (a digestive juice) from liver cells. The bile then builds up in the liver, impairing liver function. Symptoms typically become apparent in the third trimester of pregnancy and can include severe itching (pruritus). Occasionally, the skin and the whites of the eyes can have a yellow appearance (jaundice). ICP is additionally associated with risks to the fetus, such as premature delivery and stillbirth. Symptoms of ICP are typically limited to pregnancy. Bile flow returns to normal after delivery and the signs and symptoms of the condition disappear, however, they can return during later pregnancies.

Symptoms

The following table lists symptoms that people with this disease may have. For most diseases, symptoms will vary from person to person. People with the same disease may not have all the symptoms listed.

This chapter includes text excerpted from "Intrahepatic Cholestasis of Pregnancy," Genetic and Rare Diseases Information Center (GARD), National Center for Advancing Translational Sciences (NCATS), March 15, 2016.

Table 42.1. Medical Terms and Their Names

Medical Terms	Other Names
5% to 29% of people have these symptoms	
Autosomal recessive inheritance	
Jaundice	Yellow skin Yellowing of the skin
Percent of people who have these symptoms is not available through HPO	
Abnormal liver function tests during pregnancy	
Autosomal dominant inheritance	
Elevated hepatic transaminase	High liver enzymes
Fetal distress	
Increased serum bile acid concentration during pregnancy	
Intrahepatic cholestasis	
Premature birth	Premature delivery of affected infants Preterm delivery
Pruritus	Itching Itchy skin Skin itching

Causes

Largely, the cause of ICP is unknown. ICP is present in approximately one percent of pregnancies in the United States. It is thought to be caused by a mixture of genetic, hormonal, and environmental factors. Risk factors include:

- Personal or family history of cholestasis of pregnancy

- History of liver disease

- Multiple gestation pregnancies (twins, triplets, etc.)

Approximately 15 percent of women with ICP have a mutation in either the *ABCB11* or *ABCB4* gene. Mutations within these genes increase the likelihood that a woman will develop ICP.

Diagnosis

ICP is suspected during pregnancy when symptoms of itching (pruritus) present after 25 weeks of gestation with the absence of a rash or underlying maternal liver disease. The diagnosis is typically confirmed with the finding of elevated serum bile acids. In the presence of a family history of ICP and/or known mutations in either the *ABCB11* or *ABCB4* genes, genetic testing is available.

Treatment

Treatment for intrahepatic cholestasis of pregnancy aims to relieve itching and prevent complications. Medications utilized to relieve itching might include ursodiol (Actigall, Urso), which helps decrease the level of bile in the mother's bloodstream, relieves itchiness, and may reduce complications for the fetus. To prevent pregnancy complications, close monitoring of the fetus might be recommended. Even if prenatal tests appear normal, induction of early labor might be recommended.

Chapter 43

Gestational Diabetes

Gestational diabetes is a type of diabetes that can develop during pregnancy in women who do not already have diabetes. Every year, 2 to 10 percent of pregnancies in the United States are affected by gestational diabetes. Managing gestational diabetes will help make sure you have a healthy pregnancy and a healthy baby.

Causes

Gestational diabetes occurs when your body can't make enough insulin during your pregnancy. Insulin is a hormone made by your pancreas that acts as a key to let blood sugar into the cells in the body and use as energy.

During pregnancy, your body makes more hormones and goes through other changes, such as weight gain. These changes cause your body's cells to use insulin less effectively, a condition called "insulin resistance." Insulin resistance increases your body's need for insulin.

All pregnant women have some insulin resistance during late pregnancy. However, some women have insulin resistance even before they get pregnant. They start pregnancy with an increased need for insulin and are more likely to have gestational diabetes.

This chapter includes text excerpted from "Gestational Diabetes," Centers for Disease Control and Prevention (CDC), July 25, 2017.

Symptoms and Risk Factors

Gestational diabetes typically does not have any symptoms. Your medical history and whether you have any risk factors may suggest to your doctor that you could have gestational diabetes, but you will need to be tested to know for sure.

Complications

Having gestational diabetes can increase your risk of high blood pressure during pregnancy. It can also increase your risk of having a large baby that needs to be delivered by cesarean section (C-section).

If you have gestational diabetes, your baby is at higher risk of:

- Being very large (9 pounds or more), which can make delivery more difficult

- Being born early, which can cause breathing and other problems

- Having low blood sugar

- Developing type 2 diabetes later in life

Gestational diabetes usually goes away after your baby is born. However, about 50 percent of women with gestational diabetes go on to develop type 2 diabetes. You can lower your risk by reaching a healthy body weight after delivery. Visit your doctor to have your blood sugar tested 6 to 12 weeks after your baby is born and then every 1 to 3 years to make sure your levels are on target.

Getting Tested

It is important to get tested for gestational diabetes so you can begin treatment to protect your health and the fetus's health.

Gestational diabetes usually develops around the 24th week of pregnancy, so you will probably be tested between 24 and 28 weeks.

If you're at higher risk for gestational diabetes, your doctor may test you earlier. Blood sugar that's higher than normal early in your pregnancy may indicate you have type 1 or type 2 diabetes rather than gestational diabetes.

Prevention

Before you get pregnant, you may be able to prevent gestational diabetes by losing weight if you are overweight and getting regular physical activity.

Don't try to lose weight if you are already pregnant. You will need to gain some weight—but not too quickly—for your baby to be healthy. Talk to your doctor about how much weight you should gain for a healthy pregnancy.

Treatment

You can do a lot to manage your gestational diabetes. Go to all your prenatal appointments and follow your treatment plan, including:

- **Checking your blood sugar** to make sure your levels stay in a healthy range.

- **Eating healthy food in the right amounts at the right times.** Follow a healthy eating plan created by your doctor or dietitian.

- **Being active.** Regular physical activity that is moderately intense (such as brisk walking) lowers your blood sugar and makes you more sensitive to insulin so your body would not need as much. Make sure to check with your doctor about what kind of physical activity you can do and if there are any kinds you should avoid.

- **Monitoring the fetus.** Your doctor will check the fetus's growth and development.

Chapter 44

Gestational Hypertension

When high blood pressure (HBP) occurs during pregnancy and is not appropriately treated, it may negatively affect the health of both the mother and the fetus during pregnancy, during delivery, or after delivery. High blood pressure, also known as "hypertension" (HTN), is a common and treatable health condition that occurs in 6 to 8 percent of all pregnancies among women ages 20 to 44 years in the United States.

For the mother, any hypertensive conditions, regardless of whether they were first diagnosed before (chronic HTN) or during (gestational HTN) pregnancy, may be linked to preeclampsia, eclampsia, stroke, pregnancy induction (speeding up the pregnancy to give birth), and placental abruption (the placenta separating from the wall of the uterus).

For the fetus, high blood pressure during pregnancy may affect the mother's blood vessels—including the ones in the umbilical cord. When the blood vessels tighten, it becomes more difficult for the fetus to get enough oxygen and nutrients to grow, and may result in preterm delivery (birth that occurs before 37 weeks of pregnancy) and low birth weight (when a baby is born weighing less than 5 pounds, 8 ounces).

The good news is that this is a preventable issue. Poor outcomes may be detected early and/or avoided by increasing awareness, improving

This chapter includes text excerpted from "High Blood Pressure during Pregnancy Fact Sheet," Centers for Disease Control and Prevention (CDC), May 16, 2018.

patient education and counseling, and providing appropriate treatment of any high blood pressure conditions before, during, or after pregnancy.

What Should Women with High Blood Pressure Do before, during, and after Pregnancy?

Before Pregnancy

- Make a plan for pregnancy and talk with a healthcare provider about the following:

  - Review medical conditions and current medicines. Women planning to become pregnant should discuss the need for any medicine before becoming pregnant and should make sure that they are taking only medicines that are necessary.

  - Find ways to reach and maintain a healthy weight through healthy eating and regular physical activity.

During Pregnancy

- Engage early in regular prenatal care and attend scheduled healthcare provider appointments.

- Discuss current medicines and which medicines are considered to be safe with a healthcare provider. Pregnant women should not stop or start taking any type of medicine that they need, including over-the-counter (OTC) medicines, without consulting a healthcare provider.

- Keep track of blood pressure routinely by using a home blood pressure monitor. Contact a healthcare provider if blood pressure becomes higher than usual or if you experience any other signs and symptoms of preeclampsia (e.g., headache, dizziness, blurry vision).

- Continue to maintain a healthy lifestyle and track weight during pregnancy.

After Pregnancy

- Continue to monitor for symptoms of preeclampsia during the postpartum period. Contact a healthcare provider if symptoms continue or become worse so that immediate medical care can be given.

Types of High Blood Pressure Conditions before, during, and after Pregnancy

High blood pressure can appear as many different conditions at various times before or during pregnancy. Your healthcare provider (doctor or nurse) should look for these conditions before and during pregnancy:

Preeclampsia / Eclampsia
In Middle, Late, or after Pregnancy

Preeclampsia is defined as the new onset of high blood pressure (more than or equal to 140/90 mmHg)* on two occasions, at least 4 hours apart, or blood pressure readings of more than or equal to 160/110 mmHg in a woman with previously normal blood pressure (BP).

Risk factors for preeclampsia include:

• Primiparity (giving birth for the first time)

• Preeclampsia during a previous pregnancy

• Chronic hypertension, chronic renal (kidney) disease, or both

• History of thrombophilia (an abnormal condition that increases the risk of blood clots in blood vessels)

• Multiple babies in one pregnancy (e.g., twins, triplets)

• In vitro fertilization

• Family history of preeclampsia

• Type 1 or type 2 diabetes

• Obesity

• Lupus (an autoimmune disease)

• Advanced maternal age (older than 40 years)

Preeclampsia is accompanied by protein in the urine (proteinuria) and possibly other organ problems. These problems could include:

• Low blood platelet count

• Abnormal kidney or liver function, resulting in sudden weight gain, swelling of face or hands, or upper abdominal pain

• Fluid in the lungs, causing difficulty breathing

369

- Changes in vision, including seeing spots or changes in eyesight

- Severe headache, nausea, or vomiting

Preeclampsia is typically diagnosed after 20 weeks of pregnancy and most often closer to delivery. It can occur together with another high blood pressure condition (e.g., chronic hypertension with superimposed preeclampsia). Preeclampsia affects 4 percent of pregnancies in the United States.

On rare occasions, preeclampsia can occur after childbirth. This is a serious medical condition known as "postpartum preeclampsia." It may develop in women without any history of preeclampsia. The symptoms for postpartum preeclampsia are similar to the symptoms and signs of preeclampsia, and it is typically diagnosed within 48 hours after delivery but can occur up to six weeks later.

When preeclampsia is associated with seizures (without the mother having epilepsy), it is known as "eclampsia."

Chronic Hypertension
Before or in Early Pregnancy

In this condition, a woman develops high blood pressure (more than or equal to 140/90 mmHg)* before conception or before 20 weeks of pregnancy.

Chronic Hypertension with Superimposed Preeclampsia
In the Early, Middle, or Late Pregnancy

This condition happens when there are elevated blood pressure readings of less than 160/110 mmHg in pregnant women who develop protein in their urine after 20 weeks of pregnancy or before 20 weeks of pregnancy with protein in urine and accompanying organ problems.

Gestational Hypertension
In Middle or Late Pregnancy

This condition happens when high blood pressure (more than or equal to 140/90 mmHg)* happens only during pregnancy, without the

---

* In November 2017, the American College of Cardiology (ACC) and the American Heart Association (AHA) updated the definition of chronic hypertension to be more than or equal to 130/80 mmHg instead of more than or equal to 140/90 mmHg.

presence of protein in the urine. It is typically diagnosed after 20 weeks of pregnancy or close to delivery. Gestational hypertension usually goes away after childbirth; however, affected women have an increased risk of developing chronic hypertension in the future.

Chapter 45

Hyperemesis Gravidarum (Severe Nausea and Vomiting)

Know What Morning Sickness Is

Experiencing bouts of nausea and vomiting is called "morning sickness," although unpleasant, it is considered a normal part of a healthy pregnancy. For most women, it occurs during the first trimester of pregnancy, i.e., around the sixth week of pregnancy, and subsequently improves or disappears around week 14. Despite the name "morning sickness," it can occur any time of the day or night. It usually needs no treatment and resolves or subsides on its own.

Know What Is Not Normal and What It Is Called

When morning sickness becomes severe, with persistent nausea and multiple episodes of vomiting per day (more than 50 times per day for some unfortunates), this medical condition needs treatment. The condition of excessive (hyper) vomiting (emesis) during pregnancy (gravidarum) is termed medically as "hyperemesis gravidarum (HG)."

"Hyperemesis Gravidarum (Severe Nausea and Vomiting)," © 2019 Omnigraphics. Reviewed February 2019.

About Hyperemesis Gravidarum

This is a rare pregnancy-related condition that follows a similar timeline to morning sickness (i.e., it begins between week 4 and 5 and lasts throughout the entire pregnancy). Sadly, health histories say that it may continue to happen in subsequent pregnancies for women who experience it during their first pregnancy. If left untreated, it can interfere with a woman's health, as well as the fetus's ability to thrive. There are many ways to manage this condition and minimize the risk of having a low-birth-weight baby.

Why Some Women Get Hyperemesis Gravidarum and Others Do Not

The exact etiology (cause) is still unknown, but "hormonal changes" and "hereditary reasons" are to blame.

- Human chorionic gonadotropin (HCG), when present at the highest level in a pregnant woman's body, can cause nausea.

- Hyperemesis gravidarum (HG) is commonly evident in a woman whose close family members, such as mothers and sisters, have had it. This is why researchers believe the condition might be hereditary.

A risk factor is something that increases a person's chances of getting the disease or condition, but does not mean that the person will necessarily develop that particular condition. In some cases, the following can put a woman into a high-risk category:

- Carrying multiples (twins, triplets, etc.)
- History of HG in previous pregnancy(ies)
- History of motion sickness
- History of migraine headaches with nausea and vomiting episodes

Know the Symptoms and Notice the Signs

- Prolonged nausea and vomiting (increasing in severity as pregnancy progresses)
- Food aversion/being unable to eat food (leading to more than 10-pound weight loss)

- Feeling dizzy and lightheaded (fainting) due to hypotension (low blood pressure) when standing

- Being unable to drink fluids (becoming dehydrated)

- Extreme fatigue and depression (leading to confusion and headaches)

Other possible symptoms one may experience in addition to the main symptoms are:

- Heightened sense of smell

- Ptyalism (excessive saliva production)

- Ketosis (buildup of acidic chemicals in blood and urine)

- Constipation, headaches, and decrease in urination (due to dehydration)

- Urinary incontinence due to bladder pressure caused by excessive vomiting in combination with relaxin hormone

- Rapid heart rate

- Loss of skin elasticity

- Pressure sores if one is bed-bound due to sickness

In addition to feeling unwell with some of the mentioned symptoms, you may also feel anxious about going out and about because of the need to vomit. This can result in feelings of isolation as some people may not fully understand what you are going through and question whether you can cope with the rest of the pregnancy.

Get It Diagnosed and Treated

Healthcare providers may take your medical history, inquire about your symptoms, perform a physical exam, and order some blood tests to diagnose HG. During the initial stage, they may recommend:

- Consuming a bland diet—with strict avoidance of spicy and fatty foods

- Eating frequent small meals, as well as dry crackers in the morning—as high-protein snacking will help maintain nutrition

- Complete bed rest—to provide comfort (but being bed-bound for a long time should be avoided as this may cause muscle loss and bed sores)

- Acupressure—applying pressure to some locations on the body to gently reduce nausea. These points are located three finger lengths away from the crease of the wrist, at the middle of the inner wrist, and between the two tendons. Three-minute pressure sessions and sea bands (pressure-point wrist bands available at a local drug store) can be of help.

- Herbs—using ginger or peppermint, especially in tea, might help

- Homeopathic remedies—these are usually effective and nontoxic medicines

- Hypnosis—to give mental strength and reduce depression and anxiety

Some cases of HG are severe and will not settle with above-mentioned treatment or lifestyle modifications, requiring hospitalization. Hospital treatment includes:

- Using tube feeding for a short period of time (not eating by mouth to rest gastrointestinal system). There are two types of tube feeding:

  - Nasogastric tube feeding, in which nutrients will be passed through a tube that passes through the nose into the stomach

  - Percutaneous endoscopic gastrostomy, in which nutrients will be passed through the abdomen into the stomach via a surgical method

- Intravenous (IV) fluids—to hydrate and restore electrolytes, nutrients, and vitamins

- Medications—such as antihistamines, metoclopramide, Promethazine, Meclizine, Droperidol, and other antireflux medications. It is always inadvisable to self-medicate with over-the-counter (OTC) drugs; have a doctor prescribe the proper dose and remedy instead.

One can feel better, reduce symptoms, and sometimes complete resolve symptoms with appropriate treatment.

References

1. "Hyperemesis Gravidarum," American Pregnancy Association, July 27, 2018.

2. Ben-Joseph, Elana Pearl MD. "Severe Morning Sickness (Hyperemesis Gravidarum)," KidsHealth®/The Nemours Foundation, April 2014.

3. "Hyperemesis Gravidarum (Severe Nausea and Vomiting during Pregnancy)," Cleveland Clinic, November 4, 2016.

Chapter 46

Placental Complications

Placenta and Its Role in Pregnancy

The placenta is a flat, circular organ attached to the wall of the womb (uterus) and the umbilical cord. The umbilical cord is a long muscular organ that links the fetus to the placenta. Normally, the placenta grows on the upper part of the uterus and can be seen in an ultrasound around week 18. It stays there until the fetus is delivered.

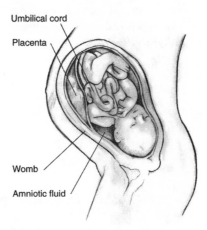

Figure 46.1. *Placenta* (Source: "NIDDK Image Library," National Institute of Diabetes and Digestive and Kidney Diseases (NIDDK).)

"Placental Complications," © 2019 Omnigraphics. Reviewed February 2019.

Some of the significant functions of the placenta are:

- It acts as a filter between the mother and fetus. It filters nutrients and oxygen from the mother's blood before reaching the fetus, as well as waste products, such as carbon dioxide, from the fetus to the mother's bloodstream for disposal. However, an intermingling of maternal and fetal blood does not occur here; in other words, it also maintains "no blood-to-blood contact" between the mother and fetus.

- It produces hormones that help the fetus grow and develop.

- It can protect the fetus against bacterial infections but cannot protect against viral infections.

- Towards the end of the pregnancy, it also passes some of the mother's antibodies to the fetus in order to give immunity to the fetus for about three months after birth.

How Is the Placenta Delivered?

If the fetus is delivered through the birth canal (vagina), it is called "vaginal/normal delivery." In such cases, the placenta will also be delivered vaginally. During the last (third) stage of labor (after childbirth), the uterine contractions continue and push the placenta to the vagina. On occasions, the healthcare provider might massage the lower abdomen to encourage uterine contractions in order to expel the placenta, and the mother might be asked to push again to deliver the placenta. When the placenta separates from the wall of the uterus and comes out of the vagina it is called "afterbirth."

If the fetus is delivered by cesarean section, then the healthcare provider will remove the placenta in its entirety from the uterus during the surgical procedure. They will examine the placenta to make sure it is intact and, if it is not intact, they remove any remaining fragments from the uterus completely in order to prevent bleeding and infection.

What Are the Factors That Affect Placental Health?

- Maternal age, if older than 35 (becoming pregnant after 40 years of age)

- High blood pressure in pregnant women (developed either before pregnancy or during pregnancy)

- Premature rupture of the membranes (the fluid-filled membrane that surrounds and cushions the fetus leaking or breaking before labor)

- Twin or other multiple pregnancies (if carrying more than one fetus)

- Substance abuse/misuse (smoking and illegal drug usage, such as cocaine, etc., during pregnancy).

- Trauma to the abdomen, such as a fall

- Previous surgery on the uterus, such as cesarean section or surgery to remove fibroids.

- Placental problem during the previous pregnancy

- Blood-clotting disorders (conditions that increase the likelihood of clotting)

Some drugs, alcohol, and nicotine can cross the placenta and cause damage to the fetus when used during pregnancy. So, it is best for pregnant women to be cautious and follow the healthcare provider's instructions.

What Are the Most Common Placental Complications?

The following are the complications that can affect the placenta during pregnancy or childbirth:

- **Placenta previa**—Also called "low-lying placenta." This is when the placenta develops low in the uterus and obstructs the passageway of childbirth. In such cases, vaginal delivery becomes impossible, necessitating a cesarean section. Risk factors include pregnancy after the age of 35, having scarring from a previous cesarean section or abortion, smoking or tobacco use during pregnancy, and having more than one delivery. Also, women with placenta previa may have placenta accreta; therefore, seeing the placenta positioned low in an ultrasound can be a red flag for placenta previa, or placenta accreta.

- **Invasive placenta**—This is when all or part of the placenta attaches deeply to the myometrium (muscular layer of the uterine wall). Based on the depth of the attachment, it is classified into three grades:

  - **Placenta accreta:** A deep and strong attachment of the placenta to the wall of the uterus, but without penetration.

- **Placenta increta:** A deeper attachment of the placenta, with penetration, to the muscle wall of the uterus.

- **Placenta percreta:** The placenta attaches itself to the uterus and grows through the uterus, sometimes invading/ extending itself to other organs such as the urinary bladder orrectum. Thisraises the complication of placenta attachment to other organs, such as the rectum, urinary bladder, etc.

This condition makes it difficult for the placenta to completely detach from the uterus during delivery or childbirth, leading to life-threatening excessive bleeding. During the ultrasound scan, if there is an unusually high blood flow of the uterus, it is considered as a sign of placenta accreta.

- **Placental insufficiency**—This is when the placenta is not providing adequate nutrients and/or blood flow to the fetus, leading to an increased likelihood of preeclampsia/toxemia (characterized by high blood pressure that occurs after 20 weeks of pregnancy) and infant developmental issues. Blood-related conditions, such as diabetes or hypertension, in the mother increases the risk of placental insufficiency.

- **Placental abruption**—This is an early detachment of the placenta from the wall of the uterus before delivery/childbirth and causes abdominal and/or uterine pain along with bloody-pregnancy discharge, contractions, and fast fetal heart rate. It commonly happens during the third trimester, but can happen anytime during pregnancy. The degree of detachment can range from mild (resolves with rest and monitoring) to severe (requires emergency delivery). If vaginal bleeding is evident at any point of pregnancy, contact the healthcare professional immediately.

- **Placental infarcts**—This is when areas of dead tissues called "infarcts" are present in the placenta, resulting in reduced blood flow. It is mainly caused by pregnancy-induced hypertension (gestational hypertension). In certain cases of severe hypertension, this blood flow reduction can be injurious to the fetus and, in extreme cases, leads to fetal death. Care should be taken to keep the blood pressure under control to avoid such scenarios.

How to Reduce the Risk of Placental Complications?

If pregnant women experience any of the following symptoms, it may be a sign of a placental health problem:

- Abdominal pain

- Uterine contraction

- Intolerable back pain

- Vaginal bleeding

Most of the placental problems cannot be prevented directly; however, one can take steps to promote placental health as a part of achieving a healthy pregnancy. For example:

- Regular follow-ups throughout the pregnancy as instructed by the healthcare provider, as they will note the position and size of the placenta in the subsequent follow-up ultrasound scans in order to rule out any abnormality and prevent further complications.

- Close monitoring, if the mother has any ongoing health conditions, such as high blood pressure, and being compliant with the advised treatment plan.

- Avoidance of smoking and other illegal drug/substance usage during pregnancy.

- If the mother had a placental problem during a previous pregnancy, it is appropriate to consult the healthcare provider regarding ways to reduce the risk of experiencing the same problem in the current pregnancy.

- Keeping the healthcare provider informed about any previous surgeries the mother had, especially in the abdomen or uterus.

References

1. "Complications of the Placenta," KidsHealth®/The Nemours Foundation, September 11, 2009.

2. "Pregnancy Complications," American Pregnancy Association, April 26, 2017.

3. "Types of Placental Disorders," Beth Israel Deaconess Medical Center, April 22, 2011.

Chapter 47

Rh Incompatibility

Rh incompatibility is a condition that occurs during pregnancy if a woman has Rh-negative blood and the fetus has Rh-positive blood. "Rh-negative" and "Rh-positive" refers to whether your blood has Rh factor. Rh factor is a protein on red blood cells (RBCs). If you have Rh factor, you are Rh-positive. If you do not have it, you are Rh-negative. Rh factor is inherited (passed from parents to children through the genes). Most people are Rh-positive. Rh factor does not affect your general health, whether you have it or not; however, it can cause problems during pregnancy.

With prompt and proper prenatal care and screening, you can prevent the problems of Rh incompatibility. Screening tests allow your doctor to find out early in your pregnancy whether you are at risk for the condition. If you are at risk, your doctor will carefully check on you and the fetus throughout your pregnancy and prescribe treatment as needed.

Injections of a medicine called "Rh immune globulin" can keep your body from making Rh antibodies. This medicine helps prevent the problems of Rh incompatibility. If you are Rh-negative, you will need this medicine every time you have a baby with Rh-positive blood.

Other events also can expose you to Rh-positive blood, which could affect a pregnancy. Examples include a miscarriage or blood transfusion. If you are treated with Rh immune globulin right after these

This chapter includes text excerpted from "Rh Incompatibility," National Heart, Lung, and Blood Institute (NHLBI), November 8, 2008. Reviewed February 2019.

events, you may be able to avoid Rh incompatibility during your next pregnancy.

Causes

A difference in blood type between a pregnant woman and the fetus causes Rh incompatibility. The condition occurs if a woman is Rh-negative and the fetus is Rh-positive. When you are pregnant, blood from the fetus can cross into your bloodstream, especially during delivery. If you are Rh-negative and the fetus is Rh-positive, your body will react to the fetus's blood as a foreign substance. Your body will create antibodies (proteins) against the fetus's Rh-positive blood. These antibodies can cross the placenta and attack the fetus's red blood cells. This can lead to hemolytic anemia in the fetus.

Rh incompatibility usually does not cause problems during a first pregnancy. The baby often is born before many of the antibodies develop. However, once you have formed Rh antibodies, they remain in your body. Thus, the condition is more likely to cause problems in second or later pregnancies (if the baby is Rh-positive).

With each pregnancy, your body continues to make Rh antibodies. As a result, each Rh-positive fetus becomes more at risk for serious problems, such as severe hemolytic anemia.

Risk Factors

An Rh-negative woman who conceives a child with an Rh-positive man is at risk for Rh incompatibility.

Rh factor is inherited (passed from parents to children through the genes). If you are Rh-negative and the father of the fetus is Rh-positive, the fetus has a 50 percent or more chance of having Rh-positive blood.

Simple blood tests can show whether you and the father of the fetus are Rh-positive or Rh-negative. If you are Rh-negative, your risk of problems from Rh incompatibility is higher if you were exposed to Rh-positive blood before the pregnancy. This may have happened during:

- An earlier pregnancy (usually during delivery). You also may have been exposed to Rh-positive blood if you had bleeding or abdominal trauma (for example, from a car accident) during the pregnancy.

- An ectopic pregnancy, a miscarriage, or an induced abortion (an ectopic pregnancy is a pregnancy that starts outside of the uterus, or womb)

- A mismatched blood transfusion or blood and marrow stem cell transplant

- An injection or puncture with a needle or other object containing Rh-positive blood

Certain tests also can expose you to Rh-positive blood. Examples include amniocentesis and chorionic villus sampling (CVS).

Amniocentesis is a test that you may have during pregnancy. Your doctor uses a needle to remove a small amount of fluid from the sac around the fetus. The fluid is then tested for various reasons.

CVS also may be done during pregnancy. For this test, your doctor threads a thin tube through the vagina and cervix to the placenta. She or he removes a tissue sample from the placenta using gentle suction. The tissue sample is tested for various reasons.

Unless you were treated with the medicine that prevents Rh antibodies (Rh immune globulin) after each of these events, you are at risk for Rh incompatibility during current and future pregnancies.

Screening and Prevention

Rh incompatibility can be prevented with Rh immune globulin, as long as the medicine is given at the correct times. Once you have formed Rh antibodies, the medicine will no longer help.

Thus, a woman who has Rh-negative blood must be treated with Rh immune globulin during and after each pregnancy or after any other event that allows her blood to mix with Rh-positive blood.

Early prenatal care also can help prevent some of the problems linked to Rh incompatibility. For example, your doctor can find out early whether you are at risk for the condition. If you are at risk, your doctor can closely monitor your pregnancy. She or he will watch for signs of hemolytic anemia in the fetus and provide treatment as needed.

Signs, Symptoms, and Complications

Rh incompatibility does not cause signs or symptoms in a pregnant woman. In a fetus, the condition can lead to hemolytic anemia. Hemolytic anemia is a condition in which red blood cells are destroyed faster than the body can replace them. Red blood cells contain hemoglobin, an iron-rich protein that carries oxygen to the body. Without enough red blood cells and hemoglobin, the fetus would not get enough oxygen. Hemolytic anemia can cause mild to severe signs and symptoms in a newborn, such as jaundice and a buildup of fluid.

Jaundice is a yellowish color of the skin and whites of the eyes. When red blood cells die, they release hemoglobin into the blood. The hemoglobin is broken down into a compound called "bilirubin." This compound gives the skin and eyes a yellowish color. High levels of bilirubin can lead to brain damage in the fetus.

The buildup of fluid is a result of heart failure. Without enough hemoglobin-carrying red blood cells, the fetus's heart has to work harder to move oxygen-rich blood through the body. This stress can lead to heart failure. Heart failure can cause fluid to build up in many parts of the body. When this occurs in a fetus or newborn, the condition is called "hydrops fetalis."

Severe hemolytic anemia can be fatal to a newborn at the time of birth or shortly after.

Diagnosis

Rh incompatibility is diagnosed with blood tests. To find out whether a fetus is developing hemolytic anemia and how serious it is, doctors may use more advanced tests, such as ultrasound.

Specialists Involved

An obstetrician will screen for Rh incompatibility. This is a doctor who specializes in treating pregnant women. The obstetrician also will monitor the pregnancy and the fetus for problems related to hemolytic anemia. She or he also will oversee treatment to prevent problems with future pregnancies.

A pediatrician or hematologist treats newborns who have hemolytic anemia and related problems. A pediatrician is a doctor who specializes in treating children. A hematologist is a doctor who specializes in treating people who have blood diseases and disorders.

Diagnostic Tests

If you are pregnant, your doctor will order a simple blood test at your first prenatal visit to learn whether you are Rh-positive or Rh-negative.

If you are Rh-negative, you also may have another blood test called an "antibody screen." This test shows whether you have Rh antibodies in your blood. If you do, it means that you were exposed to Rh-positive blood before and you are at risk for Rh incompatibility.

If you are Rh-negative and you do not have Rh antibodies, the father also will be tested to find out his Rh type. If he is Rh-negative too, the fetus has no chance of having Rh-positive blood. Thus, there is no risk of Rh incompatibility.

However, if the father is Rh-positive, the fetus has a 50 percent or more chance of having Rh-positive blood. As a result, you are at high risk of developing Rh incompatibility.

If the father is Rh-positive, or if it is not possible to find out his Rh status, your doctor may do a test called "amniocentesis."

For this test, your doctor inserts a hollow needle through your abdominal wall into your uterus. She or he removes a small amount of fluid from the sac around the fetus. The fluid is tested to learn whether the fetus is Rh-positive. (Rarely, an amniocentesis can expose you to Rh-positive blood). Your doctor also may use this test to measure bilirubin levels of the fetus. Bilirubin builds up as a result of red blood cells dying too quickly. The higher the level of bilirubin is, the greater the chance that the fetus has hemolytic anemia.

If Rh incompatibility is known or suspected, you will be tested for Rh antibodies one or more times during your pregnancy. This test often is done at least once at your sixth or seventh month of pregnancy. The results from this test also can suggest how severe the fetus's hemolytic anemia has become. Higher levels of antibodies suggest more severe hemolytic anemia.

To check the fetus for hemolytic anemia, your doctor also may use a test called "Doppler ultrasound." She or he will use this test to measure how fast blood is flowing through an artery in the fetus's head.

Doppler ultrasound uses sound waves to measure how fast blood is moving. The faster the blood flow is, the greater the risk of hemolytic anemia. This is because the anemia will cause the fetus's heart to pump more blood.

Treatment

The goals of treating Rh incompatibility are to ensure that the fetus is healthy and to lower your risk for the condition in future pregnancies. Rh incompatibility is treated with a medicine called "Rh immune globulin." Treatment for a fetus who has hemolytic anemia will vary based on the severity of the condition.

Treatment for Rh Incompatibility

If Rh incompatibility is diagnosed during your pregnancy, you will receive Rh immune globulin in your seventh month of pregnancy and again within 72 hours of delivery.

You also may receive Rh immune globulin if the risk of blood transfer between you and the fetus is high (e.g., if you have had a miscarriage, ectopic pregnancy, or bleeding during pregnancy).

Rh immune globulin contains Rh antibodies that attach to the Rh-positive blood cells in your blood. When this happens, your body does not react to the fetus's Rh-positive cells as a foreign substance. As a result, your body does not make Rh antibodies. Rh immune globulin must be given at the correct times to work properly.

Once you have formed Rh antibodies, the medicine will no longer help. That is why a woman who has Rh-negative blood must be treated with the medicine with each pregnancy or any other event that allows her blood to mix with Rh-positive blood.

Rh immune globulin is injected into the muscle of your arm or buttock. Side effects may include soreness at the injection site and a slight fever. The medicine also may be injected into a vein.

Treatment for Hemolytic Anemia

Several options are available for treating hemolytic anemia in a fetus. In mild cases, no treatment may be needed. If treatment is needed, the fetus may be given a medicine called "erythropoietin" and iron supplements. These treatments can prompt the body to make red blood cells.

If the hemolytic anemia is severe, the fetus may get a blood transfusion through the umbilical cord. If the hemolytic anemia is severe and the fetus is almost full-term, your doctor may induce labor early. This allows the baby's doctor to begin treatment right away.

A newborn who has severe anemia may be treated with a blood exchange transfusion. The procedure involves slowly removing the newborn's blood and replacing it with fresh blood or plasma from a donor.

Newborns also may be treated with special lights to reduce the amount of bilirubin in their blood. These babies may have jaundice (a yellowish color of the skin and whites of the eyes). High levels of bilirubin cause jaundice.

Reducing the blood's bilirubin level is important because high levels of this compound can cause brain damage. High levels of bilirubin often are seen in babies who have hemolytic anemia. This is because the compound forms when red blood cells break down.

Chapter 48

Umbilical Cord Abnormalities

A narrow tube-like structure, the umbilical cord, serves as the primary connection between the mother and the fetus. It connects the developing fetus to the placenta. The cord is also called the fetus's "supply line" as it delivers oxygen and nutrients to the fetus, carries blood back and forth between the fetus and the placenta, and removes the fetus's waste products.

After a woman conceives, the umbilical cord starts to develop after 5 weeks of conception. It gradually becomes longer, until 28 weeks of pregnancy, reaching 22 to 24 inches in length. The cord comprises three blood vessels: two arteries and one vein. The waste is removed from the fetus to the placenta by the arteries (waste is transferred to the mother's blood and is disposed of by her kidneys). The vein transports oxygen and nutrients from the placenta (connected to mother's blood supply) to the developing fetus. Wharton's jelly, a gelatin-like tissue, protects these blood vessels. The cord is literally the fetus's lifeline, and it cannot survive the gestational period without the umbilical cord. However, there are several cord abnormalities that can occur that are medical emergencies and need immediate medical attention.

There are numerous cord abnormalities from false knots that do not have adverse effects on the fetus or mom to vasa previa, which often leads to fetal death. Problems of the cord can occur

---

"Umbilical Cord Abnormalities," © 2017 Omnigraphics. Reviewed February 2019.

during pregnancy or during labor and delivery. In a few cases, they are found before delivery through an ultrasound; but they are usually found only during delivery when there is direct examination of the cord. Some common umbilical cord abnormalities are discussed below.

Umbilical Cord Prolapse

The prolapse happens when the umbilical cord slips through the cervix into the vagina before the fetus descends into the birth canal. Normally, the fetus comes out first through the birth canal trailing the umbilical cord behind it. The prolapse can cause the cord to be wrapped around the fetus's body or get trapped in the birth canal that leads to further complications. The fetus's oxygen supply may decrease as the pressure on the cord reduces or cuts off blood flow from the placenta to the fetus. Around 1 in 300 births experience cord prolapse. Some common reasons for the prolapse include:

- Breech delivery (foot-first) position

- Preterm labor

- Excessive amount of amniotic fluid

- The umbilical cord is unusually long

- Healthcare provider ruptures the membranes to speed up labor

The cord prolapse is a medical emergency and needs immediate medical attention; the doctor can confirm the prolapse by doing a pelvic examination. After the membranes (bag of waters) have ruptured, if the healthcare provider detects heart rate abnormalities in the fetus, umbilical cord prolapse may be a possibility. Pressure on the cord must be lifted immediately, and the mother should be made ready for prompt cesarean delivery in the case of emergency.

Single Umbilical Artery

In this particular cord abnormality, the umbilical cord has only two blood vessels instead of three. There is only one artery and one vein; mostly the left artery is absent. About 1 percent of cords in singletons and 5 percent of cords in multiple pregnancies (twins, triplets, and more) have this abnormality, the cause of which is unknown. Central nervous system problems, urinary tract defects, and heart and chromosomal abnormalities are some of the risks in single umbilical artery for infants. An ultrasound helps to identify the abnormality, and healthcare providers may suggest certain prenatal tests to rule out birth defects; tests can include a detailed ultrasound and echocardiography (fetal heart evaluation through special ultrasound).

Vasa Previa

The terms "vasa" and "previa" mean "vessels" and "before," respectively, in Latin. Vasa previa occurs when blood vessels from the cord or placenta crosses the cervix below the fetus's positioning. The blood vessels may tear when the membrane ruptures or the cervix dilates as they are unprotected by the Wharton's jelly in the cord or tissue in the placenta. Even if they do not tear, the pressure on the blood vessels may make the fetus suffer due to lack of oxygen.

This condition occurs in 1 of 2,500 births; it can be diagnosed during pregnancy by doing an ultrasound. Fetal deaths can be prevented by performing a cesarean section at about 35 weeks of gestation. However, most of the affected babies are stillborn when vasa previa is diagnosed at delivery.

Painless vaginal bleeding can occur in pregnant woman with vasa previa; hence, when the bleeding happens, a healthcare provider needs to be consulted to avoid future complications. The risk for vasa previa can be increased if a pregnant woman:

- Is expecting multiple pregnancies (twins, triplets, or more)

- Has a velamentous insertion (instead of insertion of umbilical cord in the center of the placenta, the cord is inserted into the fetal membranes)

- Has placenta previa (low-lying placenta)

Umbilical Cord Knots

Umbilical cord knots happen during pregnancy or delivery. Knot formation during pregnancy can happen while the fetus moves around in the amniotic fluid. If the umbilical cord is long, knots can occur. If the knot remains loose the fetus is unaffected; however, if the knots tighten then the fetus's oxygen supply can get cut off, leading to heart rate abnormalities. It can also result in miscarriage and stillbirth. Knots can form during the delivery when the fetus with a nuchal loop (umbilical cord wrapped around the fetus's neck) is pulled through the loop.

Umbilical Cord Cyst

An abnormal growth on the umbilical cord is known as the "umbilical cord cyst." There are true and false cysts.

- True cysts are remaining cells from fetal development

- False cysts are filled with fluid

Research suggests that both types of cysts can lead to birth defects—they include kidney defects, abdominal defects, and chromosomal abnormalities. The healthcare provider may conduct tests to rule out birth defects after an ultrasound confirms umbilical cord cysts. They are usually detected and treated during the first trimester.

Nuchal Cord

The nuchal cord is the umbilical cord wrapped around the fetus's neck. Also known as nuchal loops, they rarely cause any problems. Almost 25 percent of the fetuses are born with a nuchal loop, and they are generally healthy. An ultrasound may show some heart rate abnormalities during labor and delivery for fetuses with a nuchal cord because of the pressure on the cord. However, the pressure is not serious to cause fetal death or other major complications. Even if the nuchal cord is wrapped around other parts of the fetus's body, it causes no harm. Rarely a cesarean delivery is required for fetuses with a nuchal loop.

Cord Stricture

Cord stricture is a sharp narrowing of the umbilical cord, which is a common cause of fetal death during second trimester before birth. The cause of this condition is unknown. An early detection in cord stricture is difficult; hence the risk of fetal death is increased.

However, even if the baby survives, a few medical conditions such as septal defects, cleft lip, and trisomy 18 can occur.

References

1. "Complications and Loss—Umbilical Cord Abnormalities," March of Dimes, February 2008.

2. Beall, Marie Helen; Isaacs, Christine. "Umbilical Cord Complications," Medscape, September 9, 2015.

3. Jick, Bryan. "Umbilical Cord Abnormalities," Pregnancy Corner, June 2017.

4. "Umbilical Cord Problems," Birth Injury Guide, n.d.

Chapter 49

Sexually Transmitted Diseases during Pregnancy

Chapter Contents

Section 49.1

Sexually Transmitted Diseases Can Complicate Pregnancy

This section includes text excerpted from "STDs during Pregnancy—CDC Fact Sheet (Detailed)," Centers for Disease Control and Prevention (CDC), February 11, 2016.

Sexually transmitted diseases (STDs) can complicate pregnancy and may have serious consequences for both a woman and the fetus. Healthcare providers caring for pregnant women, play a key role in safeguarding the health of both a mother and the fetus.

A critical component of appropriate prenatal care is ensuring that pregnant patients are tested for STDs. Pregnant women should be tested for STDs early in their pregnancy with tests being repeated close to delivery when needed. Have open, honest conversations with your healthcare providers and your sex partners about symptoms they have experienced or are currently experiencing and any high-risk sexual behaviors in which they engage. The table below outlines screening recommendations from the Centers for Disease Control and Prevention (CDC) for healthcare providers, so you can be sure of what to expect.

Table 49.1. Screening Recommendations for Pregnant Women

Disease	CDC Recommendation
Chlamydia	First prenatal visit: Screen all pregnant women <25 years of age and older pregnant women at increased risk for infection. Third trimester: Rescreen if <25 years of age or at continued high risk. Risk factors: • New or multiple sex partners • Sex partner with concurrent partners • Sex partner who has a sexually transmitted disease (STD) **NOTE:** Pregnant women found to have chlamydial infection should have a test-of-cure three to four weeks after treatment and then be retested within three months.
Gonorrhea	First prenatal visit: Screen all pregnant women <25 years of age and older pregnant women at increased risk for gonorrhea at first prenatal visit. Third trimester: Rescreen for women at continued high risk. Risk factors: • Living in a high-morbidity area

Table 49.1. Continued

Disease	CDC Recommendation
	• Previous or coexisting STI • New or multiple sex partners • Inconsistent condom use among persons not in mutually monogamous relationships • Exchanging sex for money or drugs
Syphilis	First prenatal visit: Screen all pregnant women. Early third trimester: Rescreen women who are • At high risk for syphilis, • Who live in areas with high numbers of syphilis cases, and/or • Who were not previously tested, or had a positive test in the first trimester.
Bacterial Vaginosis (BV)	Evidence does not support routine screening for BV in asymptomatic pregnant women at high or low risk for preterm delivery.
Trichomoniasis	Evidence does not support routine screening for trichomoniasis in asymptomatic pregnant women.
Herpes (HSV)	Evidence does not support routine HSV-2 serologic testing among asymptomatic pregnant women.
Human Immunodeficiency Virus (HIV)	First prenatal visit: Screen all pregnant women. Third trimester: Rescreen women at high risk for acquiring HIV infection.
Hepatitis B (HBV)	First prenatal visit: Screen all pregnant women. Third trimester: Test those who were not screened prenatally, those who engage in behaviors that put them at high risk for infection, and those with signs or symptoms of hepatitis at the time of admission to the hospital for delivery. Risk factors: • Having had more than one sex partner in the previous six months • Evaluation or treatment for an STD • Recent or current injection-drug use • An HBsAg-positive sex partner
Human Papillomavirus (HPV)	There are no screening recommendations for HPV.
Hepatitis C (HCV)	First prenatal visit: Screen all pregnant women at increased risk. Risk factors: • Past or current injection-drug use • Having received a blood transfusion before July 1992 • Receipt of unregulated tattoo Long-term dialysis • Known exposure to HCV

Sexually Transmitted Diseases Impact on a Woman and the Fetus

It is crucial to be aware of the ways in which each STD can impact a pregnant woman and a fetus.

Bacterial Vaginosis

Bacterial vaginosis (BV), a common cause of vaginal discharge in women of childbearing age, is a polymicrobial clinical syndrome resulting from a change in the vaginal community of bacteria. Although, BV is often not considered an STD, it has been linked to sexual activity. Women may have no symptoms or may complain of a foul-smelling, fishy, vaginal discharge. BV during pregnancy has been associated with serious pregnancy complications, including premature rupture of the membranes surrounding the fetus in the uterus, preterm labor, premature birth, chorioamnionitis (an infection that occurs before or during labor) as well as endometritis. While there is no evidence to support screening for BV in pregnant women at high risk for preterm delivery, symptomatic women should be evaluated and treated. There are no known direct effects of BV on the newborn.

Chlamydia

Chlamydia is the most common sexually transmitted bacterium in the United States. Although, the majority of chlamydial infections (including those in pregnant women) do not have symptoms, infected women may have abnormal vaginal discharge, bleeding after sex, or itching/burning with urination. Untreated chlamydial infection has been linked to problems during pregnancy, including preterm labor, premature rupture of membranes, and low birth weight. The newborn may also become infected during delivery as the baby passes through the birth canal. Exposed newborns can develop eye and lung infections.

Gonorrhea

Gonorrhea is a common STD in the United States. Untreated gonococcal infection in pregnancy has been linked to miscarriages, premature birth and low birth weight, premature rupture of membranes, and chorioamnionitis. Gonorrhea can also infect an infant during delivery as the infant passes through the birth canal. If untreated, infants can develop eye infections. Because gonorrhea can cause problems in both the mother and the fetus, it is important for healthcare providers to accurately identify the infection, treat it with effective antibiotics, and closely follow up to make sure that the infection has been cured.

Hepatitis B

Hepatitis B is a liver infection caused by the hepatitis B virus (HBV). A mother can transmit the infection to the fetus during pregnancy. While the risk of an infected mother passing HBV to the fetus varies, depending on when she becomes infected, the greatest risk happens when mothers become infected close to the time of delivery. Infected newborns also have a high risk (up to 90%) of becoming chronic HBV carriers themselves. Infants who have a lifelong infection with HBV are at an increased risk for developing chronic liver disease or liver cancer later in life. Approximately 25 percent of infants who develop chronic HBV infection will eventually die from chronic liver disease. By being screened for the infection and treatment being provided to at-risk infants shortly after birth, steps can be taken to help prevent mother-to-child transmission of HBV.

Hepatitis C

Hepatitis C is a liver infection caused by the hepatitis C virus (HCV), and can be passed from an infected mother to the fetus during pregnancy. In general, an infected mother will transmit the infection to the fetus 10 percent of the time, but the chances are higher in certain subgroups, such as women who are also infected with HIV. In some studies, infants born to HCV-infected women have been shown to have an increased risk for being small for gestational age, premature, and having a low birth weight. Newborn infants with HCV infection usually do not have symptoms, and a majority will clear the infection without any medical help.

Herpes Simplex Virus

Herpes simplex virus (HSV) has two distinct virus types that can infect the human genital tract, HSV-1 and HSV-2. Infections of the newborn can be of either type, but most are caused by HSV-2. Generally, the symptoms of genital herpes are similar in pregnant and in nonpregnant women; however, the major concern regarding HSV infection relates to complications linked to infection of the newborn. Although transmission may occur during pregnancy and after delivery, the risk of transmission to the fetus from an infected mother is high among women who acquire genital herpes near the time of delivery and low among women with recurrent herpes or who acquire the infection during the first half of pregnancy. HSV infection can have very serious effects on newborns, especially if the mother's first outbreak occurred during the third trimester. Cesarean section is recommended for all women in labor with active genital herpes lesions or early symptoms, such as vulvar pain and itching.

Human Immunodeficiency Virus

Human immunodeficiency virus (HIV) is the virus that causes acquired immune deficiency syndrome, or acquired immunodeficiency syndrome (AIDS). HIV destroys specific blood cells that are crucial to helping the body fight diseases. According to the CDC's 2016 HIV surveillance data, women make up 24 percent of all adults and adolescents living with diagnosed HIV infection in the United States. The most common ways that HIV passes from mother to child are during pregnancy, labor and delivery, or through breastfeeding. However, when HIV is diagnosed before or during pregnancy and appropriate steps are taken, the risk of mother-to-child transmission can be lowered to less than two percent. A mother who knows early in her pregnancy that she is HIV-positive has more time to consult with her healthcare provider and decide on effective ways to protect her health and that of the fetus.

Human Papillomavirus

Human papillomaviruses (HPV) are viruses that most commonly involve the lower genital tract, including the cervix, vagina, and external genitalia. Genital warts frequently increase in number and size during pregnancy. Genital warts often appear as small cauliflower-like clusters which may burn or itch. If a woman has genital warts during pregnancy, treatment may be delayed until after delivery. When large or spread out, genital warts can complicate a vaginal delivery. In cases where there are large genital warts that are blocking the birth canal, a cesarean section may be recommended. Infection of the mother may be linked to the development of laryngeal papillomatosis in the newborn—a rare, noncancerous growth in the larynx.

Syphilis

Syphilis is primarily a sexually transmitted disease, but it may be transmitted to a fetus by an infected mother during pregnancy. Transmission of syphilis to a fetus can lead to a serious multisystem infection, known as "congenital syphilis." Recently, there has been a sharp increase in the number of congenital syphilis cases in the United States. Syphilis has been linked to premature births, stillbirths, and, in some cases, death shortly after birth. Untreated infants that survive tend to develop problems in multiple organs, including the brain, eyes, ears, heart, skin, teeth, and bones.

Trichomoniasis

Vaginal infection due to the sexually transmitted parasite Trichomonas vaginalis is very common. Although most people report no symptoms, others complain of itching, irritation, unusual odor, discharge, and pain during urination or sex. If a pregnant woman has symptoms of trichomoniasis, she will be evaluated for Trichomonas vaginalis and treated appropriately. Infection in pregnancy has been linked to premature rupture of membranes, preterm birth, and low birth-weight infants. Rarely, the female newborn can acquire the infection when passing through the birth canal during delivery and have vaginal discharge after birth.

Screening and prompt treatment are recommended at least annually for all HIV-infected women, based on the high prevalence of T. vaginalis infection, the increased risk of pelvic inflammatory disease (PID) associated with this infection, and the ability of treatment to reduce genital-tract viral load and vaginal HIV shedding. This includes HIV-infected women who are pregnant, as T. vaginalis infection is a risk factor for vertical transmission of HIV. For other pregnant women, screening may be considered at the discretion of the treating clinician, as the benefit of routine screening for pregnant women has not been established. Screening might be considered for persons receiving care in high-prevalence settings (e.g., STD clinics or correctional facilities) and for asymptomatic (showing no symptoms) persons at high risk for infection. Decisions about screening might be informed by local epidemiology of T. vaginalis infection. However, data are lacking on whether screening and treatment for asymptomatic trichomoniasis in high prevalence settings or persons at high risk can reduce any adverse health events and health disparities or reduce community burden of infection.

Sexually Transmitted Disease Treatment during Pregnancy

STDs, such as chlamydia, gonorrhea, syphilis, and trichomoniasis can all be treated and cured with antibiotics that are safe to take during pregnancy. Viral STDs, including genital herpes, hepatitis B, and HIV cannot be cured. However, in some cases these infections can be treated with antiviral medications or other preventive measures to reduce the risk of passing the infection to the fetus.

Sexually Transmitted Disease Prevention during Pregnancy

The most reliable way to avoid transmission of STDs is to abstain from oral, vaginal, and anal sex or to be in a long-term, mutually monogamous relationship with a partner known to be uninfected. For women who are being treated for an STD other than HIV (or whose partners are undergoing treatment), abstinence from sexual intercourse until completion of treatment can be helpful. Latex male condoms, when used consistently and correctly, can reduce the risk of transmitting or acquiring STDs and HIV.

Section 49.2

Sexually Transmitted Disease and Pregnancy FAQs

This section includes text excerpted from "STDs during Pregnancy—CDC Fact Sheet," Centers for Disease Control and Prevention (CDC), March 28, 2016.

If you are pregnant, you can become infected with the same sexually transmitted diseases (STDs) as women who are not pregnant. Pregnant women should ask their doctors about getting tested for STDs, since some doctors do not routinely perform these tests.

I'm Pregnant. Can I Get a Sexually Transmitted Disease?

Yes, you can. Women who are pregnant can become infected with the same STDs as women who are not pregnant. Pregnancy does not provide women or their fetus's any additional protection against STDs. Many STDs are 'silent,' or have no symptoms, so you may not know if you are infected. If you are pregnant, you should be tested for STDs, including human immunodeficiency virus (HIV), as a part of your medical care during pregnancy. The results of an STD can be more serious, even life-threatening, for you and the fetus if you become infected while pregnant. It is important that you are aware of the harmful effects of STDs and how to protect yourself and the fetus against infection. If you are diagnosed with an STD while pregnant, your sex partner(s) should also be tested and treated.

How Can Sexually Transmitted Diseases Affect Me and the Fetus?

STDs can complicate your pregnancy and may have serious effects on both you and the fetus. Some of these problems may be seen at birth; others may not be discovered until months or years later. In addition, it is well known that infection with an STD can make it easier for a person to get infected with HIV. Most of these problems can be prevented if you receive regular medical care during pregnancy. This includes tests for STDs starting early in pregnancy and repeated close to delivery, as needed.

Should I Be Tested for Sexually Transmitted Diseases during My Pregnancy?

Yes. Testing and treating pregnant women for STDs is a vital way to prevent serious health complications to both mother and fetus that may otherwise happen with infection. The sooner you begin receiving medical care during pregnancy, the better the health outcomes will be for you and the fetus. The Centers for Disease Control and Prevention's (CDC) 2015 STD Treatment Guidelines recommend screening pregnant women for STDs.

Be sure to ask your doctor about getting tested for STDs. It is also important that you have an open, honest conversation with your provider and discuss any symptoms you are experiencing and any high-risk sexual behavior that you engage in, since some doctors do not routinely perform these tests. Even if you have been tested in the past, you should be tested again when you become pregnant.

Can I Get Treated for a Sexually Transmitted Disease While I'm Pregnant?

It depends. STDs, such as chlamydia, gonorrhea, syphilis, trichomoniasis, and BV can all be treated and cured with antibiotics that are safe to take during pregnancy. STDs that are caused by viruses, such as genital herpes, hepatitis B, or HIV cannot be cured. However, in some cases these infections can be treated with antiviral medications or other preventive measures to reduce the risk of passing the infection to the fetus. If you are pregnant or considering pregnancy, you should be tested so you can take steps to protect yourself and your baby.

How Can I Reduce My Risk of Getting a Sexually Transmitted Disease While Pregnant?

The only way to avoid STDs is to not have vaginal, anal, or oral sex.

If you are sexually active, you can do the following things to lower your chances of getting chlamydia:

- Being in a long-term mutually monogamous relationship with a partner who has been tested and has negative STD test results

- Using latex condoms the right way every time you have sex

Chapter 50

Hepatitis B and Pregnancy

What Is Hepatitis B?

Hepatitis B is a liver infection caused by the hepatitis B (HBV) virus. Hepatitis B can range from a mild illness lasting a few weeks to a serious, lifelong illness.

- Acute hepatitis B is a short-term illness that occurs within the first six months after someone is exposed to the hepatitis B virus. An acute infection can range in severity from a mild illness with few or no symptoms to a serious condition requiring hospitalization. Some people, especially adults, are able to clear the virus without treatment. People who clear the virus become immune and cannot get infected with the hepatitis B virus again. Acute infection can— but does not always—lead to chronic infection.

- Chronic hepatitis B is a lifelong infection with the hepatitis B virus. Over time, chronic hepatitis B can cause serious health problems, including liver damage, cirrhosis, liver cancer, and even death.

How Is Hepatitis B Spread?

The hepatitis B virus is spread when blood, semen, or other body fluid infected with the hepatitis B virus enters the body of

This chapter includes text excerpted from "Hepatitis B Questions and Answers for the Public," Centers for Disease Control and Prevention (CDC), May 22, 2018.

a person who is not infected. People can become infected with the virus from:

- Birth (spread from an infected mother to her baby during birth)
- Sex with an infected partner
- Sharing needles, syringes, or drug preparation equipment
- Sharing items such as toothbrushes, razors, or medical equipment such as a glucose monitor with an infected person
- Direct contact with the blood or open sores of an infected person
- Exposure to blood from needlesticks or other sharp instruments of an infected person

Hepatitis B virus is not spread through food or water, sharing eating utensils, breastfeeding, hugging, kissing, hand holding, coughing, or sneezing.

Who Is at Risk for Hepatitis B?

Although anyone can get hepatitis B, some people are at greater risk:

- Infants born to infected mothers
- People who inject drugs or share needles, syringes, or other drug equipment
- Sex partners of people with hepatitis B
- Men who have sexual contact with men
- People who live with a person who has hepatitis B
- Healthcare and public safety workers exposed to blood on the job
- Hemodialysis patients

What Are the Symptoms of Acute Hepatitis B?

Symptoms of acute hepatitis B, if they appear, can include:

- Fever
- Fatigue
- Loss of appetite
- Nausea

- Vomiting
- Abdominal pain
- Dark urine
- Clay-colored bowel movements
- Joint pain
- Jaundice (yellow color in the skin or the eyes)

Can Hepatitis B Be Prevented?

Yes. The best way to prevent hepatitis B is by getting vaccinated. The hepatitis B vaccine is safe and effective. Completing the series of shots is needed for full protection.

Are There Reasons to Get Tested for Hepatitis B Immunity?

There are many different reasons for a person to get a blood test that looks for hepatitis B immunity through the presence of surface antibody (anti-HBs). The test is especially important for people who may or have been exposed to the blood of a person infected with the hepatitis B virus. This includes:

- Infants born to mothers with hepatitis B
- Healthcare Providers
- Hemodialysis patients
- Sex partners of someone with hepatitis B
- Any other people that have an ongoing risk for exposure to the blood of an infected person

The test can help determine if the person needs another dose of the hepatitis B vaccine in order to help give them further protection against infection.

Are Pregnant Women Tested for Hepatitis B?

Yes. When a pregnant woman comes in for prenatal care, she will be given a series of routine blood tests, including one that checks for the presence of hepatitis B virus infection.

If a Pregnant Woman Has Hepatitis B, Is There a Way to Prevent Her Baby from Getting Hepatitis B?

Yes, almost all cases of hepatitis B can be prevented if a baby born to an infected woman receives the necessary shots at the recommended times. The infant should receive a shot called "hepatitis B immune globulin" (HBIG) and the first dose of hepatitis B vaccine within 12 hours of birth. Two or three additional shots of vaccine are needed over the next 1 to 6 months to help prevent hepatitis B. The timing and the total number of shots will be influenced by several factors, including the type of vaccine given and the baby's age and birth weight. In addition, experts recommend that the baby get an antibody test 1 to 2 months after completion of the vaccine series at age 9 to 12 months to make sure she or he is protected from the disease. To best protect your baby, follow the advice from your baby's doctor.

What Happens If a Baby Gets Hepatitis B

Newborns who become infected with the hepatitis B virus have a 90 percent chance of developing chronic hepatitis B. This can eventually lead to serious health problems, including liver damage, liver cancer, and even death.

Why Is the Hepatitis B Vaccine Recommended for All Babies?

Hepatitis B vaccination is recommended for all babies to protect them from this serious but preventable disease. Babies and young children are at much greater risk for developing a chronic infection if infected with the hepatitis B virus, but the vaccine is highly effective in preventing the infection.

How Does the Hepatitis B Vaccine Work?

The hepatitis B vaccine stimulates your natural immune system to protect against the hepatitis B virus. After the vaccine is given, your body makes antibodies that protect you against the virus. An antibody is a substance found in the blood that is produced in response to a virus invading the body. These antibodies will fight off the infection if a person is exposed to the hepatitis B virus in the future.

Who Should Get Vaccinated against Hepatitis B?

Hepatitis B vaccination is recommended for:

- All infants
- All children and adolescents younger than 19 years of age who have not been vaccinated
- People at risk for infection by sexual exposure
- People whose sex partners have hepatitis B
  - Sexually active people who are not in a long-term, mutually monogamous relationship (for example, people with more than one sex partner during the previous 6 months)
  - People seeking evaluation or treatment for a sexually transmitted infection
  - Men who have sex with men (MSM)
- People at risk for infection by exposure to blood
- People who share needles, syringes, or other drug preparation equipment
  - People who live with a person who has hepatitis B
  - Residents and staff of facilities for developmentally disabled people
  - Healthcare and public safety workers at risk for exposure to blood or blood-contaminated body fluids on the job
  - Hemodialysis patients and predialysis, peritoneal dialysis, and home dialysis patients
  - People with diabetes aged 19 to 59 years; People with diabetes aged 60 or older should ask their healthcare professional.
- International travelers to countries where hepatitis B is common
- People with hepatitis C virus infection
- People with chronic liver disease
- People with human immunodeficiency virus (HIV) infection
- People who are in jail or prison
- All other people seeking protection from hepatitis B virus infection

411

Are Booster Doses of the Hepatitis B Vaccine Necessary?

It depends. A "booster" dose of hepatitis B vaccine is a dose that increases or extends the effectiveness of the vaccine. Booster doses are not recommended for most healthy people. Booster doses are recommended only in certain circumstances, and the need for booster doses is determined by a certain blood test that looks for hepatitis B surface antibody (anti-HBs).

Chapter 51

Mother-to-Child Transmission of Human Immunodeficiency Virus

What Is Mother-to-Child Transmission of Human Immunodeficiency Virus?

Mother-to-child transmission of human immunodeficiency virus (HIV) is the spread of HIV from a woman living with HIV to her child during pregnancy, childbirth (also called "labor and delivery"), or breastfeeding (through breast milk). Mother-to-child transmission of HIV is also called "perinatal transmission of HIV."

Can Mother-to-Child Transmission of Human Immunodeficiency Virus Be Prevented?

Yes. The use of HIV medicines and other strategies have helped to lower the risk of mother-to-child transmission of HIV to one percent or less in the United States and Europe. The risk of transmission is low when:

- HIV is detected as early as possible during pregnancy (or before a woman gets pregnant).

This chapter includes text excerpted from "Preventing Mother-to-Child Transmission of HIV," AIDS*info*, U.S. Department of Health and Human Services (HHS), December 17, 2018.

- Women with HIV receive HIV medicines during pregnancy and childbirth and, in certain situations, have a scheduled cesarean delivery (sometimes called a "C-section").

- Babies born to women with HIV receive HIV medicines for 4 to 6 weeks after birth and are not breastfed.

Is Human Immunodeficiency Virus Testing Recommended for Pregnant Women?

The Centers for Disease Control and Prevention (CDC) recommends that all women get tested for HIV before they become pregnant or as early as possible in their pregnancy. Women should be tested for HIV again during every pregnancy.

Pregnant women with HIV receive HIV medicines to reduce the risk of mother-to-child transmission of HIV and to protect their own health. HIV medicines are recommended for everyone who has HIV. HIV medicines help people with HIV live longer, healthier lives and reduce the risk of HIV transmission.

How Do Human Immunodeficiency Virus Medicines Prevent Mother-to-Child Transmission of Human Immunodeficiency Virus?

HIV medicines work by preventing HIV from multiplying, which reduces the amount of HIV in the body (also called the "viral load"). Having less HIV in the body protects a woman's health and reduces her risk of passing HIV to her child during pregnancy and childbirth.

Some HIV medicines pass from the pregnant woman to the fetus across the placenta (also called the "afterbirth"). This transfer of HIV medicines protects the fetus from HIV infection, especially during a vaginal delivery when the fetus passes through the birth canal and is exposed to any HIV in the mother's blood or other fluids. In some situations, a woman with HIV may have a cesarean delivery to reduce the risk of mother-to-child transmission of HIV during delivery.

Babies born to women with HIV receive HIV medicines for four to six weeks after birth. HIV medicines reduce the risk of infection from any HIV that may have entered a baby's body during childbirth.

Are Human Immunodeficiency Virus Medicines Safe to Use during Pregnancy?

Most HIV medicines are safe to use during pregnancy. In general, HIV medicines don't increase the risk of birth defects. Healthcare providers can explain the benefits and risks of specific HIV medicines to help women with HIV decide which HIV medicines to use during pregnancy or while they are trying to conceive.

Are There Other Ways to Prevent Mother-to-Child Transmission of Human Immunodeficiency Virus?

Because HIV can be transmitted in breast milk, women with HIV in the United States should not breastfeed their babies. In the United States, baby formula is a safe and healthy alternative to breast milk.

There are reports of children becoming infected with HIV by eating food that was previously chewed by a person with HIV. To be safe, babies should not be fed prechewed food.

Chapter 52

Group B Streptococcus

Group B streptococcus (group B strep, GBS) are bacteria that come and go naturally in the body. Most of the time the bacteria are not harmful, but they can cause serious illness in people of all ages. In fact, group B strep disease is a common cause of severe infection in newborns. While GBS disease can be deadly, there are steps pregnant women can take to help protect the fetuses.

Preventing Early-Onset Group B Strep Disease

The two most important ways to prevent early-onset group B strep (GBS) disease are:

- Testing pregnant women for GBS bacteria late in pregnancy (ideally between 35 and 37 weeks pregnant)

- Giving antibiotics during labor to women at increased risk, including those who test positive for GBS bacteria

Testing Pregnant Women

Doctors should test pregnant women for GBS bacteria when they are 35 to 37 weeks pregnant. About 1 in every 4 pregnant women

---

This chapter contains text excerpted from the following sources: Text in this chapter begins with excerpts from "Group B Strep (GBS)," Centers for Disease Control and Prevention (CDC), May 29, 2018; Text beginning with the heading "Preventing Early-Onset Group B Strep Disease" is excerpted from "Prevention in Newborns," Centers for Disease Control and Prevention (CDC), May 29, 2018.

carry GBS bacteria in their body. Women who test positive are not sick, but are at increased risk for passing the bacteria to their babies during birth.

The test is simple and does not hurt. Clinicians use a sterile swab ("Q-tip") to collect a sample from the vagina and the rectum. They send the sample to a laboratory for testing.

A woman may test positive for the bacteria at some times and not others. That is why doctors should test pregnant women between 35 to 37 weeks of every pregnancy.

Note: Clinicians do not need to test women who had a previous baby who developed GBS disease. These women should receive antibiotics no matter what.

Antibiotics during Labor

Pregnant women should receive antibiotics through the vein (IV) during labor if:

- They test positive for GBS bacteria during their current pregnancy

- They have GBS bacteria in their urine anytime during their current pregnancy

- They had a previous baby who developed GBS disease

Pregnant women who do not know if they are positive for GBS bacteria when labor starts should receive antibiotics if they have:

- Labor starting at less than 37 weeks (preterm labor)

- Prolonged membrane rupture (water breaking 18 or more hours before delivery)

- Fever during labor

Giving antibiotics to pregnant women during labor helps protect the fetus from infection. The antibiotics help during labor only, because the bacteria can grow back quickly; doctors cannot give antibiotics before labor begins. Penicillin is the most common antibiotic that doctors prescribe, but they can also give other antibiotics to women who are severely allergic to penicillin. Women should tell their doctor or nurse about any allergies during a checkup and try to make a plan for delivery. When arriving at the hospital, women should remind their doctor and any staff if they have any allergies to medicines.

Penicillin is very safe and effective at preventing the spread of GBS bacteria to newborns during birth. About 1 in every 10 women have mild side effects from receiving penicillin. There is a rare chance (about 1 in every 10,000 women) of having a severe allergic reaction that requires emergency treatment.

Preventing Late-Onset Group B Strep Disease

Researchers have not identified an effective strategy for preventing late-onset GBS disease. Unfortunately, giving women antibiotics during labor does not prevent late-onset disease.

Alternative Prevention Strategies

Currently, there is no vaccine to help pregnant women protect their newborns from GBS bacteria and disease. Researchers are working on developing a vaccine, which may become available in the future.

The following strategies are not effective at preventing GBS disease in babies:

- Taking antibiotics by mouth

- Taking antibiotics before labor begins

- Using birth canal washes with the disinfectant chlorhexidine

To date, receiving antibiotics through the vein during labor is the only proven strategy to protect a baby from early-onset GBS disease.

Chapter 53

Zika Virus and Pregnancy

Zika is a virus spread to people primarily through the bite of an infected mosquito. Zika infection during pregnancy can cause serious birth defects.

What We Know

- Zika virus can be passed from a pregnant woman to her fetus.

- Infection during pregnancy can cause a birth defect called "microcephaly" and other severe fetal brain defects.

- Zika primarily spreads through infected mosquitoes. You can also get Zika through sex without a condom with someone infected by Zika, even if that person does not show symptoms of Zika.

- There is no vaccine to prevent or medicine to treat Zika.

- Pregnant women should not travel to areas with risk of Zika.

This chapter contains text excerpted from the following sources: Text is this chapter begins with excerpts from "What We Know about Zika and Pregnancy," Centers for Disease Control and Prevention (CDC), April 24, 2018; Text under the heading "Pregnant Women and Zika" is excerpted from "Pregnant Women and Zika," Centers for Disease Control and Prevention (CDC), April 24, 2018.

What We Do Not Know

- How likely it is that Zika infection will affect your pregnancy.

- If the fetus will have birth defects if you are infected while pregnant.

- The full range of health effects that Zika virus infection during pregnancy might lead to.

Pregnant Women and Zika

The Centers for Disease Control and Prevention (CDC) recommends special precautions for pregnant women to protect themselves from Zika virus infection.

Pregnant Women Should Not Travel to an Area with Risk of Zika

- Pregnant women should not travel to areas with risk of Zika (i.e., with documented or likely Zika virus transmission).

- In 2018, no local mosquito-borne Zika virus transmission has been reported in the continental United States.

What to Do If You Live in or Travel to an Area with Risk of Zika

If you live in or must travel to one of these areas, talk to your doctor or other healthcare provider first and strictly follow steps to prevent mosquito bites and practice safe sex.

During Travel or While Living in an Area with Risk of Zika

- Take steps to prevent mosquito bites.

- Take steps to prevent getting Zika through sex by using condoms from start to finish every time you have sex (oral, vaginal, or anal) or by not having sex during your entire pregnancy.

After Travel

- Talk to a doctor or other healthcare provider after travel to an area with risk of Zika.

- If you develop a fever with a rash, headache, joint pain, red eyes, or muscle pain, talk to your doctor immediately and tell him or her about your travel.

- Take steps to prevent mosquito bites for 3 weeks after returning.

- Take steps to prevent passing Zika through sex by using condoms from start to finish every time you have sex (oral, vaginal, or anal) or by not having sex.

Table 53.1. Zika Testing for Pregnant Women

If You...	When to Be Tested
Traveled to an area with risk of Zika or had sex with a partner who lived in or traveled to one of these areas	• You should be tested if you have symptoms of Zika or if an ultrasound shows that your fetus has abnormalities that might be related to Zika infection. • Routine testing is not recommended for pregnant women exposed to these areas who do not have symptoms. However, your doctor may offer testing based on your individual situation.
Live in or frequently travel (daily or weekly) to an area with risk of Zika	• If you have symptoms of Zika at any time during your pregnancy, you should be tested for Zika. • If you do not have symptoms, you should be offered testing at your first prenatal care visit, followed by two additional rounds of testing at regular prenatal care visits during your pregnancy.

Risk of Zika Infection on Future Pregnancies

Based on the available evidence, Zika virus infection in a woman who is not pregnant would not pose a risk for birth defects in future pregnancies after the virus has cleared from her blood. Knowing from similar infections, once a person has been infected with Zika virus, he or she is likely to be protected from a future Zika infection.

If you're thinking about having a baby in the near future and you or your partner live in or traveled to an area with risk of Zika, talk with your doctor or other healthcare provider.

Chapter 54

Pregnancy Loss: Ectopic Pregnancy, Miscarriage, and Stillbirth

Chapter Contents

Section 54.1

Ectopic Pregnancy

What Is an Ectopic Pregnancy?

Normally, a fertilized egg gets implanted and develops in the main uterine cavity. However, sometimes a fertilized egg implants itself in another place, often the fallopian tubes (the structures leading from the ovaries to the uterus). This is called an "ectopic pregnancy" or "tubular pregnancy." Ectopic pregnancies can also occur in the ovaries, cervix, or the abdominal cavity. Since these other anatomical structures lack the space and nourishing environment of the uterus, an ectopic pregnancy will not be viable. Also, ectopic pregnancies must be removed immediately, because, if not treated, the growing embryonic tissue will damage the mother's reproductive organs, resulting in serious and potentially life-threatening blood loss.

What Are the Risk Factors for an Ectopic Pregnancy?

All women have a slight risk of ectopic pregnancy. However, the risk increases with the following factors:

- Becoming pregnant over the age of 35
- History of
  - Ectopic pregnancy
  - Endometriosis
  - Pelvic surgery, abdominal surgery, or multiple abortions
  - Sexually transmitted diseases (STDs)
- Structural abnormalities in the fallopian tubes that restrict the movement of eggs
- Conception that occurs in spite of tubal ligation or intrauterine device
- Conception assisted by fertility drugs or procedures
- Hormonal imbalances

- Smoking
- Abnormal development of a fertilized egg

What Are the Symptoms of an Ectopic Pregnancy?

The symptoms of an ectopic pregnancy are similar to those in the early stages of a normal pregnancy. As with a normal pregnancy, a woman will experience a missed period, nausea, and tenderness in the breasts. A pregnancy test will be positive. However, an ectopic pregnancy does not proceed normally. The first indication is slight vaginal bleeding or brown watery discharge accompanied by dull pelvic pain. However, the pain in the pelvis may spread to the abdomen and become sharp and stabbing. A woman may also experience shoulder pain or an urge to move her bowels if blood has leaked from the fallopian tube and pooled in the abdominal cavity where it irritates related nerves. If the fallopian tube is completely ruptured, resulting in heavy bleeding in the abdominal cavity, lightheadedness, fainting, and shock will occur.

When Should You Call for Emergency Help?

Given the potential life-threatening complications of an ectopic pregnancy, emergency help should be sought out immediately should you experience:

- Severe pain in the abdomen and pelvic areas accompanied by vaginal bleeding
- Fainting and lightheadedness
- Pain in the shoulders

How Is an Ectopic Pregnancy Diagnosed?

The doctor will perform an initial pregnancy test and pelvic examination. Since an ectopic pregnancy cannot be detected by a physical examination alone, the doctor will also order an ultrasound test. When the pregnancy is too early to see via imaging, the doctor will monitor the patient using blood tests until the condition can be confirmed using an ultrasound. One of the ultrasound tests frequently used is a transvaginal ultrasound, which uses a wand-like device placed in the vagina to produce images of the uterus and fallopian tubes to detect an ectopic pregnancy.

How Is an Ectopic Pregnancy Treated?

An ectopic pregnancy is treated by removing the implanted embryo via the following methods:

- **Medication.** If the ectopic pregnancy has been detected early, doctors will use an injection of the drug methotrexate to stop cell growth in the embryo and dissolve the tissue. They will then monitor levels of the pregnancy hormone chorionic gonadotropin (HCG) in the patient's blood. If the levels are high, indicating that the fetal tissue has not been completely removed, the doctor will administer a second injection of the same drug.

- **Surgery.** Doctors can also use laparoscopic surgery to remove an ectopic embryo. An incision is made in or near the navel, and a tube is inserted with surgical tools and a camera with a light source. The embryo is then removed and any damage to the fallopian tube repaired. If heavy bleeding and heavy damage to the fallopian tube has occurred, the surgeon may remove the fallopian tube as well. After surgery, the patient is monitored for levels of HCG to confirm that all ectopic tissue was removed. Otherwise, a methotrexate injection is administered.

How Can an Ectopic Pregnancy Be Prevented?

An ectopic pregnancy cannot be prevented but the risk factors can be controlled.

- Limit the number of sexual partners.
- Do not engage in unprotected sex.
- Quit smoking.

What Is the Outlook after an Ectopic Pregnancy?

The outlook after an ectopic pregnancy depends on what effect it has had on the fallopian tubes or other reproductive organs. If the fallopian tubes are intact and damage has been minimal, the chances of having a normal pregnancy in the future are good. You will be advised to wait for two to three months before trying to get pregnant again. About 65 percent of women who have undergone treatment for ectopic pregnancy successfully become pregnant within 18 months of treatment. In some cases, in vitro fertilization (IVF) treatment may be necessary. The risk for a repeat ectopic pregnancy exists but is significantly less at 10 percent.

How Can You Cope after an Ectopic Pregnancy?

The loss of a pregnancy is devastating. It is important to recognize the loss and give yourself time to grieve. Seek the support of your partner, friend, or loved one. Contact a support group, grief counselor, or a mental health provider for support if needed.

Women who have been treated for ectopic pregnancies often go on to have healthy pregnancies later. If one fallopian tube was removed during treatment, the other fallopian tube can still function as part of a normal pregnancy. IVF treatment could be an option for women who have lost both fallopian tubes due to ectopic pregnancies.

Plan your pregnancy ahead of time and discuss it with your doctor. You can be reassured of a normal pregnancy with the help of blood tests and ultrasound imaging early in your pregnancy.

References

1. Johnson, Traci C., MD. "What to Know about Ectopic Pregnancy," WebMD, LLC, January 21, 2017.

2. "Ectopic Pregnancy," NHS Choices, March 2, 2016.

3. Selner, Marissa, Nall, Rachel. "Ectopic Pregnancy," Healthline, October 13, 2015.

4. "Ectopic Pregnancy," Mayo Foundation for Medical Education and Research (MFMER), January 20, 2015.

Section 54.2

What Is a Miscarriage?

This section includes text excerpted from "About Pregnancy Loss (before 20 Weeks of Pregnancy)," *Eunice Kennedy Shriver* National Institute of Child Health and Human Development (NICHD), September 1, 2017.

Pregnancy loss is the unexpected loss of a fetus before the 20th week of pregnancy. It is sometimes called "miscarriage," "early pregnancy loss," "mid-trimester pregnancy loss," "fetal demise," or "spontaneous abortion."

Healthcare providers use a different term—stillbirth—to describe the loss of a fetus after 20 weeks of pregnancy.

Pregnancy loss may occur so early that a woman may not know she was pregnant.

Researchers can only estimate the number of women who experience pregnancy loss, because some losses occur before a woman's pregnancy is confirmed by a healthcare provider or pregnancy test. But the American College of Obstetricians and Gynecologists (ACOG) estimates that early pregnancy loss is common, occurring in about 10 percent of confirmed pregnancies.

What Are the Symptoms of Pregnancy Loss (Before 20 Weeks of Pregnancy)?

Symptoms of pregnancy loss may include:

- Bleeding from the vagina

- Pain or cramps in the lower stomach area (abdomen)

- Low back pain

- Fluid, tissue, or clot-like material coming out of the vagina

However, bleeding from the vagina during pregnancy doesn't always mean a miscarriage. Many pregnant women have spotting and cramping in early pregnancy but do not miscarry. Your healthcare provider might call this pregnancy "threatened." In any case, pregnant women who have any of the symptoms of miscarriage should contact their healthcare provider immediately.

Some women do not experience any symptoms of pregnancy loss.

Although this is rare in the United States, some women who have a miscarriage may get an infection in the uterus, which can be life threatening. Women who have the following symptoms more than 24 hours after treatment should call 911:

- A fever higher than 100.4 degrees Fahrenheit on more than two occasions

- Severe pain in the lower abdomen

- Bloody discharge from the vagina (which can include pus and be foul smelling)

430

Recent research has also found that morning sickness—nausea and vomiting during pregnancy—is linked to lower risk of pregnancy loss. *Eunice Kennedy Shriver* National Institute of Child Health and Human Development (NICHD) researchers are continuing to look for other factors that may indicate lower risk of pregnancy loss.

What Are the Causes of and Risks for Pregnancy Loss (Before 20 Weeks of Pregnancy)?

Pregnancy loss may occur for many reasons, and sometimes the cause remains unknown even after additional tests are completed.

Possible Causes

Pregnancy loss often happens when a pregnancy doesn't develop normally.

In many cases, miscarriages result from a problem with the chromosomes in the fetus. The number of chromosomes the fetus has—too many or too few—can affect survival.

Other possible causes of pregnancy loss include:

- Being exposed to toxins in the environment

- Problems of the placenta, cervix, or uterus

- Problems with the father's sperm

In many cases, though, healthcare providers can't identify a cause or causes for pregnancy loss.

Risk Factors

Problems with chromosomes happen more often in the fetuses of older parents, particularly among women who are older than 35. For this reason, risk for pregnancy loss increases as the parents age; it is much higher at age 45 than at age 35.

Women who have had previous miscarriages are also at a higher risk for pregnancy loss.

Health issues, such as chronic diseases, in the mother that can also increase risk for pregnancy loss include:

- Chronic diseases, such as high blood pressure, diabetes, thyroid disease, or polycystic ovary syndrome (PCOS)

- Problems with the immune system, such as an autoimmune disorder

- Infections (such as untreated gonorrhea or Zika)

- Hormone problems

- Extremes in weight, such as obesity or being too thin

- Lifestyle factors, such as using drugs or alcohol, smoking, or consuming more than 200 milligrams of caffeine per day (equal to about one 12-ounce cup of coffee)

Findings from an NICHD study suggest that women who are at higher risk for pregnancy loss because of two or more previous losses may increase their chances of carrying the pregnancy to term by taking a low-dose aspirin every day if they have high levels of inflammation.

Recent research has also found that morning sickness is linked to lower risk of pregnancy loss. The NICHD researchers are continuing their research to find other factors that may indicate lower risk of pregnancy loss.

How Do HealthCare Providers Diagnose and Treat Pregnancy Loss (Before 20 Weeks of Pregnancy)?

If a pregnant woman has any of the symptoms of pregnancy loss, such as abdominal cramps, back pain, light spotting, or bleeding, she should contact her healthcare provider immediately. Remember that vaginal bleeding during pregnancy does not definitely mean a pregnancy loss is occurring.

Diagnosing Pregnancy Loss

Depending on how far along the pregnancy is, healthcare providers may use different methods to determine whether a pregnancy loss has occurred:

- A blood test to check the level of human chorionic gonadotropin (hCG), the pregnancy hormone

- A pelvic exam to see whether the woman's cervix is dilated or thinned, which can be a sign of pregnancy loss

- An ultrasound test, which allows the provider to look at the pregnancy, uterus, and placenta

If a woman has had more than one miscarriage, she may want to have a healthcare provider check her blood for chromosome problems, hormone problems, or immune system disorders that may be contributing to pregnancy loss.

Treating Pregnancy Loss

Treatments for pregnancy loss focus on ensuring that the nonviable pregnancy leaves the woman's body safely and completely. Women going through pregnancy loss are at risk for bleeding, pain, and infection, especially if some of the pregnancy tissue remains behind in the uterus.

The specific treatment used depends on how far along the pregnancy was, the woman's overall health, her age, and other factors.

In many cases, pregnancy loss before 20 weeks may not require any special treatment. The bleeding that occurs with pregnancy loss empties the uterus without any further problems.

Women who have heavy bleeding during pregnancy loss should contact a healthcare provider immediately. For reference, heavy bleeding refers to soaking at least two maxi pads an hour for at least two hours in a row.

Some women may need a surgical procedure called a "dilation and curettage" (D and C) to remove any pregnancy tissue that is still in the uterus. A D and C is recommended if a woman is bleeding heavily or if an ultrasound shows pregnancy tissue still in the uterus. D and C may also be used if a woman has any signs of infection, such as a fever, or if she has other health problems, such as cardiovascular disease or a bleeding disorder.

Some women are treated with a medication called "misoprostol," which helps the tissue pass out of the uterus and controls the resulting bleeding. Research shows that misoprostol is safe and effective in most cases.

Women who lose a pregnancy may also need other treatments to control mild to moderate bleeding, prevent infection, relieve pain, and help with emotional support.

Although this is rare in the United States, some women who have a miscarriage may get an infection in the uterus, which can be life threatening. Women who have the following symptoms more than 24 hours after treatment should call 911:

- A fever higher than 100.4 degrees Fahrenheit on more than two occasions

- Severe pain in the lower abdomen

- Bloody discharge from the vagina that includes pus or is foul smelling

433

Is There a Way to Prevent Pregnancy Loss (Before 20 Weeks of Pregnancy)?

There is currently no known way to prevent pregnancy loss before 20 weeks from occurring, nor is there a way to stop pregnancy loss once it has started.

There are ways to lower the risk of general pregnancy complications, but none of them definitely prevent pregnancy loss. Some ways to lower overall risk include:

- Staying in good health before becoming pregnant and getting regular care during pregnancy

- Diagnosing any health conditions, such as diabetes or thyroid disorders, and taking steps to manage or treat the condition before getting pregnant

- Avoiding environmental hazards, such as exposure to radiation, pollution, or toxic chemicals

- Avoiding alcohol and drugs, including high levels of caffeine in both partners

- Protecting yourself from certain infections by not traveling to certain areas and by preventing mosquito bites

An NICHD study found that women who are at higher risk for pregnancy loss because of two or more previous losses may increase their chances of carrying the pregnancy to term by taking a low-dose aspirin every day if they have high levels of inflammation.

Section 54.3

What Is a Stillbirth?

This section includes text excerpted from "Facts about Stillbirth," Centers for Disease Control and Prevention (CDC), August 16, 2018.

A stillbirth is the death or loss of a fetus before or during delivery. Both miscarriage and stillbirth describe pregnancy loss, but they differ according to when the loss occurs. In the United States, a miscarriage is usually defined as loss of a fetus before the 20th week of pregnancy, and a stillbirth is loss of a fetus after 20 weeks of pregnancy.

Stillbirth is further classified as either early, late, or term.

- An early stillbirth is a fetal death occurring between 20 and 27 completed weeks of pregnancy

- A late stillbirth occurs between 28 and 36 completed pregnancy weeks

- A term stillbirth occurs between 37 or more completed pregnancy weeks

How Many Babies Are Stillborn?

Stillbirth effects about one percent of all pregnancies, and each year about 24,000 babies are stillborn in the United States. That is about the same number of babies that die during the first year of life, and it is more than 10 times as many deaths as the number that occur from sudden infant death syndrome (SIDS).

Because of advances in medical technology over the last 30 years, prenatal care (medical care during pregnancy) has improved, which has dramatically reduced the number of late and term stillbirth. However, the rate of early stillbirth has remained about the same over time.

What Increases the Risk of Stillbirth

The causes of many stillbirths are unknown. Therefore, families are often left grieving without answers to their questions. Stillbirth is not a cause of death, but rather a term that means a fetus's death during the pregnancy. Some women blame themselves, but rarely are these deaths caused by something a woman did or did not do. Known contributors to stillbirth generally fall into one of three broad categories:

- Problems with the fetus (birth defects or genetic problems)

- Problems with the placenta or umbilical cord (this is where the mother and the fetus exchange oxygen and nutrients)

- Certain conditions in the mother (for example, uncontrolled diabetes, high blood pressure, or obesity)

Stillbirth with an unknown cause is called "unexplained stillbirth." Having an unexplained stillbirth is more likely to occur the further along a woman is in her pregnancy.

Although stillbirth occurs in families of all races, ethnicities, and income levels, and to women of all ages, some women are at higher risk for having a stillbirth. Some of the factors that increase the risk for a stillbirth include the mother:

- Being of Black race

- Being a teenager

- Being 35 years of age or older

- Being unmarried

- Being obese

- Smoking cigarettes during pregnancy

- Having certain medical conditions, such as high blood pressure or diabetes

- Having multiple pregnancies

- Having had a previous pregnancy loss

These factors are also associated with other poor pregnancy outcomes, such as preterm birth.

State laws require the reporting of fetal deaths, and federal law supports national collection and publication of fetal death data.

What Can Be Done?

The Centers for Disease Prevention and Control (CDC) works to learn more about who might have a stillbirth and why. The CDC does this by tracking how often stillbirth occurs and researching what causes stillbirth and how to prevent it. Knowledge about the potential causes of stillbirth can be used to develop recommendations, policies, and services to help prevent stillbirth. While the CDC continues to learn more about stillbirth, much work remains.

Section 54.4

Stillbirths due to Placental Complications

This section includes text excerpted from "Most Stillbirths Caused
by Placental, Pregnancy Conditions," National Institutes of
Health (NIH), December 19, 2011. Reviewed February 2019.

Half of all stillbirths result from pregnancy disorders and conditions
that affect the placenta, according to a report. Risk factors already
known at the start of pregnancy—such as previous pregnancy loss or
obesity—accounted for only a small proportion of the overall risk of
stillbirth.

Stillbirth is the death of the fetus during the second half of pregnancy—at or after the 20th week of gestation. It occurs in 1 out of 160
pregnancies nationwide. Some risk factors had previously been linked
to stillbirth, including maternal diabetes or high blood pressure. But
the underlying causes of stillbirth remain unknown in as many as
half of stillbirths.

Most Stillbirths Caused by Placental, Pregnancy Conditions

To learn more about the origins and prevention of stillbirth,
National Institutes of Health (NIH) created the Stillbirth Collaborative
Research Network (SCRN). With support from NIH's *Eunice Kennedy
Shriver* National Institute of Child Health and Human Development
(NICHD), the network enrolled more than 600 women who delivered a
stillbirth in certain regions of the country. The findings were reported
in a pair of papers published in the *Journal of the American Medical
Association* (JAMA) on December 14, 2011.

In one of the studies, the researchers compared 614 stillbirths
with 1,816 live births. They searched for factors at the start of pregnancy that might raise the risk for stillbirth. The analysis strongly
linked stillbirth with several reproductive features, including being a
first-time mother or having stillbirth or miscarriage in earlier pregnancies. Other maternal factors linked with stillbirth include being
overweight or obese, age 40 or older, AB blood type, a history of drug
addiction and smoking three months prior to pregnancy. Still, these
early risk factors represented little of the overall risk, and so they have
limited usefulness as predictors of stillbirth.

The analysis confirmed earlier findings that African American women are at greater risk for stillbirth compared to White or Hispanic women. The stillbirth risk for African Americans was greatest for deliveries before the 24th week of pregnancy. Further analyses of early pregnancy may yield insights for reducing the racial disparity in stillbirth rates.

In the other study, researchers completed comprehensive medical evaluations of 512 stillborn babies to identify the causes of death. Evaluation included an autopsy, examination of the placenta, a karyotype test to check for abnormalities in the baby's chromosomes, and a review of the medical records.

The detailed medical evaluations allowed scientists to identify a probable cause of death in 61 percent of cases and a probable or possible cause of death in 76 percent of cases. Earlier studies, which typically were limited to analyzing medical records, could identify a cause of death in only about half of the cases.

The researchers found that pregnancy or birth-related complications contributed to the largest proportion of stillbirths (29%). These complications include preterm labor or premature rupture of membranes that hold the amniotic fluid. Another such complication is abruption of the placenta, in which the placenta separates from the wall of the uterus. Other identified causes included abnormalities of the placenta (24% of cases), genetic conditions or birth defects (14%), infection (13%), problems with the umbilical cord (10%), and maternal high blood pressure (9%).

"Our study showed that a probable cause of death—more than 60 percent—could be found by a thorough medical evaluation," says study co-author Dr. Uma M. Reddy of NICHD. "Greater availability of medical evaluation of stillborn infants, particularly autopsy, placental exam, and karyotype, would provide information to better understand the causes of stillbirth."

Section 54.5

Coping with Pregnancy Loss

This section includes text excerpted from "Pregnancy Loss,"
Office on Women's Health (OWH), U.S. Department of
Health and Human Services (HHS), January 30, 2019.

Why Pregnancy Loss Happens

As many as 10 to 15 percent of confirmed pregnancies are lost. The
true percentage of pregnancy losses might even be higher as many take
place before a woman even knows that she is pregnant. Most losses
occur very early on—before eight weeks. Pregnancy that ends before
20 weeks is called "miscarriage." Miscarriage usually happens because
of genetic problems in the fetus. Sometimes, problems with the uterus
or cervix might play a role in miscarriage. Health problems, such as
polycystic ovary syndrome, might also be a factor.

After 20 weeks, losing a pregnancy is called "stillbirth." Stillbirth
is much less common. Some reasons stillbirth occur include problems
with the placenta, genetic problems in the fetus, poor fetal growth,
and infections. Almost half of the time, the reason for stillbirth is not
known.

Coping with Loss

After the loss, you might be stunned or shocked. You might be
asking, "Why me?" You might feel guilty that you did or did not do
something to cause your pregnancy to end. You might feel cheated and
angry. Or you might feel extremely sad as you come to terms with the
baby that will never be. These emotions are all normal reactions to
loss. With time, you will be able to accept the loss and move on. You
will be able to put this chapter behind you and look forward to life
ahead. To help get you through this difficult time, try some of these
ideas:

- Turn to loved ones and friends for support. Share your feelings
  and ask for help when you need it.

- Talk to your partner about your loss. Keep in mind that men and
  women cope with loss in different ways.

- Take care of yourself. Eating healthy foods, keeping active, and
  getting enough sleep will help restore energy and well-being.

- Join a support group. A support group might help you to feel less alone.

- Do something in remembrance of your baby.

- Seek help from a grief counselor, especially if your grief doesn't ease with time.

Trying Again

Give yourself plenty of time to heal emotionally. It could take a few months or even a year. Once you and your partner are emotionally ready to try again, confirm with your doctor that you are in good physical health and that your body is ready for pregnancy. Following a miscarriage, most healthy women do not need to wait before trying to conceive again. You might worry that pregnancy loss could happen again, but take heart in knowing that most women who have gone through pregnancy loss go on to have healthy children.

Chapter 55

Preterm and Postterm Labor and Birth

Chapter Contents

Section 55.1

What Is Preterm Labor?

This section includes text excerpted from "Preterm
Labor and Birth: Condition Information," *Eunice Kennedy
Shriver* National Institute of Child Health and Human
Development (NICHD), January 31, 2017.

Preterm Labor and Birth

In general, a normal human pregnancy is about 40 weeks long (9.2
months). Healthcare providers now define "full-term" birth as birth
that occurs between 39 weeks and 40 weeks and six days of pregnancy.
Infants born during this time are considered full-term infants.

Infants born in the 37th and 38th weeks of pregnancy—previously
called "term" but now referred to as "early term"—face more health
risks than do those born at 39 or 40 weeks.

Deliveries before 37 weeks of pregnancy are considered "preterm"
or premature:

- Labor that begins before 37 weeks of pregnancy is preterm or
  premature labor

- A birth that occurs before 37 weeks of pregnancy is a preterm or
  premature birth

- An infant born before 37 weeks in the womb is a preterm
  or premature infant. (These infants are commonly called
  "preemies" as a reference to being born prematurely.)

"Late preterm" refers to 34 weeks through 36 weeks of pregnancy.
Infants born during this time are considered late preterm infants, but
they face many of the same health challenges as preterm infants. More
than 70 percent of preterm infants are born during the late preterm
time frame.

Preterm birth is the most common cause of infant death and is
the leading cause of long-term disability in children. Many organs,
including the brain, lungs, and liver, are still developing in the final
weeks of pregnancy. The earlier the delivery, the higher the risk of
serious disability or death.

Infants born prematurely are at risk for cerebral palsy (a group
of nervous system disorders that affect control of movement and posture and limit activity), developmental delays, and vision and hearing
problems.

Late preterm infants typically have better health outcomes than those born earlier, but they are still three times more likely to die in the first year of life than are full-term infants. Preterm births can also take a heavy emotional and economic toll on families.

What Are the Symptoms of Preterm Labor?

Preterm labor is any labor that occurs from 20 weeks through 36 weeks of pregnancy. Here are the symptoms:

- Contractions (tightening of stomach muscles, or birth pains) every 10 minutes or more often

- Change in vaginal discharge (leaking fluid or bleeding from the vagina)

- Feeling of pressure in the pelvis (hip) area

- Low, dull backache

- Cramps that feel like menstrual cramps

- Abdominal cramps with or without diarrhea

It is normal for pregnant women to have some uterine contractions throughout the day. It is not normal to have frequent uterine contractions, such as six or more in one hour. Frequent uterine contractions, or tightenings, may cause the cervix to begin to open.

If a woman thinks that she might be having preterm labor, she should call her doctor or go to the hospital to be evaluated.

What Causes Preterm Labor and Birth

The causes of preterm labor and premature birth are numerous, complex, and only partly understood. Medical, psychosocial, and biological factors may all play a role in preterm labor and birth.

There are three main situations in which preterm labor and premature birth may occur:

- **Spontaneous preterm labor and birth.** This term refers to unintentional, unplanned delivery before the 37th week of pregnancy. This type of preterm birth can result from a number of causes, such as infection or inflammation, although the cause of spontaneous preterm labor and delivery is usually not known. A history of delivering preterm is one of the strongest predictors for subsequent preterm births.

443

- **Medically indicated preterm birth.** If a serious medical condition—such as preeclampsia—exists, the healthcare provider might recommend a preterm delivery. In these cases, healthcare providers often take steps to keep the fetus in the womb as long as possible to allow for additional growth and development, while also monitoring the mother and fetus for health issues. Providers also use additional interventions, such as steroids, to help improve outcomes for the baby.

- **Nonmedically indicated (elective) preterm delivery.** Some late preterm births result from inducing labor or having a cesarean delivery even though there is not a medical reason to do so, even though this practice is not recommended. Research indicates that even babies born at 37 or 38 weeks of pregnancy are at higher risk for poor health outcomes than are babies born at 39 weeks of pregnancy or later. Therefore, unless there are medical problems, healthcare providers should wait until at least 39 weeks of pregnancy to induce labor or perform a cesarean delivery to prevent possible health problems.

The National Child and Maternal Health Education Program (NCMHEP), led by the *Eunice Kennedy Shriver* National Institute of Child Health and Human Development (NICHD) in collaboration with 33 other agencies, organizations, and groups focused on maternal and child health, offers videos and other information about why it's best to wait until at least 39 weeks of pregnancy to deliver unless there is a medical reason.

What Are the Risk Factors for Preterm Labor and Birth?

There are several risk factors for preterm labor and premature birth, including ones that researchers have not yet identified. Some of these risk factors are "modifiable," meaning they can be changed to help reduce the risk. Other factors cannot be changed.

Healthcare providers consider the following factors to put women at high risk for preterm labor or birth:

- Women who have delivered preterm before, or who have experienced preterm labor before, are considered to be at high risk for preterm labor and birth.

- Being pregnant with twins, triplets, or more (called "multiple gestations") or the use of assisted reproductive technology is associated with a higher risk of preterm labor and birth. One study showed that more than 50 percent of twin births occurred preterm, compared with only 10 percent of births of single infants.

- Women with certain abnormalities of the reproductive organs are at greater risk for preterm labor and birth than are women who do not have these abnormalities. For instance, women who have a short cervix (the lower part of the uterus) or whose cervix shortens in the second trimester (fourth through sixth months) of pregnancy instead of the third trimester are at high risk for preterm delivery.

Certain medical conditions, including some that occur only during pregnancy, also place a woman at higher risk for preterm labor and delivery. Some of these conditions include:

- Urinary tract infections

- Sexually transmitted infections (STIs)

- Certain vaginal infections, such as bacterial vaginosis and trichomoniasis

- High blood pressure

- Bleeding from the vagina

- Certain developmental abnormalities in the fetus

- Pregnancy resulting from in vitro fertilization

- Being underweight or obese before pregnancy

- Short time period between pregnancies (less than 6 months between a birth and the beginning of the next pregnancy)

- Placenta previa, a condition in which the placenta grows in the lowest part of the uterus and covers all or part of the opening to the cervix

- Being at risk for rupture of the uterus (when the wall of the uterus rips open). Rupture of the uterus is more likely if you have had a prior cesarean delivery or have had a uterine fibroid removed.

- Diabetes (high blood sugar) and gestational diabetes (which occurs only during pregnancy)

- Blood clotting problems

Other factors that may increase the risk for preterm labor and premature birth include:

- Ethnicity. Preterm labor and birth occur more often among certain racial and ethnic groups. For example, infants of African American mothers are more likely to be born preterm than infants of White mothers. American Indian/Alaska Native mothers are also more likely to give birth preterm than are White mothers.

- Age of the mother

- Women younger than age 18 are more likely to have a preterm delivery.

- Women older than age 35 are also at risk of having preterm infants because they are more likely to have other conditions (such as high blood pressure and diabetes) that can cause complications requiring preterm delivery.

- Certain lifestyle and environmental factors, including:

- Late or no healthcare during pregnancy

- Smoking

- Drinking alcohol

- Using illegal drugs

- Domestic violence, including physical, sexual, or emotional abuse

- Lack of social support

- Stress

- Long working hours with long periods of standing

- Exposure to certain environmental pollutants

Section 55.2

Preterm Labor Prediction and Prevention

This section includes text excerpted from "Is It Possible to Predict Which Women Are More Likely to Have Preterm Labor and Birth?" *Eunice Kennedy Shriver* National Institute of Child Health and Human Development (NICHD), January 31, 2017.

Is It Possible to Predict Which Women Are More Likely to Have Preterm Labor and Birth?

Currently, there is no definitive way to predict preterm labor or premature birth. Many research studies are focusing on this important issue. By identifying which women are at increased risk, healthcare providers may be able to provide early interventions, treatments, and close monitoring of these pregnancies to prevent preterm delivery or to improve health outcomes.

However, in some situations, healthcare providers know that a preterm delivery is very likely. Some of these situations are described below.

Shortened Cervix

As a preparation for birth, the cervix (the lower part of the uterus) naturally shortens late in pregnancy. However, in some women, the cervix shortens prematurely, around the fourth or fifth month of pregnancy, increasing the risk for preterm delivery.

In some cases, a healthcare provider may recommend measuring a pregnant woman's cervical length, especially if she previously had preterm labor or a preterm birth. Ultrasound scans may be used to measure cervical length and identify women with a shortened cervix.

"Incompetent" Cervix

The cervix normally remains closed during pregnancy. In some cases, the cervix starts to open early, before a fetus is ready to be born. Healthcare providers may refer to a cervix that begins to open as an "incompetent" cervix. The process of cervical opening is painless and unnoticeable, without labor contractions or cramping.

To try to prevent preterm birth, a doctor may place a stitch around the cervix to keep it closed. This procedure is called "cervical cerclage." Research supported by the *Eunice Kennedy Shriver* National Institute of Child Health and Human Development (NICHD) has found that, in women with a prior preterm birth who have a short cervix, cerclage may improve the likelihood of a full-term delivery.

How Do Healthcare Providers Diagnose Preterm Labor?

If a woman is concerned that she could be showing signs of preterm labor, she should call her healthcare provider or go to the hospital to be evaluated. In particular, a woman should call if she has more than six contractions in an hour or if fluid or blood is leaking from the vagina.

Physical Exam

If a woman is experiencing signs of labor, the healthcare provider may perform a pelvic exam to see if:

• The membranes have ruptured

• The cervix is beginning to get thinner (efface)

• The cervix is beginning to open (dilate)

Any of these situations could mean the woman is in preterm labor.

Providers may also do an ultrasound exam and use a monitor to electronically record contractions and the fetal heart rate.

Fetal Fibronectin Test

Fetal fibronectin (fFN) test is used to detect whether the protein fetal fibronectin is being produced. fFN is like a biological "glue" between the uterine lining and the membrane that surrounds the fetus.

Normally fFN is detectable in the pregnant woman's secretions from the vagina and cervix early in the pregnancy (up to 22 weeks, or about 5 months) and again toward the end of the pregnancy (1 to 3 weeks before labor begins). It is usually not present between 24 and 34 weeks of pregnancy (5½ to 8½ months). If fFN is detected during this time, it may be a sign that the woman may be at risk of preterm labor and birth.

In most cases, the fFN test is performed on women who are showing signs of preterm labor. Testing for fFN can help predict which pregnant women showing signs of preterm labor will have a preterm delivery. It is typically used for its negative predictive value, meaning that if

448

it is negative, it is unlikely that a woman will deliver within the next seven days.

Section 55.3

Preterm Labor Risk Reduction Methods That Work and Do Not Work

This section includes text excerpted from "What Treatments Can Reduce the Chances of Preterm Labor and Birth?" *Eunice Kennedy Shriver* National Institute of Child Health and Human Development (NICHD), January 31, 2017.

What Treatments Can Reduce the Chances of Preterm Labor and Birth?

If a pregnant woman is showing signs of preterm labor, her doctor will often try treatments to stop labor and prolong the pregnancy until the fetus is more fully developed. Treatments include therapies to try to stop labor (tocolytics) and medications administered before birth to improve outcomes for the infant if born preterm (antenatal steroids to improve the respiratory outcomes and neuroprotective medications such as magnesium sulfate).

Medications to Delay Labor

Drugs called "tocolytics" can be given to many women with symptoms of preterm labor. These drugs can slow or stop contractions of the uterus and may prevent labor for 2 to 7 days. One common treatment for delaying labor is magnesium sulfate, given to the pregnant woman intravenously through a needle inserted in an arm vein.

Medications to Speed Development of the Fetus

Tocolytics may provide the extra time for treatment with corticosteroids to speed up development of the fetus's lungs and some other organs or for the pregnant woman to get to a hospital that offers specialized care for preterm infants. Corticosteroids can be particularly effective if the pregnancy is between 24 and 34 weeks (between 5½ and 7¾ months) and the woman's healthcare provider suspects that the birth may occur within the next week. Intravenously delivered magnesium sulfate may also reduce the risk of cerebral palsy if the child is born early.

What Methods Do Not Work to Prevent Preterm Labor?

Researchers have found that some methods for trying to stop preterm labor are not as effective as once thought. These include:

- Home uterine monitors

- Routine screening of all asymptomatic women for bacterial vaginosis (*Trichomonas vaginalis*) infection. Routine screening and treatment with antibiotics did not reduce preterm birth; in fact, the latter increased the risk of preterm birth.

Section 55.4

Overdue/Postdue Pregnancy

This section contains text excerpted from the following sources: Text in this section begins with excerpts from "Postterm Pregnancy," U.S. National Library of Medicine (NLM), 2012. Reviewed February 2019; Text under the heading "Inducing Labor" is excerpted from "Labor and Birth," Office on Women's Health (OWH), U.S. Department of Health and Human Services (HHS), June 6, 2018.

Postterm pregnancy is a pregnancy that extends to 42 weeks of gestation or beyond. Fetal, neonatal, and maternal complications associated with this condition have always been underestimated. It is not well understood why some women become postterm although, in obesity, hormonal, and genetic factors have been implicated. The management of postterm pregnancy constitutes a challenge to clinicians: knowing who to induce, who will respond to induction, and who will require a cesarean section (CS). The current definition and management of postterm pregnancy have been challenged in several studies as the emerging evidence demonstrates that the incidence of complications associated with postterm pregnancy also increases prior to 42 weeks of gestation. For example, the incidence of stillbirth increases from 39 weeks onwards with a sharp rise after 40 weeks of gestation. Induction of labor before 42 weeks of gestation has the potential to prevent these complications; however, both patients and clinicians alike are concerned about risks associated with induction of labor such as failure of induction and increases in CS rates. There is a strong body of evidence; however, that demonstrates that induction of labor at term and prior to 42 weeks of gestation (particularly between 40 and 42 weeks) is associated with a reduction in perinatal complications without an associated increase in CS rates. It seems, therefore, that a policy of induction of labor at 41 weeks in postterm women could be beneficial with potential improvement in perinatal outcome and a reduction in maternal complications.

Inducing Labor

Sometimes, a doctor or midwife might need to induce (bring about) labor. The decision to induce labor often is made when a woman is past her due date but labor has not yet begun or when there is concern about the fetus or mother's health. Some specific reasons why labor might be induced include:

- A woman's water has broken (ruptured membranes), but labor has not begun on its own

- Infection inside the uterus

- The fetus is growing too slowly

- Complications that arise when the mother's Rh factor is negative and the fetus's is positive

- Not enough amniotic fluid

- Complications, such as high blood pressure or preeclampsia

- Health problems in the mother, such as kidney disease or diabetes

The doctor or midwife can use medicines and other methods to open a pregnant woman's cervix, stimulate contractions, and prepare for vaginal birth.

Elective labor induction has become more common in recent years. This is when labor is induced at term but for no medical reason. Some doctors may suggest elective induction due to a woman's discomfort, scheduling issues, or concern that waiting may lead to complications. But the benefits and harms of elective induction are not well understood. For instance, it's not known if elective labor induction leads to higher or lower rates of cesarean delivery compared to waiting for labor to start on its own. Yet, doctors have ways to assess risk of cesarean delivery, such as a woman's age, whether it is her first pregnancy, and the status of her cervix. Elective induction (not before 39 weeks) does not appear to affect the health of the fetus.

If your doctor suggests inducing labor, talk to your doctor about the possible harms and benefits for both mother and the fetus, such as the risk of c-section and the risk of low birth weight. You will want to be sure the benefits of inducing labor outweigh the risks of induction and the risks of continuing the pregnancy.

Chapter 56

Birth Defects and Developmental Disabilities

Chapter Contents

Section 56.1

Birth Defects That May Be Diagnosed during Pregnancy

This section contains text excerpted from the following sources: Text under the heading "What Are Birth Defects?" is excerpted from "What Are Birth Defects?" Centers for Disease Control and Prevention (CDC), June 19, 2018; Text under the heading "Diagnosis of Birth Defects" is excerpted from "Diagnosis of Birth Defects" Centers for Disease Control and Prevention (CDC), November 21, 2017.

What Are Birth Defects?

Birth defects are common, costly, and critical conditions that affect 1 in every 33 babies born in the United States each year. Every 4 ½ minutes, a baby is born with a birth defect in the United States. That means nearly 120,000 babies are affected by birth defects each year.

Birth defects are structural changes present at birth that can affect almost any part or parts of the body (e.g., heart, brain, foot). They may affect how the body looks, works, or both. Birth defects can vary from mild to severe. The well-being of each child affected with a birth defect depends mostly on which organ or body part is involved and how much it is affected. Depending on the severity of the defect and what body part is affected, the expected lifespan of a person with a birth defect may or may not be affected.

Causes of Birth Defects

Birth defects can occur during any stage of pregnancy. Most birth defects occur in the first three months of pregnancy, when the organs of the fetus are forming. This is a very important stage of development. However, some birth defects occur later in pregnancy. During the last six months of pregnancy, the tissues and organs continue to grow and develop.

For some birth defects, like fetal alcohol syndrome (FAS), the cause is known. But for most birth defects, the causes are not known. For most birth defects, they are caused by a complex mix of factors. These factors include our genes (information inherited from our parents), our behaviors, and things in the environment. But, it's not fully understood how these factors might work together to cause birth defects.

While there is still more work to do, a lot about birth defects are learned through past research. For example, some things might increase the chances of having a baby with a birth defect, such as:

- Smoking, drinking alcohol, or taking certain "street" drugs during pregnancy

- Having certain medical conditions, such as being obese or having uncontrolled diabetes before and during pregnancy

- Taking certain medications, such as isotretinoin (a drug used to treat severe acne)

- Having someone in your family with a birth defect. To learn more about your risk of having a baby with a birth defect, you can talk with a clinical geneticist or a genetic counselor.

- Being an older mother, typically over the age of 34 years

Having one or more of these risks doesn't mean you'll have a pregnancy affected by a birth defect. Also, women can have a baby born with a birth defect even when they don't have any of these risks. It is important to talk to your doctor about what you can do to lower your risk.

Identifying Birth Defects

A birth defect can be found before birth, at birth, or any time after birth. Most birth defects are found within the first year of life. Some birth defects (such as cleft lip) are easy to see, but others (such as heart defects or hearing loss) are found using special tests, such as echocardiograms (an ultrasound picture of the heart), X-rays, or hearing tests.

Diagnosis of Birth Defects

Birth defects can be diagnosed during pregnancy or after the baby is born, depending on the specific type of birth defect.

During Pregnancy: Prenatal Testing
Screening Tests

A screening test is a procedure or test that is done to see if a woman or the fetus might have certain problems. A screening test does not provide a specific diagnosis—that requires a diagnostic test. A screening test can sometimes give an abnormal result even when there is nothing wrong with the mother or the fetus. Less often, a screening test result can be normal and miss a problem that does exist. During pregnancy, women are usually offered these screening tests to check for birth defects or other problems for the woman or the fetus. Talk to your doctor about any concerns you have about prenatal testing.

First Trimester Screening

First trimester screening is a combination of tests completed between weeks 11 and 13 of pregnancy. It is used to look for certain birth defects related to the fetus's heart or chromosomal disorders, such as Down syndrome. This screen includes a maternal blood test and an ultrasound.

- Maternal blood screen. The maternal blood screen is a simple blood test. It measures the levels of two proteins, human chorionic gonadotropin (hCG) and pregnancy-associated plasma protein A (PAPP-A). If the protein levels are abnormally high or low, there could be a chromosomal disorder in the fetus.

- Ultrasound. An ultrasound creates pictures of the fetus. The ultrasound for the first trimester screen looks for extra fluid behind the fetus's neck. If there is increased fluid found on the ultrasound, there could be a chromosomal disorder or heart defect in the fetus.

Second Trimester Screening

Second-trimester screening tests are completed between weeks 15 and 20 of pregnancy. They are used to look for certain birth defects in the fetus. Second trimester screening tests include a maternal serum screen and a comprehensive ultrasound evaluation of the fetus looking for the presence of structural anomalies (also known as an "anomaly ultrasound").

- Maternal serum screen. The maternal serum screen is a simple blood test used to identify if a woman is at increased risk for having a baby with certain birth defects, such as neural-tube defects or chromosomal disorders, such as Down syndrome. It is also known as a "triple screen" or "quad screen" depending on the number of proteins measured in the mother's blood. For example, a quad screen tests the levels of 4 proteins AFP (alpha-fetoprotein), hCG, estriol, and inhibin-A. Generally, the maternal serum screen is completed during the second trimester.

- Anomaly ultrasound. An ultrasound creates pictures of the fetus. This test is usually completed around 18 to 20 weeks of pregnancy. The ultrasound is used to check the size of the fetus and looks for birth defects or other problems with the fetus.

Diagnostic Tests

If the result of a screening test is abnormal, doctors usually offer further diagnostic tests to determine if birth defects or other possible problems with the fetus are present. These diagnostic tests are also offered to women with higher risk pregnancies, which may include women who are 35 years of age or older; women who have had a previous pregnancy affected by a birth defect; women who have chronic diseases such as lupus, high blood pressure, diabetes, or epilepsy; or women who use certain medications.

High Resolution Ultrasound

An ultrasound creates pictures of the fetus. This ultrasound, also known as a level II ultrasound, is used to look in more detail for possible birth defects or other problems with the fetus that were suggested in the previous screening tests. It is usually completed between weeks 18 and 22 of pregnancy.

Chorionic Villus Sampling

Chorionic villus sampling (CVS) is a test where the doctor collects a tiny piece of the placenta, called "chorionic villus," which is then tested to check for chromosomal or genetic disorders in the fetus. Generally, a CVS test is offered to women who received an abnormal result on a first-trimester screening test or to women who could be at higher risk. It is completed between 10 and 12 weeks of pregnancy, earlier than an amniocentesis.

Amniocentesis

An amniocentesis is a test where the doctor collects a small amount of amniotic fluid from the area surrounding the fetus. The fluid is then tested to measure the fetus's protein levels, which might indicate certain birth defects. Cells in the amniotic fluid can be tested for chromosomal disorders, such as Down syndrome, and genetic problems, such as cystic fibrosis or Tay-Sachs disease (TSD). Generally, an amniocentesis is offered to women who received an abnormal result

457

on a screening test or to women who might be at higher risk. It is completed between 15 and 18 weeks of pregnancy. Below are some of the proteins for which an amniocentesis tests.

- AFP. AFP stands for alpha-fetoprotein, a protein the fetus produces. A high level of AFP in the amniotic fluid might mean that the fetus has a defect indicating an opening in the tissue, such as a neural-tube defect (anencephaly or spina bifida), or a body wall defect, such as omphalocele or gastroschisis.

- AChE. AChE stands for acetylcholinesterase, an enzyme that the fetus produces. This enzyme can pass from the fetus to the fluid surrounding the fetus if there is an opening in the neural tube.

After the Baby Is Born

Certain birth defects might not be diagnosed until after the baby is born. Sometimes, the birth defect is immediately seen at birth. For other birth defects including some heart defects, the birth defect might not be diagnosed until later in life.

When there is a health problem with a child, the primary care provider might look for birth defects by taking a medical and family history, doing a physical exam, and sometimes recommending further tests. If a diagnosis cannot be made after the exam, the primary care provider might refer the child to a specialist in birth defects and genetics. A clinical geneticist is a doctor with special training to evaluate patients who may have genetic conditions or birth defects. Even if a child sees a specialist, an exact diagnosis might not be reached.

Section 56.2

Developmental Disabilities

This section includes text excerpted from "Facts about Developmental Disabilities," Centers for Disease Control and Prevention (CDC), April 17, 2018.

Developmental disabilities are a group of conditions due to an impairment in physical, learning, language, or behavior areas. These conditions begin during the developmental period, may impact day-to-day functioning, and usually last throughout a person's lifetime.

Developmental Milestones

Skills such as taking a first step, smiling for the first time, and waving "bye-bye" are called "developmental milestones." Children reach milestones in how they play, learn, speak, behave, and move (for example, crawling and walking).

Children develop at their own pace, so it's impossible to tell exactly when a child will learn a given skill. However, the developmental milestones give a general idea of the changes to expect as a child gets older.

As a parent, you know your child best. If your child is not meeting the milestones for his or her age, or if you think there could be a problem with your child's development, talk with your child's doctor or healthcare provider and share your concerns. Don't wait.

If You're Concerned

If your child is not meeting the milestones for his or her age, or you are concerned about your child's development, talk with your child's doctor and share your concerns. Don't wait!

Developmental Monitoring and Screening

A child's growth and development are followed through a partnership between parents and healthcare professionals. At each well-child visit, the doctor looks for developmental delays or problems and talks with the parents about any concerns the parents might have. This is called "developmental monitoring."

Any problems noticed during developmental monitoring should be followed up with developmental screening. Developmental screening

459

is a short test to tell if a child is learning basic skills when he or she should, or if there are delays.

If a child has a developmental delay, it is important to get help as soon as possible. Early identification and intervention can have a significant impact on a child's ability to learn new skills, as well as reduce the need for costly interventions over time.

Causes and Risk Factors

Developmental disabilities begin anytime during the developmental period and usually last throughout a person's lifetime. Most developmental disabilities begin before a baby is born, but some can happen after birth because of injury, infection, or other factors.

Most developmental disabilities are thought to be caused by a complex mix of factors. These factors include genetics; parental health and behaviors (such as smoking and drinking) during pregnancy; complications during birth; infections the mother might have during pregnancy or the baby might have very early in life; and exposure of the mother or child to high levels of environmental toxins, such as lead. For some developmental disabilities, such as fetal alcohol syndrome, which is caused by drinking alcohol during pregnancy, the cause is known. But for most, it's not.

The following are some examples of what are known about specific developmental disabilities:

- At least 25 percent of hearing loss among babies is due to maternal infections during pregnancy, such as cytomegalovirus (CMV) infection; complications after birth; and head trauma.

- Some of the most common known causes of intellectual disability include fetal alcohol syndrome; genetic and chromosomal conditions, such as Down syndrome and fragile X syndrome; and certain infections during pregnancy.

- Children who have a sibling with autism are at a higher risk of also having an autism spectrum disorder.

- Low birthweight, premature birth, multiple birth, and infections during pregnancy are associated with an increased risk for many developmental disabilities.

- Untreated-newborn jaundice (high levels of bilirubin in the blood during the first few days after birth) can cause a type of brain damage known as "kernicterus." Children with kernicterus are more likely to have cerebral palsy, hearing and vision problems, and problems with their teeth. Early detection and treatment of newborn jaundice can prevent kernicterus.

The Study to Explore Early Development (SEED) is a multiyear study funded by the Centers for Disease Control and Prevention (CDC). It is currently the largest study in the United States to help identify factors that may put children at risk for autism spectrum disorders and other developmental disabilities.

Who Is Affected?

Developmental disabilities occur among all racial, ethnic, and socio-economic groups. Recent estimates in the United States show that about one in six, or about 15 percent, of children aged 3 through 17 years have a one or more developmental disabilities, such as:

- Attention deficit hyperactivity disorder (ADHD)
- Autism spectrum disorder
- Cerebral palsy
- Hearing loss
- Intellectual disability
- Learning disability
- Vision impairment
- Other developmental delays

Living with a Developmental Disability

Children and adults with disabilities need healthcare and health programs for the same reasons anyone else does—to stay well, active, and a part of the community.

Having a disability does not mean a person is not healthy or that he or she cannot be healthy. Being healthy means the same thing for all of us—getting and staying well so we can lead full, active lives. That includes having the tools and information to make healthy choices and knowing how to prevent illness. Some health conditions, such as asthma, gastrointestinal symptoms, eczema and skin allergies, and migraine headaches, have been found to be more common among children with developmental disabilities. Thus, it is especially important for children with developmental disabilities to see a healthcare provider regularly.

The CDC does not study education or treatment programs for people with developmental disabilities, nor does it provide direct services to people with developmental disabilities or to their families. However, the CDC has put together a list of resources for people affected by developmental disabilities.

Part Six

Labor and Delivery

Chapter 57

All about Labor and Delivery

Chapter Contents

Section 57.1

Signs of True Labor

This section includes text excerpted from "When Does Labor Usually Start?" *Eunice Kennedy Shriver* National Institute of Child Health and Human Development (NICHD), September 1, 2017.

When Does Labor Usually Start?

For most women, labor begins sometime between week 37 and week 42 of pregnancy. Labor that occurs before 37 weeks of pregnancy is considered premature, or preterm.

Just as pregnancy is different for every woman, the start of labor, the signs of labor, and the length of time it takes to go through labor vary from woman to woman and even from pregnancy to pregnancy.

Signs of Labor

The primary sign of labor is a series of contractions (tightening and relaxing of the uterus) that arrive regularly. Over time, they become stronger, last longer, and are more frequent. Some women may experience false labor, when contractions are weak or irregular or stop when the woman changes positions. Women who have regular contractions every 5 to 10 minutes for an hour should let their healthcare provider know.

It is important to discuss labor and signs of labor with a healthcare provider early in pregnancy before labor begins. Some providers may want a woman to wait until she has multiple signs of labor or is in "active" labor before coming to the hospital or birthing center.

Other signs of labor include:

- "Lightening." This term refers to when the fetus "drops," or moves lower in the uterus. This may happen several weeks or only a few hours before labor begins. Not all fetuses drop before birth. Lightening gets its name from the feeling of lightness or relief that some women experience when the fetus moves from the rib cage to the pelvic area. It allows some women to breathe more easily, more deeply and may provide relief from heartburn.

- Increase in vaginal discharge. Called "show" or "the bloody show," the discharge can be clear, pink, or slightly bloody. This discharge occurs as the cervix begins to open (dilate) and can happen several days before labor or just as labor begins.

Labor contractions before 37 weeks of pregnancy are a sign of preterm labor. Women who notice regular, frequent contractions at any point in pregnancy should notify a provider or go to the hospital. Providers can check for changes in the cervix to see whether labor has begun. As needed, providers can also give women in preterm labor specialized care. Among women who experience preterm labor, only about 10 percent go on to give birth within a week.

Other signs of labor include:

- Change in vaginal discharge

- Pain or pressure around the front of the pelvis or the rectum

- Low, dull backache

- Cramps that feel like menstrual cramps, with or without diarrhea

- A gush or trickle of fluid, which is a sign of water breaking

Sometimes, if the health of the mother or the fetus is at risk, a woman's healthcare provider will recommend inducing or causing labor using medically-supervised methods, such as medication.

Unless earlier delivery is medically necessary or occurs on its own, waiting until at least 39 weeks before delivering gives the mother and the fetus the best chance for healthy outcomes. During the last few weeks of pregnancy, the fetus's lungs, brain, and liver are still developing.

Section 57.2

What Is False Labor and Braxton Hicks Contractions

This section includes text excerpted from "Other Labor and Delivery FAQs," *Eunice Kennedy Shriver* National Institute of Child Health and Human Development (NICHD), September 1, 2017.

"False labor" refers to irregular contractions that sometimes happen before true labor begins. These contractions are also called "Braxton Hicks contractions." It can be hard to tell the difference between Braxton Hicks contractions and true labor contractions.

The following chart, from the American Congress of Obstetricians and Gynecologists (ACOG), shows some ways that Braxton Hicks contractions differ from true labor contractions.

Table 57.1. Difference between True and False Labor

Type of Change	False Labor	True Labor
Timing of contractions	Contractions do not come regularly and do not get closer together.	Contractions come at regular times and get closer together over time. Each lasts about 30 to 70 seconds.
Effect of movement	Contractions may stop when the woman walks or rests, or they may stop when the woman changes position.	Contractions continue despite movement.
Strength of contractions	Contractions are usually weak and do not get much stronger or they may start strong and get weaker.	Contractions get steadily stronger.
Pain of contractions	The woman usually feels pain only in the front.	Pain usually starts in the back and moves to the front.

How Are Labor and Delivery Different for a Woman Having Multiples?

When women carry multiple fetuses—twins, triplets, or quadruplets, for example—labor and delivery proceed through the same stages as with a single infant. But labor and delivery with multiples has some important differences. For example, women having multiples are more likely to have certain complications. The most common are preterm labor and preterm birth.

Preterm labor is labor that starts before 37 weeks of pregnancy. It can result in preterm birth. More than half of all twins are born preterm. Preterm infants can have problems with breathing and eating and may have to stay in the hospital longer than other infants.

In a pregnancy with multiples, providers look to see whether the woman has one or more than one placenta, which direction(s) the fetuses are facing, and where the umbilical cords lie. In addition, they closely monitor the woman's health, because carrying multiples can increase a woman's risk of gestational diabetes and preeclampsia. These factors can all affect when and how a provider recommends delivering the babies. Some of these complications may require a cesarean (C-section) delivery to resolve. Multiples are about 2.5 times more likely to be delivered by C-section than singletons are.

What Is the Apgar Test?

The Apgar test, performed 1 minute and 5 minutes after birth, gauges an infant's overall health. A healthcare provider assesses the following aspects of an infant's health:

- Skin color
- Heart rate
- Reflexes (response to stimulation, such as a mild pinch)
- Muscle tone
- Breathing

Based on this examination, the healthcare provider gives the infant an Apgar score of 1 to 10. The higher the score, the better the infant is doing.

Are There Added Labor and Delivery Risks for Older Women?

Women older than 35 are at higher risk for preterm labor and preterm birth. Preterm infants can have serious short- and long-term health problems.

Older women are also more likely to have a stillbirth, which is when a fetus dies in the uterus after 20 weeks of pregnancy.

Women in their 30s are also more likely than younger women to need a cesarean delivery.

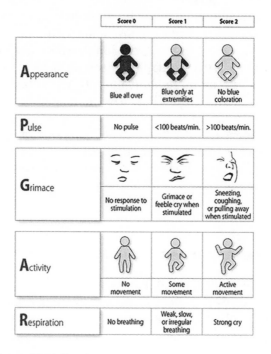

Figure 57.1. *Apgar Test Scoring*

What Should Women Consider When Choosing Where to Deliver?

Although most women give birth in hospitals, some families choose a homebirth or birth in an out-of-hospital birthing center. The American Academy of Pediatrics (AAP) and the American College of Obstetricians and Gynecologists (ACOG) recommend births in hospitals or birthing centers as the safest options.

Talk to your healthcare provider about where you want to deliver your baby. If possible, schedule a time to visit the hospital, birthing center, or other settings before you make your decision. Consider the risks and benefits of each as you make your decision.

Women who are good candidates for homebirth:

- Are generally in good health

- Have not had a previous cesarean delivery

- Do not have pregnancy-related health problems or illness
- Do not have multiples
- Have a fetus with good size and health
- Have a fetus in the head-down position
- Go into labor at 37 weeks or later

Planned homebirths benefit from having the following resources in place:

- A certified nurse-midwife, certified midwife, or practicing physician
- At least one appropriately trained individual whose primary responsibility is the care of the newborn infant
- Quick access to healthcare providers who can provide consultation if complications happen
- A reliable plan for safe and fast transportation to a nearby hospital in case of an emergency

Is Giving Birth in Water Beneficial?

Some women report that being immersed in water during early labor shortened their labor and reduced their pain. However, these and other benefits of giving birth in water are unconfirmed by research evidence. Also, water births carry risks, including infections and drowning. The American College of Obstetricians and Gynecologists (ACOG) notes that allowing women to labor in a birthing pool may have benefits, but it recommends against giving birth in water.

What Are Preterm Labor and Birth?

Labor and birth are considered preterm, or "premature," if they occur before 37 weeks of pregnancy. Preterm labor and birth share many features with regular labor and delivery, but they also have unique features. For this reason, preterm labor and preterm birth are addressed in a separate topic.

Chapter 58

Maternity Care Practices

Maternity Practices in Infant Nutrition and Care

In the United States, nearly all infants are born in a hospital. Their stay is typically very short, but events during this time have lasting effects. Experiences with breastfeeding in the first hours and days of life significantly influence an infant's later feeding. Several key supportive hospital practices can improve breastfeeding outcomes. Birth facility policies and practices that create a supportive environment for breastfeeding begin prenatally and continue through discharge, and include:

- **Hospital policies**—Written hospital policies support breastfeeding and are communicated to staff and patients.

- **Staff training**—Hospital requires breastfeeding education, clinical training, and competency verification for all maternity staff who work with breastfeeding families.

- **Immediate skin-to-skin contact**—Newborns are placed skin-to-skin with their mothers immediately after birth, with no bedding or clothing between them, allowing enough uninterrupted time (at least one hour) for mother and baby to start breastfeeding well.

This chapter includes text excerpted from "Overview: Maternity Care Practices," Centers for Disease Control and Prevention (CDC), February 6, 2019.

- **Early and frequent breastfeeding**—Hospital staff help mothers and babies start breastfeeding as soon as possible after birth, with many opportunities to practice throughout the hospital stay.

- **Teaching about breastfeeding**—Hospital staff teach mothers and babies how to breastfeed and to recognize and respond to feeding cues.

- **Exclusive breastfeeding**—Hospital staff follow current evidence-based protocols for breastfeeding infants, and provide supplementary feedings only when medically necessary.

- **Rooming-in**—Hospital staff encourage mothers and babies to room together and teach families the benefits of this kind of close contact, including more opportunities to practice breastfeeding and learn their infant's feeding cues.

- **Followup after discharge**—Hospital staff schedule follow-up visits for mothers and babies after they go home and connect families to community breastfeeding resources.

Chapter 59

Birth Partners

Chapter Contents

Section 59.1

Tip Card for Expectant Dads

This section includes text excerpted from "Tip Card for Expectant Dads," National Responsible Fatherhood Clearinghouse (NRFC), Office of Family Assistance (OFA), January 13, 2017.

Did You Know?

When dads are involved as supportive partners during pregnancy, it is good for their babies, good for moms, and good for dads.

When their partner supports them, pregnant women are more likely to get regular prenatal care and eat and live healthily, which increases the likelihood of positive health outcomes for their baby.[1]

Dads who are there for mom and baby during the pregnancy are better prepared for their role as a new dad. They feel more involved, and their baby has more opportunities to get to know their dad.[2]

Moms who have calm and supportive birth partners have better labor experiences.[3]

Figure 59.1. *Fatherhood*

[1]*MenCare (2015), State of the World's Fathers. (sowf.men-care.org/wp-content/uploads/sites/4/2015/06/State-of-the-Worlds-Fathers_23June2015-1.pdf; Fatherhood Institute (2014), FI Research Summary: Supportive Fathers, Healthy Mothers. (www.fatherhoodinstitute.org/wp-content/uploads/2014/04/FI-Research-Summary- Supportive-Fathers-Healthy-Mothers.pdf)*
[2]*NRFC Webinar (2013), Working with Dads: Encouraging and Supporting Father Involvement from Birth through Adolescence. (www.fatherhood.gov/webinars)*
[3]*Fatherhood Institute (2014), Making the Most of Fathers to Improve Maternal and Infant Health. (www.fatherhoodinstitute.org/wp-content/uploads/2014/11/Making-the-most-of-fathers-to-.-.-.-Improve-maternal-and-infant-health.pdf)*

What You Can Do?

- Talk with your partner about expectations and feelings: what is she expecting from you as a dad? What are you feeling and expecting?

- Take a childbirth class; go to prenatal and doctor visits with your partner—get to know the people who are going to be delivering your baby.

- Recognize that pregnancy can be stressful for you and your partner. Besides supporting and helping her, you also need to find time to focus on yourself.

- Talk with other dads and ask how they prepared for the birth of their children.

- Start taking on extra responsibilities around the house—pick things up, clean the house, make some meals, go shopping.

- Prepare for the birth.

  - Get things ready for your new baby—you'll need a crib, diapers, car seat, and stroller.

  - Map out a route to the hospital.

  - Help your partner prepare a bag that will be ready with a change of clothes and other essentials to take with you.

- If you are employed, talk with your employer about taking family leave or working flexible time after the birth so you can help care for your new baby.

Section 59.2

Doula Services

This section includes text excerpted from "Doulas' Perceptions on Single Mothers' Risk and Protective Factors, and Aspirations Relative to Child-Birth," Education Resources Information Center (ERIC), U.S. Department of Education (ED), April 30, 2017.

Doulas provide services to other women during pregnancy, childbirth, and the postpartum period. The content of their services is compromised of continuous nonmedical social, physical, and emotional support. Doulas' role is recognized as a "sister-like," "woman-to-woman," "mother-to-daughter," or "friend-to-friend" relationship. Doulas often encourage young mothers to explore their goals. In traditional societies, relatives and elderly women (e.g., mothers, grandmothers) are acknowledged as young mothers' role models to teach childbearing skills from one generation to another. Contrary to traditional societies, in individualistic cultures, the help of family members is barely available to young mothers. Due to the lack of partners of family members, doulas take the role of these extended family members in individualistic cultures. For example, doulas help mothers by providing 24-hour call availability at prebirth, labor, delivery, and postpartum period, individual counseling, and transportation provision to mothers. While providing services and accompanying mothers, all doulas respect each woman's uniqueness, diverse religious, and cultural beliefs.

The main role of doulas is to care for the mothers in early pregnancy through the transition of motherhood. Doulas professionally assist the mother through all of her child's development and meet their needs. The role of doulas is to help women have a safe and empowering birthing experience. Doulas accompany women throughout labor and delivery at home and in a hospital setting. Further, doulas educate mothers, their partner, and family members about childbirth preparation and breastfeeding.

There are three types of doulas. The first one is called a "prenatal doula." Prenatal doulas promote health, build healthy relationships, encourage receiving good medical care, educate the mother about the baby, and teach about labor and delivery. The other one is called a "birth doula" (intrapartum) that provides comfort, assists in the birth progress, and nurtures the family interaction. After the birth, doulas make home visits to teach breastfeeding techniques, nurture the family connection, educate the new parents on childbearing, and help new mothers for transportation. The third one is classified as a "postpartum doula." These doulas accompany mothers to take care of their newborn babies, and teach baby care basics. Although there are three types of doulas, sometimes doulas can carry out all roles.

Finally, of the single mothers' aspirations, the most important one is to have a healthy baby while they continue their education and concentrate on career development. From the Doulas perspective, family support and doula support are salient protective factors especially for single mothers relative to childbirth. Family connectedness and professional support may provide young mothers many benefits, such as a sense of belonging, higher expectations for parenting and overall achievement.

Chapter 60

Cord Blood Banking

Expecting a baby can be a very exciting time for soon-to-be parents. It can also be very confusing, with many decisions to make. One choice prospective parents often face is whether to donate, bank, or discard their baby's cord blood. Did you know that the U.S. Food and Drug Administration (FDA) regulates cord blood? Here is some information for expectant parents about the regulations in place designed to help ensure the safety of cord blood for transplantation.

What Is Cord Blood?

Cord blood is the blood contained in the placental blood vessels and umbilical cord, which connects an unborn baby to the mother's womb. Cord blood contains hematopoietic progenitor cells. At birth, cord blood can be collected (or "recovered") from the umbilical cord.

What Are Hematopoietic Progenitor Cells?

Hematopoietic progenitor cells (HPCs) are blood-forming stem cells. HPCs are found in bone marrow, peripheral blood, and cord blood. These types of stem cells are routinely used to treat patients with cancers such as leukemia or lymphoma, and other disorders of the blood and immune systems.

This chapter contains text excerpted from the following sources: Text in this chapter begins with excerpts from "Cord Blood Banking—Information for Consumers," U.S. Food and Drug Administration (FDA), March 27, 2018; Text under the heading "Tips for Consumers" is excerpted from "Cord Blood: What You Need to Know," U.S. Food and Drug Administration (FDA), September 10, 2018.

479

How Are Patients and Donated Cord Blood Units "Matched" So That a Unit of Cord Blood Can Be Used for Patient Transplant?

Human leukocyte antigen (HLA) typing is used to match patients and donors for cord blood transplants. HLAs are proteins found on most cells in the body. A person's immune system uses these proteins as markers to recognize which cells belong in their body and which do not. A close match between the patient's and the donor's HLA markers can reduce the risk that the patient's immune cells will attack the donor's cells, or that the donor's immune cells will attack the patient's body after the transplant.

How Are Hematopoietic Progenitor Cells from Cord Blood Different Than Hematopoietic Progenitor Cells from Other Sources?

There is evidence that cord blood HPCs may not require as exact a match as HPCs from bone marrow or the bloodstream because the antigens in cord blood are less mature. This suggests that transplants involving compatible HPCs from cord blood may be less likely to cause adverse reactions because the donor's cells are less likely to see the patient's cells as foreign bodies and attack them.

What Are the Options for Cord Blood Banking?

Cord blood can be donated to a public cord blood bank, where it will be stored for potential future use by anyone who may need it. Alternatively, parents may arrange for the cord blood to be stored in a private cord bank, for potential use if it is later needed for treatment of the child from whom it was recovered, or for use in first- or second-degree relatives. Information on cord blood donation options may be found on the Health Resources and Services Administration (HRSA) website (www.hrsa.gov).

You may also wish to consult your healthcare provider about the options.

How Does the U.S. Food and Drug Administration Regulate Cord Blood Stored for Personal or Family Use?

Cord blood stored for personal use and for use in first- or second-degree relatives that also meets other criteria in the FDA's regulations does not require approval before use. Private cord banks must still comply with other FDA requirements, including establishment registration and listing, donor screening and testing for infectious diseases (except when used for the original donor), reporting and labeling requirements, and compliance with current good tissue practice regulations.

How Does the U.S. Food and Drug Administration Regulate Cord Blood Intended for Use in Patients Unrelated to the Donor (i.e., Cord Blood Stored in Public Banks)?

Cord blood stored for potential future use by a patient unrelated to the donor meets the definition of "drug" under the Food, Drug, and Cosmetic Act (FDCA) and "biological product" under Section 351 of the Public Health Service Act. Cord blood in this category must meet additional requirements and be licensed under a biologics license application (BLA), or subject to an investigational new drug application (IND) before use.

Are There Any U.S. Food and Drug Administration-Approved Uses for Cord Blood?

Cord blood can be used in hematopoietic stem cell transplantation procedures in patients with some disorders affecting the hematopoietic (blood forming) system. For example, cord blood transplants have been used to treat patients with certain blood cancers and some inherited metabolic and immune system disorders.

If a Cord Blood Bank Is Registered with the U.S. Food and Drug Administration, Does That Mean That the Cord Bank Is the U.S. Food and Drug Administration Approved?

Establishments that perform any of the manufacturing steps for cord blood must register with the FDA and list their products and each of the manufacturing steps they perform. Registration with the FDA doesn't mean a firm is "endorsed" by the agency, it simply means the firm has notified the FDA that it is performing one or more manufacturing steps.

Does the U.S. Food and Drug Administration Inspect Facilities That Store Cord Blood?

Yes. Registered establishments are subject to FDA inspection to ensure they are complying with the regulations. The inspections of private banks are designed to ensure prevention of infectious disease transmission.

Where Can I Get More Information about Donating My Baby's Cord Blood?

To make your baby's cord blood available for use by anyone who needs a cord blood transplant, you may donate it to a public cord blood bank. Information on donating cord blood to a public cord blood bank is also found on the HRSA website.

Where Can I Get More Information about Banking My Baby's Cord Blood?

To make your baby's cord blood available for use by the child from whom it was recovered, or for use in first- or second-degree relatives, you may bank it with a private cord blood bank. Information on banking cord blood with a private cord blood bank is also found on the HRSA website.

For some diseases, such as genetically heritable diseases, in the event that your child would need treatment, it is possible that the cord blood would not be recommended for such use.

Tips for Consumers

If you're considering donating to a cord blood bank, you should look into your options during your pregnancy to have enough time to decide before your baby is born. For public banking, ask whether your delivery hospital participates in a cord blood banking program.

If you have questions about collection procedures and risks, or about the donation process, ask your healthcare provider.

The FDA also offers a searchable database that maintains information on registered cord blood banks.

Be skeptical of claims that cord blood is a miracle cure—it is not. Some parents may consider using a private bank as a form of "insurance" against future illness. But remember that, the only approved use of cord blood is for treatment of blood-related illnesses.

Also know that in some cases your stored cord blood may not be suitable for use in the child who donated it. "For instance, you can't cure some diseases or genetic defects with cord blood that contains the same disease or defect," Karandish says.

Parents from minority ethnic groups may especially want to consider donation to a public bank, says Wonnacott, because more donations from these populations will help more minority patients who need a stem cell transplant. (The recipients must be "matched" to donors, so doctors are more likely to find a good match among donors from the recipient's ethnic group.)

"When it comes to public banking, there's a proven need for cord blood," Wonnacott says. "And there's a need especially among minorities to have stem cell transplants available. Cord blood is an excellent source for stem cell transplants."

And these transplants can be life-changing for patients.

Chapter 61

Pain Relief during Labor

The amount of pain felt during labor and delivery is different for every woman. The level of pain depends on many factors, including the size and position of the fetus, the woman's level of comfort with the process, and the strength of her contractions.

There are two general ways to relieve pain during labor and delivery: using medications and using "natural" methods (no medications). Some women choose one way or another, while other women rely on a combination of the two.

A woman should discuss the many aspects of labor with her healthcare provider well before labor begins to ensure that she understands all of the options, risks, and benefits of pain relief during labor and delivery before making a decision. It might also be helpful to put all the decisions in writing to clarify things for all those who might be involved with delivering the baby.

Pain-Relieving Medications

Pain-relief drugs fall into two categories: analgesics and anesthetics Each category has different forms of medications. Some of these medications carry risks. It is important for women to discuss medications with their healthcare provider before going into labor to ensure that they are making informed decisions about pain relief.

This chapter includes text excerpted from "What Are the Options for Pain Relief during Labor and Delivery?" *Eunice Kennedy Shriver* National Institute of Child Health and Human Development (NICHD), September 1, 2017.

Analgesics

Analgesics relieve pain without causing total loss of feeling or muscle movement. These drugs do not always stop pain completely, but they reduce it.

- Systemic analgesics affect the whole nervous system rather than a single area. They ease pain but do not cause the patient to go to sleep. Systemic analgesics are often used in early labor. They are not given right before delivery, because they may slow the baby's breathing and reflexes. They are given in three ways:

  - Injected into a muscle or vein

  - Administered through a small tube placed in a vein. The woman can often control the amount of analgesic flowing through the tube.

  - Inhaled or breathed in with a mixture of oxygen. The woman holds a mask to her face, so she decides how much or how little analgesic she receives for pain relief.

- Regional analgesics relieve pain in one region of the body. In the United States, regional analgesia is the most common way to relieve pain during labor. Several types of regional analgesia can be given during labor:

  - Epidural analgesia, also called an "epidural block" or an "epidural" causes loss of feeling in the lower body while the patient stays awake. The drug starts working about 10 minutes to 20 minutes after it is given. A healthcare provider injects the drug near the spinal cord. A small tube (catheter) is placed through the needle. The needle is then withdrawn, but the tube stays in place. Small amounts of the drug can then be given through the catheter throughout labor without the need for another injection.

  - A spinal block is an injection of a much smaller amount of the drug into the sac of spinal fluid around the spine. The drug starts working right away, but it lasts for only one to two hours. Usually, a spinal block is given only once during labor, to help with pain during delivery.

  - A combined spinal-epidural block also called a "walking epidural," gives the benefits of an epidural block and a spinal block. The spinal part relieves pain immediately. The epidural part allows drugs to be given throughout labor. Some women may be able to walk around after a combined spinal-epidural block.

Anesthetics

Anesthetics block all feeling, including pain.

- General anesthesia causes the patient to go to sleep. The patient does not feel pain while asleep.

- Local anesthesia removes all feeling, including pain, from a small part of the body while the patient stays awake. It does not lessen the pain of contractions. Healthcare providers often use it when performing an episiotomy, a surgical cut made in the region between the vagina and anus to widen the vaginal opening for delivery or when repairing vaginal tears that happen during birth.

Natural Pain-Relief Methods (Natural Childbirth)

Women who choose natural childbirth rely on a number of ways to ease pain without taking medication. These include:

- The company of others who offer reassurance, advice, or other help throughout labor, also known as "continuous labor support"

- Relaxation techniques, such as deep breathing, music therapy, or biofeedback

- A soothing atmosphere

- Moving and changing positions frequently

- Using a birthing ball

- Massage

- Yoga

- Taking a bath or shower

- Hypnosis

- Using soothing scents (aromatherapy)

- Acupuncture or acupressure

- Applying small doses of electrical stimulation to nerve fibers to activate the body's own pain-relieving substances (called "transcutaneous electrical nerve stimulation," or TENS)

- Injecting sterile water into the lower back, which can relieve the intense discomfort and pain in the lower back known as "back labor"

Chapter 62

Vaginal and Cesarean Childbirths

Chapter Contents

Section 62.1

Vaginal/Natural Childbirth

This section includes text excerpted from "Labor and Birth,"
Office on Women's Health (OWH), U.S. Department of
Health and Human Services (HHS), June 6, 2018.

Spot the Signs of Labor

As you approach your due date, you will be looking for any little sign that labor is about to start. You might notice that your fetus has "dropped" or moved lower into your pelvis. This is called "lightening." If you have a pelvic exam during your prenatal visit, your doctor might report changes in your cervix that you cannot feel, but that suggest your body is getting ready. For some women, a flurry of energy and the impulse to cook or clean, called "nesting," is a sign that labor is approaching.

Some signs suggest that labor will begin very soon. Call your doctor or midwife if you have any of the following signs of labor. Call your doctor even if it's weeks before your due date—you might be going into preterm labor. Your doctor or midwife can decide if it's time to go to the hospital or if you should be seen at the office first.

- You have contractions that become stronger at regular and increasingly shorter intervals.

- You have lower back pain and cramping that does not go away.

- Your water breaks (can be a large gush or a continuous trickle).

- You have a bloody (brownish or red-tinged) mucus discharge. This is probably the mucus plug that blocks the cervix. Losing your mucus plug usually means your cervix is dilating (opening up) and becoming thinner and softer (effacing). Labor could start right away or may still be days away.

Did My Water Break?

It's not always easy to know. If your water breaks, it could be a gush or a slow trickle of amniotic fluid. Rupture of membranes is the medical term for your water breaking. Let your doctor know the time your water breaks and any color or odor. Also, call your doctor if you think your water broke, but are not sure. An easy test can tell your doctor if the leaking fluid is urine (many pregnant women leak urine) or amniotic fluid. Often a woman will go into labor soon after her water breaks. When this doesn't happen, her doctor may want to induce (bring about) labor. This is because once your water breaks, your risk of getting an infection goes up as labor is delayed.

Stages of Labor

Labor occurs in three stages. When regular contractions begin, the baby moves down into the pelvis as the cervix both effaces (thins) and dilates (opens). How labor progresses and how long it lasts is different for every woman. But each stage features some milestones that are true for every woman.

First Stage

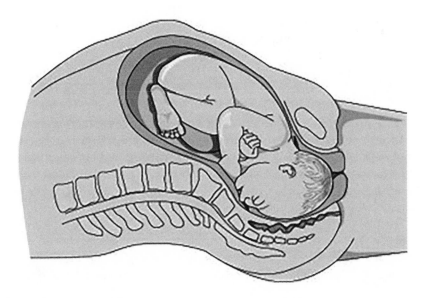

Figure 62.1. *First Stage*

Most babies' heads enter the pelvis facing to one side and then rotate to face down.

The first stage begins with the onset of labor and ends when the cervix is fully opened. It is the longest stage of labor, usually lasting about 12 to 19 hours. Many women spend the early part of this first stage at home. You might want to rest, watch TV, hang out with family, or even go for a walk. Most women can drink and eat during labor, which can provide needed energy later. Yet some doctors advise laboring women to avoid solid food as a precaution should a cesarean delivery be needed. Ask your doctor about eating during labor. While at home, time your contractions and keep your doctor up to date on your progress. Your doctor will tell you when to go to the hospital or birthing center.

At the hospital, your doctor will monitor the progress of your labor by periodically checking your cervix, as well as the fetus's position and station (location in the birth canal). Most fetus's heads enter the pelvis facing to one side and then rotate to face down. Sometimes, a fetus will be facing up, towards the mother's abdomen. Intense back labor often goes along with this position. Your doctor might try to rotate the fetus, or the fetus might turn on its own.

As you near the end of the first stage of labor, contractions become longer, stronger, and closer together. Many of the positioning and relaxation tips you learned in childbirth class can help now. Try to find the most comfortable position during contractions and to let your muscles go limp between contractions. Let your support person know how she or he can be helpful, such as by rubbing your lower back, giving you ice chips to suck, or putting a cold washcloth on your forehead.

Sometimes, medicines and other methods are used to help speed up labor that is progressing slowly. Many doctors will rupture the membranes. Although this practice is widely used, studies show that doing so during labor does not help shorten the length of labor.

Your doctor might want to use an electronic fetal monitor to see if blood supply to the fetus is okay. For most women, this involves putting two straps around the mother's abdomen. One strap measures the strength and frequency of your contractions. The other strap records how the fetus's heartbeat reacts to the contraction.

The most difficult phase of this first stage is the transition. Contractions are very powerful, with very little time to relax in between, as the cervix stretches the last, few centimeters. Many women feel shaky or nauseated. The cervix is fully dilated when it reaches 10 centimeters.

Second Stage

The second stage involves pushing and delivery of your baby. It usually lasts 20 minutes to two hours. You will push hard during contractions, and rest between contractions. Pushing is hard work, and a support person can really help keep you focused. A woman can give birth in many positions, such as squatting, sitting, kneeling, or lying back. Giving birth in an upright position, such as squatting, appears to have some benefits, including shortening this stage of labor and helping to keep the tissue near the birth canal intact. You might find pushing to be easier or more comfortable one way, and you should be allowed to choose the birth position that feels best to you.

When the top of your baby's head fully appears (crowning), your doctor will tell you when to push and deliver your baby. Your doctor may make a small cut, called an "episiotomy," to enlarge the vaginal opening. Most women in childbirth do not need an episiotomy. Sometimes, forceps (tool shaped like salad-tongs) or suction is used to help guide the baby through the birth canal. This is called "assisted vaginal delivery." After your baby is born, the umbilical cord is cut. Make sure to tell your doctor if you or your partner would like to cut the umbilical cord.

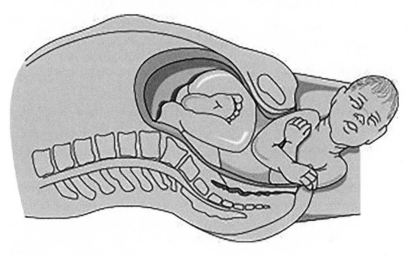

Figure 62.2. *Second Stage*

The baby twists and turns through the birth canal.

Third Stage

The third stage involves the delivery of the placenta (afterbirth). It is the shortest stage, lasting five to 30 minutes. Contractions will begin five to 30 minutes after birth, signaling that it's time to deliver the placenta. You might have chills or shakiness. Labor is over once the placenta is delivered. Your doctor will repair the episiotomy and any tears you might have.

Managing Labor Pain

Virtually all women worry about how they will cope with the pain of labor and delivery. Childbirth is different for everyone. So no one can predict how you will feel. The amount of pain a woman feels during labor depends partly on the size and position of the fetus, the size of her pelvis, her emotions, the strength of the contractions, and her outlook.

Some women do fine with natural methods of pain relief alone. Many women blend natural methods with medications that relieve pain. Building a positive outlook on childbirth and managing fear may also help some women cope with the pain. It is important to realize that labor pain is not like pain due to illness or injury. Instead, it is caused by contractions of the uterus that are pushing your baby down and out of the birth canal. In other words, labor pain has a purpose.

Try the following to help you feel positive about childbirth:

- Take a childbirth class. Call the doctor, midwife, hospital, or birthing center for class information.

- Get information from your doctor or midwife. Write down your questions and talk about them at your regular visits.

- Share your fears and emotions with friends, family, and your partner.

Section 62.2

Cesarean Section

This section includes text excerpted from "Labor and Birth,"
Office on Women's Health (OWH), U.S. Department of
Health and Human Services (HHS), June 6, 2018.

Cesarean delivery, also called "C-section," is surgery to deliver a baby. The baby is taken out through the mother's abdomen. Most cesarean births result in healthy babies and mothers. But C-section is major surgery and carries risks. Healing also takes longer than with vaginal birth.

Most healthy pregnant women with no risk factors for problems during labor or delivery have their babies vaginally. Still, the cesarean birth rate in the United States has risen greatly in recent decades. Today, nearly one in three women have babies by C-section in this country. The rate was one in five in 1995.

Public health experts think that many C-sections are unnecessary. So it is important for pregnant women to get the facts about C-sections before they deliver. Women should find out what C-sections are, why they are performed, and the pros and cons of this surgery.

Reasons for Cesarean Sections

Your doctor might recommend a C-section if she or he thinks it is safer for you or your baby than vaginal birth. Some C-sections are planned. But most C-sections are done when unexpected problems happen during delivery. Even so, there are risks of delivering by C-section. Limited studies show that the benefits of having a C-section may outweigh the risks when:

- The mother is carrying more than one baby (twins, triplets, etc.)

- The mother has health problems including HIV infection, herpes infection, and heart disease

- The mother has dangerously high blood pressure

- The mother has problems with the shape of her pelvis

- There are problems with the placenta

- There are problems with the umbilical cord

- There are problems with the position of the fetus, such as breech

- The fetus shows signs of distress, such as a slowed heart rate

- The mother has had a previous C-section

Patient-Requested Cesarean Section: Can a Woman Choose?

A growing number of women are asking their doctors for C-sections when there is no medical reason. Some women want a C-section because they fear the pain of childbirth. Others like the convenience of being able to decide when and how to deliver their baby. Still, others fear the risks of vaginal delivery including tearing and sexual problems.

But is it safe and ethical for doctors to allow women to choose C-section? The answer is unclear. Only more research on both types of deliveries will provide the answer. In the meantime, many obstetricians feel it is their ethical obligation to talk women out of elective C-sections. Others believe that women should be able to choose a C-section if they understand the risks and benefits.

Experts who believe C-sections should only be performed for medical reasons point to the risks. These include infection, dangerous bleeding, blood transfusions, and blood clots. Babies born by C-section have more breathing problems right after birth. Women who have C-sections stay at the hospital for longer than women who have vaginal births. Plus, recovery from this surgery takes longer and is often more painful than that after a vaginal birth. C-sections also increase the risk of problems in future pregnancies. Women who have had C-sections have a higher risk of uterine rupture. If the uterus ruptures, the life of the baby and mother is in danger.

Supporters of elective C-sections say that this surgery may protect a woman's pelvic organs, reduces the risk of bowel and bladder problems, and is as safe for the baby as vaginal delivery.

The National Institutes of Health (NIH) and American College of Obstetricians (ACOG) agree that a doctor's decision to perform a C-section at the request of a patient should be made on a case-by-case basis and be consistent with ethical principles. ACOG states that "if the physician believes that (cesarean) delivery promotes the overall health and welfare of the woman and her fetus more than vaginal birth, he or she is ethically justified in performing" a C-section. Both organizations also say that C-section should never be scheduled before a pregnancy is 39 weeks, or the lungs are mature, unless there is medical need.

The Cesarean Section Experience

Most C-sections are unplanned. So, learning about C-sections is important for all women who are pregnant. Whether a C-section is planned or comes up during labor, it can be a positive birth experience for many women. The overview that follows will help you to know what to expect during a nonemergency C-section and what questions to ask.

Before Surgery

Cesarean delivery takes about 45 to 60 minutes. It takes place in an operating room. So if you were in a labor and delivery room, you will be moved to an operating room. Often, the mood of the operating room is unhurried and relaxed. A doctor will give you medicine through an epidural or spinal block, which will block the feeling of pain in part of your body but allow you to stay awake and alert. The spinal block works right away and completely numbs your body from the chest down. The epidural takes away pain, but you might be aware of some tugging or pushing. Medicine that makes you fall asleep and lose all awareness is usually only used in emergency situations. Your abdomen will be cleaned and prepped. You will have an IV for fluids and medicines. A nurse will insert a catheter to drain urine from your bladder. This is to protect the bladder from harm during surgery. Your heart rate, blood pressure, and breathing also will be monitored. Questions to ask:

- Can I have a support person with me during the operation?
- What are my options for blocking pain?
- Can I have music played during the surgery?
- Will I be able to watch the surgery if I want?

During Surgery

The doctor will make two incisions. The first is about 6 inches long and goes through the skin, fat, and muscle. Most incisions are made side to side and low on the abdomen called a "bikini incision." Next, the doctor will make an incision to open the uterus. The opening is made just wide enough for the baby to fit through. One doctor will use a hand to support the baby while another doctor pushes the uterus to help push that baby out. Fluid will be suctioned out of your baby's mouth and nose. The doctor will hold up your baby for you to see. Once your baby is delivered, the umbilical cord is cut, and the placenta is removed. Then, the doctor cleans and stitches up the uterus and abdomen. The repair takes up most of the surgery time. Questions to ask:

- Can my partner cut the umbilical cord?
- What happens to my baby right after delivery?
- Can I hold and touch my baby during the surgery repair?
- When is it okay for me to try to breastfeed?
- When can my partner take pictures or video?

After Surgery

You will be moved to a recovery room and monitored for a few hours. You might feel shaky, nauseated, and very sleepy. Later, you will be brought to a hospital room. When you and your baby are ready, you can hold, snuggle, and nurse your baby. Many people will be excited to see you. But don't accept too many visitors. Use your time in the hospital, usually about four days, to rest and bond with your baby.

C-section is major surgery, and recovery takes about six weeks (not counting the fatigue of new motherhood). In the weeks ahead, you will need to focus on healing, getting as much rest as possible, and bonding with your baby. Be careful about taking on too much and accept help as needed. Questions to ask:

- Can my baby be brought to me in the recovery room?

- What are the best positions for me to breastfeed?

Section 62.3

Vaginal Birth after Cesarean Delivery or Repeat Cesarean Section

This section includes text excerpted from "What Is Vaginal Birth after Cesarean (VBAC)?" *Eunice Kennedy Shriver* National Institute of Child Health and Human Development (NICHD), September 1, 2017.

What Is Vaginal Birth after Cesarean?

Vaginal birth after cesarean (VBAC) refers to vaginal delivery of a baby after a previous pregnancy was delivered by cesarean delivery.

In the past, pregnant women who had one cesarean delivery would automatically have another. But research shows that for many women who had prior cesarean deliveries, attempting to give birth vaginally—called a "trial of labor after cesarean delivery" (TOLAC)—and VBAC might be safe options in certain situations.

In fact, *Eunice Kennedy Shriver* National Institute of Child Health and Human Development (NICHD) research shows that among appropriate candidates, about 75 percent of VBAC attempts are successful. A National Institutes of Health (NIH) Consensus Development Conference on VBAC evaluated available data and determined that VBAC was a reasonable option for many women.

Women should discuss VBAC and TOLAC with their healthcare providers early in pregnancy to learn whether these options are appropriate for them. Providers are encouraged to discuss plans for VBAC or refer women to a facility that can support VBAC when it is medically safe to consider.

When Is Vaginal Birth after Cesarean Appropriate?

VBAC may be safe and appropriate for some women, including those:

- Whose prior cesarean incision was across the uterus toward its base (called a "low-transverse incision")—the most common type of incision. Note that the incision on the uterus is different than the incision on the skin.

- With two previous low-transverse cesarean incisions

- Who are carrying twins

- With an unknown type of uterine incision

Benefits of VBAC include:

- No abdominal surgery

- A lower risk of hemorrhage and infection compared with a C-section

- Faster recovery

- Potential to avoid the risks of many cesarean deliveries, such as hysterectomy, bowel and bladder injury, blood transfusion, infection, and abnormal placenta conditions

- Greater likelihood of being able to have more children in the future

If labor fails to progress or if there is another problem, a woman may need a C-section after trying TOLAC. Most risks associated with C-section after TOLAC are similar to those associated with choosing a repeat cesarean. They include:

- Uterine rupture

- Maternal hemorrhage and infection

- Blood clots

- Need for a hysterectomy

Chapter 63

Problems during Childbirth

Labor and Childbirth: An Overview

Towards the end of the pregnancy, i.e., around 37 to 42 weeks, the womb (uterus) contracts in a rhythmic way to push the fetus and placenta. This is called "labor."

The fetus and the placenta coming out of the birth canal (vagina) is called "delivery." Altogether this process is called "childbirth."

A mixture of "pain and pressure" sensation naturally develops in the mother, which pushes the fetus and the placenta out of the vagina. This method is termed as "normal delivery/vaginal delivery." When complications develop, an alternative to vaginal delivery may be needed, which include:

- Operative vaginal delivery (use of forceps or vaginal extractor to take the baby out).

- Cesarean delivery (surgical method of taking the fetus out of the uterus).

Problems One Can Expect during the Childbirth

Most childbirth occurs without complications if planned appropriately; however, unexpected problems can happen during the childbirth and they are:

Timing of Labor

- **Preterm labor:** Labor that starts too early (before 37 weeks).

- **Protracted labor:** Also known as prolonged labor or failure to progress. Abnormally slow progression of active labor with slow cervical dilatation or slow fetal descent.

- **Precipitous labor:** Also known as rapid labor/short labor. Fetus comes out in a short period of time like 3 hours whereas normal considerable time between the labor onset and delivery is 12 to 18 hours.

- **Past due/post-term pregnancy:** Prolonged pregnancy that lasts more than 42 weeks.

Possible Fetal Problems

- **Cephalopelvic disproportion (CPD):** Condition of the fetal head being too large to pass through the birth canal.

- **Fetopelvic disproportion (FPD):** The body of the fetus is too large to pass through the birth canal. In other words, size mismatch, i.e., small birth canal being unable to pass the large fetus.

- **Shoulder dystocia:** Fetus gets stuck in the birth canal as the shoulder of the fetus lodges against the woman's pubic bone.

- **Perinatal asphyxia:** Fetus fails to initiate and sustain breathing during birth. It can happen before, during, and immediately after delivery due to the poor/inadequate oxygen supply necessitating mechanical breathing or medications.

- **Abnormal fetal position and presentation:**"Presentation" means the part of the fetus proceeding towards the birth canal. Cephalic presentation "head first," is the normal one, and all the following presentations are considered abnormal.

  - Breech presentation—buttocks of the fetus in the birth canal

  - Compound presentation—hands of the fetus in the birth canal

  - Shoulder presentation—shoulder of the fetus in the birth canal

  - Transverse lie presentation—lying horizontally (exactly diagonally opposite than normal)

Possible Maternal Problems

- **Problems related to umbilical cord**

  - **Umbilical cord prolapse:** Tube-like muscular structure that connects the placenta and fetus (umbilical cord) comes out of the birth canal while the fetus is still inside the womb (uterus).

  - **Nuchal cord:** Wrapping of umbilical cord around the neck of the fetus or body of the fetus.

- **Problems related to amniotic fluid**

  - **Preterm/premature rupture of the membranes:** Watery (amniotic) fluid surrounding the unborn fetus is contained in a bag (sac) that breaks open early. Usually, a woman notices painless steady leakage or a large gush of fluid from the vagina that wets their undergarments or bed sheets.

  - **Amniotic fluid embolism:** Fluid that surrounds fetus enters the mother's bloodstream causing blood clots (life-threatening).

- **Problems related to placenta**

  - **Placenta accreta:** When all or part of the placenta attaches to the uterine wall and does not detach during the childbirth causing excessive bleeding.

  - **Placenta previa:** When the placenta blocks the birth passage making it impossible for the fetus to come out of the birth canal.

  - **Placental abruption:** Placenta separates from the uterus before the time of delivery causing excessive bleeding.

- **Problems related to the perineum**

  - **Perineal trauma:**The area between the birth canal and opening through which stool passes out of the body (anus) is called perineum. Perineum becomes traumatized due to tearing, which can happen naturally during childbirth when the fetus' head/fetus is large. There are four types of tear and they are:

  - First-degree tear—minor tear that needs few to no stitches and causes minimal pain.

- Second-degree tear—involves tearing of the muscular layer needing stitches in place and 5 to 7 days for recovery.

- Third-degree and fourth-degree tears—extend to the anal sphincter (the string which controls the stool/fecal movement) and is a very rare situation, which needs surgical correction. Perineal massage during delivery can be of some help and prevent higher degree tears.

- Episiotomy: Healthcare provider manually tears the perineum (perineal incision) to widen the birth canal so that the fetus can come out of the birth passage easily. This process is called "episiotomy." The torn perineum will be stitched mostly using absorbable sutures; however, women have to accept some uncertainty as the healing may be uncomfortable even with the use of over-the-counter painkillers and antibiotics (as prevention or if infected). This procedure of episiotomy is usually done during:

  - Operative vaginal delivery

  - Shoulder dystocia

  - Fetal heart rate abnormalities

Problems One Can Expect Immediately after Childbirth

Some problems occur immediately after the delivery of the fetus, i.e., during the phase of placental delivery, and they are:

- **Postpartum hemorrhage:** Excessive uterine bleeding due to placental problems such as placenta accreta and others.

- **Inverted uterus:** Uterus turning inside out—also known as the retroverted uterus, tilted uterus or tipped uterus, which heals with manipulation, and on occasion need other treatments.

- **Uterine rupture:** A very rare condition in which the uterus of the mother tears and the fetus slips into the abdomen causing severe bleeding to the mother and suffocation for the fetus.

- **Fetal distress and respiratory distress:**Occurs when the fetus has not been getting enough oxygen in some situations like:

  - Fetus passing the first stool inside the womb that gets mixed with the amniotic fluid (meconium) which causes difficulty breathing.

- Rapid labor of the mother
- Prolonged pregnancy

Techniques Handled by Healthcare Providers

Healthcare providers handle the complications that occur during delivery by:

- Changing mothers position to ease the delivery (changing maneuver).
- Bed rest to avoid rapid labor.
- Maintaining oxygenation for the mother to avoid fainting.
- Increasing maternal hydration using intravenous administration of dextrose to avoid rupture of the uterus.
- Amnioinfusion (insertion of fluid into the amniotic cavity) to relieve pressure on the umbilical cord.
- Tocolysis (temporary stoppage of contractions) to delay preterm labor.
- Artificial induction of labor to initiate delivery in prolonged pregnancies.
- Opting for an immediate cesarean section if the vaginal delivery is complicated enough to harm either the mother or the fetus.

Some problems can be life-threatening, but with appropriate medical help, the outlook is normally good.

References

1. Moldenhauer, Julie S MD. "Introduction to Abnormalities and Complications of Labor and Delivery," MSD Manual, June 2018.
2. "Labor and Delivery," Mayoclinic, September 1, 2016.
3. "Obstetrics and Gynecology," Medscape, November 16, 2016.

Chapter 64

Disaster Safety for Expecting and New Parents

Disasters, such as wildfires, hurricanes, and floods, can be unpredictable and devastating. Learn general tips to get prepared before a disaster and what to do in case of a disaster to help keep you and your family safe and healthy.

Get Prepared for an Emergency or Disaster

Disasters can be scary and stressful, especially if you are expecting or have a baby. You can take the following steps now to help you prepare for an emergency and better cope if an emergency happens.

- Talk to your doctor or other healthcare provider about where you will get prenatal care or deliver your baby if your doctor's office or hospital is closed.

- If you are close to your due date, learn the signs of labor and talk to your healthcare provider about what to do in case of an emergency.

- Be informed—check with your local emergency management agency to find out how to get emergency alerts (such as text alerts).

This chapter includes text excerpted from "Disaster Safety for Expecting and New Parents," Centers for Disease Control and Prevention (CDC), September 4, 2018.

- Make a family communication plan for how you and your family will contact one another and what steps you will take in different types of situations.

- Prepare an emergency kit that includes a 3-day supply of food and water, health supplies including medications, baby care and safety supplies, electronics, and important documents, such as emergency telephone numbers.

- Plan ahead to help your baby sleep safely if you have to evacuate your home. Your baby is safest sleeping on his or her back in his or her own sleep area (e.g., a portable crib or bassinet) that does not have pillows, blankets, or toys.

What to Do during and Just after Disaster
Expectant Parents

Pregnant women have special medical needs. If you're pregnant or think you may be pregnant, you and your partner can take the following steps to help you stay safe and healthy in the event of a disaster.

- If you have any signs of labor, call your healthcare provider, or go to the hospital immediately if it is safe to leave.

- If you have to evacuate your home, be prepared to leave quickly and have your emergency kit ready to go.

- If staying at a shelter or in temporary housing, tell the staff as soon as possible that you are pregnant and if you have any health problems.

- If you have your prenatal vitamins or prescription medicines with you, continue taking them as directed.

- Once you are out of immediate danger, continue your prenatal care, even if it is not with your primary doctor. Tell the doctor or other healthcare provider if you have any health problems and if you need help getting your prenatal vitamins or medications.

- Protect yourself from infections by washing your hands often and staying away from people who are sick. If you do get sick, talk with a healthcare provider right away.

- During disasters, harmful chemicals from businesses and other places may be released into the environment. Listen to announcements from emergency officials about chemical safety and actions you may need to take to protect yourself. If you have questions about exposure to harmful chemicals during pregnancy, call MotherToBaby (mothertobaby.org) at 866-626-6847. To reach the nationwide poison control center, call 800-222-1222.

- To help with physical stress, drink plenty of clean water and rest as often as you can. To help relieve emotional stress, talk to a healthcare provider, friend, or family member about your concerns and feelings.

Parents of Infants

A disaster can make it difficult to access necessary supplies and healthcare. Parents and caregivers of infants can take the following steps to help keep their families safe and healthy in the event of a disaster.

- If you have to evacuate, be prepared to leave quickly and have your emergency kit that includes infant care supplies, such as baby food and a portable crib, ready to go.

- If you breastfeed your baby, continue to do so. If you feed your baby formula, use ready-to-feed formula if possible. Clean water may not be available for mixing formula or washing bottles.

- If staying at a shelter or in temporary housing, tell the staff as soon as possible that you have a newborn.

- If you are away from your home during a disaster, take these actions to help your baby sleep safely.

  - If you or your baby use prescription medicines and you have them with you, continue taking or giving them as directed.

  - As soon as it is safe to do so, get a postpartum checkup if you are due for a visit, even if it is not with your usual doctor. Tell them if you need help getting your prescription medications. If you're not ready to get pregnant, you can ask for several months' supply of the pill, patch, or ring or consider using a birth control method that will prevent pregnancy for an extended period of time.

  - As soon as it is safe to do so, see a doctor or other healthcare provider for well-baby checkups or if you're concerned about a health problem, even if it is not with your baby's usual doctor.

Tell them if you need help getting your baby's prescription medications.

• To help relieve emotional stress, talk to a healthcare provider, friend, or family member about your concerns and feelings.

Part Seven

Postpartum and Newborn Care

Chapter 65

Recovering from Delivery: Physical and Emotional Concerns

Right now, you are focused on caring for your new baby. But new mothers must take special care of their bodies after giving birth and while breastfeeding, too. Doing so will help you to regain your energy and strength. When you take care of yourself, you are able to best care for and enjoy your baby.

Getting Rest

The first few days at home after having your baby are a time for rest and recovery—physically and emotionally. You need to focus your energy on yourself and on getting to know your new baby. Even though you may be very excited and have requests for lots of visits from family and friends, try to limit visitors and get as much rest as possible. Do not expect to keep your house perfect. You may find that all you can do is eat, sleep, and care for your baby. And that is perfectly okay. Learn to pace yourself from the first day that you arrive back home. Try to lie down or nap while the baby naps. Do not try to do too much around

---

This chapter includes text excerpted from "Recovering from Birth," Office on Women's Health (OWH), U.S. Department of Health and Human Services (HHS), June 6, 2018.

the house. Allow others to help you and do not be afraid to ask for help with cleaning, laundry, meals, or with caring for the baby.

Physical Changes

After the birth of your baby, your doctor will talk with you about things you will experience as your body starts to recover.

- You will have vaginal discharge called "lochia." It is the tissue and blood that lined your uterus during pregnancy. It is heavy and bright red at first, becoming lighter in flow and color until it goes away after a few weeks.

- You might also have swelling in your legs and feet. You can reduce swelling by keeping your feet elevated when possible.

- You might feel constipated. Try to drink plenty of water and eat fresh fruits and vegetables.

- Menstrual-like cramping is common, especially if you are breastfeeding. Your breast milk will come in within three to six days after your delivery. Even if you are not breastfeeding, you can have milk leaking from your nipples, and your breasts might feel full, tender, or uncomfortable.

- Follow your doctor's instructions on how much activity, like climbing stairs or walking, you can do for the next few weeks.

Your doctor will check your recovery at your postpartum visit, about six weeks after birth. Ask about resuming normal activities, as well as eating and fitness plans to help you return to a healthy weight. Also ask your doctor about having sex and birth control. Your period could return in six to eight weeks, or sooner if you do not breastfeed. If you breastfeed, your period might not resume for many months. Still, using reliable birth control is the best way to prevent pregnancy until you want to have another baby.

Some women develop thyroid problems in the first year after giving birth. This is called "postpartum thyroiditis." It often begins with overactive thyroid, which lasts two to four months. Most women then develop symptoms of an underactive thyroid, which can last up to a year. Thyroid problems are easy to overlook as many symptoms, such as fatigue, sleep problems, low energy, and changes in weight, are common after having a baby. Talk to your doctor if you have symptoms that do not go away. An underactive thyroid needs to be treated. In most cases, thyroid function returns to normal as the thyroid heals.

But some women develop permanent underactive thyroid disease, called "Hashimoto disease," and need lifelong treatment.

Regaining a Healthy Weight and Shape

Both pregnancy and labor can affect a woman's body. After giving birth, you will lose about 10 pounds right away and a little more as body fluid levels decrease. Do not expect or try to lose additional pregnancy weight right away. Gradual weight loss over several months is the safest way, especially if you are breastfeeding. Nursing mothers can safely lose a moderate amount of weight without affecting their milk supply or their babies' growth.

A healthy eating plan along with regular physical fitness might be all you need to return to a healthy weight. If you are not losing weight or losing weight too slowly, cut back on foods with added sugars and fats, like soft drinks, desserts, fried foods, fatty meats, and alcohol. Keep in mind, nursing mothers should avoid alcohol. By cutting back on "extras," you can focus on healthy, well-balanced food choices that will keep your energy level up and help you get the nutrients you and your baby need for good health. Make sure to talk to your doctor before you start any type of diet or exercise plan.

Feeling Blue

After childbirth you may feel sad, weepy, and overwhelmed for a few days. Many new mothers have the "baby blues" after giving birth. Changing hormones, anxiety about caring for the baby, and lack of sleep all affect your emotions.

Be patient with yourself. These feelings are normal and usually go away quickly. But if sadness lasts more than two weeks, go see your doctor. Do not wait until you postpartum visit to do so. You might have a serious but treatable condition called "postpartum depression." Postpartum depression can happen any time within the first year after birth.

Signs of postpartum depression include:

- Feeling restless or irritable

- Feeling sad, depressed, or crying a lot

- Having no energy

- Having headaches, chest pains, heart palpitations (the heart being fast and feeling like it is skipping beats), numbness, or hyperventilation (fast and shallow breathing)

515

- Not being able to sleep, being very tired, or both
- Not being able to eat and weight loss
- Overeating and weight gain
- Trouble focusing, remembering, or making decisions
- Being overly worried about the baby
- Not having any interest in the baby
- Feeling worthless and guilty
- Having no interest or getting no pleasure from activities like sex and socializing
- Thoughts of harming your baby or yourself

Some women do not tell anyone about their symptoms because they feel embarrassed or guilty about having these feelings at a time when they think they should be happy. Do not let this happen to you! Postpartum depression can make it hard to take care of your baby. Infants with mothers with postpartum depression can have delays in learning how to talk. They can have problems with emotional bonding. Your doctor can help you feel better and get back to enjoying your new baby. Therapy and/or medicine can treat postpartum depression. Emerging research suggests that 1 in 10 new fathers may experience depression during or after pregnancy. Although more research is needed, having depression may make it harder to be a good father and perhaps affect the baby's development. Having depression may also be related to a mother's depression. Expecting or new fathers with emotional problems or symptoms of depression should talk to their doctors. Depression is a treatable illness.

Chapter 66

Your Baby's First Hours and Newborn Screening Tests

After months of waiting, finally, your new baby has arrived! Mothers-to-be often spend so much time in anticipation of labor, they don't think about or even know what to expect during the first hours after delivery. Read on so you will be ready to bond with your new bundle of joy.

What Newborns Look Like

You might be surprised by how your newborn looks at birth. If you had a vaginal delivery, your baby entered this world through a narrow and boney passage. It's not uncommon for newborns to be born bluish, bruised, and with a misshapen head. An ear might be folded over. Your baby may have a complete head of hair or be bald. Your baby also will have a thick, pasty, whitish coating, which protected the skin in the womb. This will wash away during the first bathing.

Once your baby is placed into your arms, your gaze will go right to her or his eyes. Most newborns open their eyes soon after birth.

This chapter contains text excerpted from the following sources: Text in this chapter begins with excerpts from "Your Baby's First Hours of Life," Office on Women's Health (OWH), U.S. Department of Health and Human Services (HHS), June 6, 2018; Text beginning with the heading "What Is Newborn Screening?" is excerpted from "What Is Newborn Screening?" Genetics Home Reference (GHR), National Institutes of Health (NIH), February 19, 2019.

Eyes will be brown or bluish-gray at first. Looking over your baby, you might notice that the face is a little puffy. You might notice small white bumps inside your baby's mouth or on her or his tongue. Your baby might be very wrinkly. Some babies, especially those born early, are covered in soft, fine hair, which will come off in a couple of weeks. Your baby's skin might have various colored marks, blotches, or rashes, and fingernails could be long. You might also notice that your baby's breasts and penis or vulva are a bit swollen.

How your baby looks will change from day to day, and many of the early marks of childbirth go away with time. If you have any concerns about something you see, talk to your doctor. After a few weeks, your newborn will look more and more like the baby you pictured in your dreams.

Bonding with Your Baby

Spending time with your baby in those first hours of life is very special. Although you might be tired, your newborn could be quite alert after birth. Cuddle your baby skin-to-skin. Let your baby get to know your voice and study your face. Your baby can see up to about two feet away. You might notice that your baby throws her or his arms out if someone turns on a light or makes a sudden noise. This is called the "startle response." Babies also are born with grasp and sucking reflexes. Put your finger in your baby's palm and watch how she or he knows to squeeze it. Feed your baby when she or he shows signs of hunger.

Medical Care for Your Newborn

Right after birth, babies need many important tests and procedures to ensure their health. Some of these are even required by law. But as long as the baby is healthy, everything but the Apgar test can wait for at least an hour. Delaying further medical care will preserve the precious first moments of life for you, your partner, and the baby. A baby who has not been poked and prodded may be more willing to nurse and cuddle. So before delivery, talk to your doctor or midwife about delaying shots, medicine, and tests. At the same time, please don't assume "everything is being taken care of." As a parent, it's your job to make sure your newborn gets all the necessary and appropriate vaccines and tests in a timely manner.

The following tests and procedures are recommended or required in most hospitals in the United States:

Apgar Evaluation

The Apgar test is a quick way for doctors to figure out if the baby is healthy or needs extra medical care. Apgar tests are usually done twice: one minute after birth and again five minutes after birth. Doctors and nurses measure five signs of the baby's condition. These are:

- Heart rate
- Breathing
- Activity and muscle tone
- Reflexes
- Skin color

Apgar scores range from 0 to 10. A baby who scores seven or more is considered very healthy. But a lower score doesn't always mean there is something wrong. Perfectly healthy babies often have low Apgar scores in the first minute of life.

In more than 98 percent of cases, the Apgar score reaches seven after five minutes of life. When it does not, the baby needs medical care and close monitoring.

Eye Care

Your baby may receive eye drops or ointment to prevent eye infections they can get during delivery. Sexually transmitted infections (STIs), including gonorrhea and chlamydia, are the main cause of newborn eye infections. These infections can cause blindness if not treated.

Medicines used can sting and/or blur the baby's vision. So you may want to postpone this treatment for a little while.

Some parents question whether this treatment is really necessary. Many women at low risk for STIs do not want their newborns to receive eye medicine. But there is no evidence to suggest that this medicine harms the baby.

It is important to note that even pregnant women who test negative for STIs may get an infection by the time of delivery. Plus, most women with gonorrhea and/or chlamydia don't know it because they have no symptoms.

Vitamin K Shot

The American Academy of Pediatrics (AAP) recommends that all newborns receive a shot of vitamin K in the upper leg. Newborns usually have low levels of vitamin K in their bodies. This vitamin is needed for the blood to clot. Low levels of vitamin K can cause a rare but serious bleeding problem. Research shows that vitamin K shots prevent dangerous bleeding in newborns.

Newborns probably feel pain when the shot is given. But afterwards, babies don't seem to have any discomfort. Since it may be uncomfortable for the baby, you may want to postpone this shot for a little while.

Newborn Metabolic Screening

Doctors or nurses prick your baby's heel to take a tiny sample of blood. They use this blood to test for many diseases. All babies should be tested because a few babies may look healthy but have a rare health problem. A blood test is the only way to find out about these problems. If found right away, serious problems like developmental disabilities, organ damage, blindness, and even death might be prevented.

All 50 states and U.S. territories screen newborns for phenylketonuria (PKU), hypothyroidism, galactosemia, and sickle cell disease. But many states routinely test for up to 30 different diseases. The March of Dimes recommends that all newborns be tested for at least 29 diseases.

You can find out what tests are offered in your state by contacting your state's health department or newborn screening program. Or, you can contact the National Newborn Screening and Genetics Resource Center (NNSGRC).

Hearing Test

Most babies have a hearing screening soon after birth, usually before they leave the hospital. Tiny earphones or microphones are used to see how the baby reacts to sounds. All newborns need a hearing screening because hearing defects are not uncommon, and hearing loss can be hard to detect in babies and young children. When problems are found early, children can get the services they need at an early age. This might prevent delays in speech, language, and thinking. Ask your hospital or your baby's doctor about newborn hearing screening.

Hepatitis B Vaccine

All newborns should get a vaccine to protect against the hepatitis B virus (HBV) before leaving the hospital. Sadly, 1 in 5 babies at risk of HBV infection leaves the hospital without receiving the vaccine and treatment shown to protect newborns, even if exposed to HBV at birth. HBV can cause a lifelong infection, serious liver damage, and even death.

The hepatitis B vaccine (HepB) is a series of three different shots. The AAP and the Centers for Disease Control and Prevention (CDC) recommend that all newborns get the first HepB shot before leaving the hospital. If the mother has HBV, her baby should also get a HBIG shot within 12 hours of birth. The second HepB shot should be given one to two months after birth. The third HepB shot should be given no earlier than 24 weeks of age, but before 18 months of age.

Complete Checkup

Soon after delivery most doctors or nurses also:

- Measure the newborn's weight, length, and head

- Take the baby's temperature

- Measure that baby's breathing and heart rate

- Give the baby a bath and clean the umbilical cord stump

What Is Newborn Screening?

Newborn screening is the practice of testing all babies in their first days of life for certain disorders and conditions that can hinder their normal development. This testing is required in every state and is typically performed before the baby leaves the hospital. The conditions included in newborn screening can cause serious health problems starting in infancy or childhood. Early detection and treatment can help prevent intellectual and physical disabilities and life-threatening illnesses.

How Is Newborn Screening Done?

Newborn screening usually begins with a blood test 24 to 48 hours after a baby is born, while she or he is still in the hospital. In some states, a second blood test is performed at a check-up appointment with the baby's pediatrician when the baby is 1 to 2 weeks old. Newborn screening is part of standard care; parents do not need to request to have the test done.

The test is performed by pricking the baby's heel to collect a few drops of blood. There are very few risks associated with this procedure, and it involves minimal discomfort to the baby. The blood is placed on a special type of paper and sent to a laboratory for analysis. Within 2 to 3 weeks, the test results are sent to the baby's doctor's office or clinic.

If a baby is born outside a hospital (for example, at home or in a birthing center), a doula or midwife may collect the blood sample needed for the newborn screening test. Otherwise, the required testing can be performed at the baby's doctor's office or at a hospital.

In addition to the blood test, most states also screen newborns for hearing loss and critical congenital heart disease. These tests are also done shortly after birth. The hearing test uses earphones and sensors to determine whether the baby's inner ear or brain respond to sound. The test for critical congenital heart disease, called "pulse oximetry," uses a sensor on the skin to measure how much oxygen is in the blood. Low oxygen levels suggest that an infant may have heart problems. The hearing and pulse oximetry tests are painless and can be done while the baby is sleeping.

What Disorders Are Included in Newborn Screening?

The disorders included in newborn screening vary from state to state. Most states test for all of the conditions specified by the Health Resources and Services Administration (HRSA) in their Recommended Uniform Screening Panel. These conditions include phenylketonuria (PKU), cystic fibrosis, sickle cell disease, critical congenital heart disease, hearing loss, and others. Some states test for additional disorders that are not part of the HRSA panel.

Most of the conditions included in newborn screening can cause serious health problems if treatment is not started shortly after birth. Prompt identification and management of these conditions may be able to prevent life-threatening complications.

Parents can ask their baby's healthcare provider about expanded (supplemental) screening if they live in a state that screens for a smaller number of disorders. Supplemental screening is typically done by commercial laboratories. It is separate from the testing done by the state, although it often uses a blood sample drawn at the same time.

Chapter 67

Newborn Health Concerns

Newborn Care[1]

If this is your first baby, you might worry that you are not ready to take care of a newborn. You are not alone. Lots of new parents feel unprepared when it is time to bring their new babies home from the hospital. You can take steps to help yourself get ready for the transition home.

Taking a newborn care class during your pregnancy can prepare you for the real thing. But feeding and diapering a baby doll isn't quite the same. During your hospital stay, make sure to ask the nurses for help with basic baby care. Do not hesitate to ask the nurse to show you how to do something more than once. Remember, practice makes perfect. Before discharge, make sure you—and your partner—are comfortable with these newborn care basics:

- Handling a newborn, including supporting your baby's neck

- Changing your baby's diaper

This chapter includes text excerpted from documents published by two public domain sources. Text under the headings marked 1 are excerpted from "Newborn Care and Safety," Office on Women's Health (OWH), U.S. Department of Health and Human Services (HHS), October 11, 2018; Text under the heading marked 2 is excerpted from "What Are Some of the Basics of Infant Health?" *Eunice Kennedy Shriver* National Institute of Child Health and Human Development (NICHD), December 1, 2016.

- Bathing your baby

- Dressing your baby

- Swaddling your baby

- Feeding and burping your baby

- Cleaning the umbilical cord

- Caring for a healing circumcision

- Using a bulb syringe to clear your baby's nasal passages

- Taking a newborn's temperature

- Tips for soothing your baby

Before leaving the hospital, ask about home visits by a nurse or healthcare worker. Many new parents appreciate somebody checking in with them and their baby a few days after coming home. If you are breastfeeding, ask whether a lactation consultant can come to your home to provide follow-up support, as well as other resources in your community, such as peer support groups.

Many first-time parents also welcome the help of a family member or friend who has "been there." Having a support person stay with you for a few days can give you the confidence to go at it alone in the weeks ahead. Try to arrange this before delivery.

Your baby's first doctor's visit is another good time to ask about any infant care questions you might have. Ask about reasons to call the doctor. Also, ask about what vaccines your baby needs and when. Infants and young children need vaccines because the diseases they protect against can strike at an early age and can be very dangerous in childhood. This includes rare diseases and more common ones, such as the flu.

What Are Some of the Basics of Infant Health?[2]

Some physical conditions and issues are very common during the first couple of weeks after birth. Many are normal, and the infant's caregivers can deal with them if they occur. Mostly, it is a matter of the caregivers learning about what is normal for their infant and getting comfortable with the new routine in the household.

New parents and caregivers often have questions about several aspects of their infant's health and well-being.

Bowel Movements

Infants' bowel movements go through many changes in color and consistency, even within the first few days after birth. It is important to keep track of your infant's bowel movements. Some things to look for include:

- **Color.** A newborn's first bowel movements usually consist of a thick, black or dark green substance called "meconium." After the meconium is passed, the stools ("poop") will turn yellow-green. The stools of breastfed infants look mustard-yellow with seed-like particles.

- **Consistency.** Until the infant starts to eat solid foods, the consistency of the stool can range from very soft to loose and runny. Formula-fed infants usually have stools that are tan or yellow in color and firmer than those of a breastfed infant. Whether your baby is breastfed or bottle-fed, hard or very dry stools may be a sign of dehydration.

- **Frequency.** Infants who are eating solid foods can become constipated if they eat too many constipating foods, such as cereal or cow's milk, before their system can handle them. The U.S. Food and Drug Administration (FDA) and the AAP do not recommend cow's milk for babies under 12 months.

Also, because an infant's stools are normally soft and a little runny, it is not always easy to tell when a young infant has mild diarrhea. The main signs are a sudden increase in the number of bowel movements (more than one per feeding) and watery stools.

Diarrhea can be a sign of intestinal infection, or it may be caused by a change in diet. If the infant is breastfeeding, diarrhea can result from a change in the mother's diet. The main concern with diarrhea is the possibility that dehydration can develop. If fever is also present and your infant is less than two months old, you should call your healthcare provider. If the infant is over two months old and the fever lasts more than a day, check the infant's urine output and rectal temperature and consult a healthcare provider. Make sure the infant continues to feed often.

Starting around the age of three to six weeks, some breastfed babies have only one bowel movement a week. This is normal because breast milk leaves very little solid waste to pass through the digestive system. Formula-fed infants should have at least one bowel movement a day. If a formula-fed infant has fewer bowel movements than this and appears to be straining because of hard stools, constipation may be the cause. Check with your healthcare provider if there are any changes in or problems with your infant's bowel movements.

Care of the Umbilicus

The umbilical cord delivers oxygen and nutrients to the fetus while it is in the womb. After delivery, the umbilical cord is cut. The remaining part of the cord dries and falls off in about 10 days, forming the belly button (navel).

Follow your healthcare provider's recommendations about how to care for the umbilicus. This care might include:

- Keeping the area clean and dry.

- Folding down the top of the diaper to expose the umbilicus to the air.

- Cleaning the umbilicus gently with a baby wipe or with a cotton swab dipped in rubbing alcohol.

Contact your healthcare provider if there is pus or redness.

Colic

Many infants are fussy in the evenings, but if the crying does not stop and gets worse throughout the day or night, it may be caused by colic. According to the AAP, about one-fifth of all infants develop colic, usually starting between two and four weeks of age. They may cry inconsolably or scream, extend or pull up their legs, and pass gas. Their stomachs may be enlarged. The crying spells can occur anytime, although they often get worse in the early evening.

The colic will likely improve or disappear by the age of three or four months. There is no definite explanation for why some infants get colic. Sometimes, in breastfeeding babies, colic is a sign of sensitivity to a food in the mother's diet. Rarely, colic is caused by sensitivity to milk protein in formula. Colic could be a sign of a medical problem, such as a hernia or some type of illness.

If your infant shows signs of colic, the first step is to consult with your healthcare provider. Sometimes changing the diet of a breastfeeding mother or changing the formula for bottle-fed infants can help. Some infants seem to be soothed by being held, rocked, or wrapped snugly in a blanket. Some like a pacifier.

Diaper Rash

A rash on the skin covered by a diaper is quite common. It is usually caused by irritation of the skin from being in contact with stool and urine. It can get worse during bouts of diarrhea. Diaper rash usually can be prevented by frequent diaper changes.

Your healthcare provider can recommend care for diaper rash, which may include:

- Rinsing the skin with warm water, using soap only after bowel movements. Because baby wipes may leave a film of bacteria on the skin, their use is often not recommended.

- Exposing the rash to air as much as possible by loosely attaching the diaper at the waist, or removing the diaper entirely during naps.

- Laying the infant on a towel to absorb urine.

Caregivers should contact a healthcare provider if the rash is not better in 3 days or if the child becomes worse.

Spitting Up / Vomiting

Spitting up is a common occurrence for newborns and is usually not a sign of a more serious problem. After feeding, try to keep the infant calm and in an upright position for a little while. Keep a burp towel handy, just in case. Contact your healthcare provider immediately if your infant:

- Is not gaining weight

- Is spitting up so forcefully that stomach contents shoot out of the infant's mouth

- Spits up green or yellow liquid, blood, or a substance that looks like coffee grounds

- Has blood in the stool

- Shows other signs of illness, such as fever, diarrhea, or difficulty with breathing

Some parents worry that their infant will spit up and choke if they are put to sleep on their backs, but this is not the case. Healthy infants naturally swallow or cough up fluids—it is a reflex all people have. Where the opening to the windpipe is located in the body makes it unlikely for fluids to cause choking. Babies may actually clear such fluids better when on their backs.

Teething

Although newborns usually have no visible teeth, baby teeth begin to appear generally about six months after birth. During the first few years, all 20 baby teeth will push through the gums, and most children will have their full set of these teeth in place by age three.

An infant's front four teeth usually appear first, at about six months of age, although some children do not get their first tooth until 12 or 14 months. As their teeth break through the gums, some infants become fussy, sleepless, and irritable; lose their appetite, or drool more than usual. If an infant has a fever or diarrhea while teething or continues to be cranky and uncomfortable, contact your baby's healthcare provider.

The FDA does not recommend gum-numbing medications with an ingredient called "benzocaine," because they can cause a potentially fatal condition in young children. Talk to your healthcare provider for advice on using these products for your teething infant. Other potential forms of relief for your infant include a chilled teething ring or gently rubbing the child's gums with a clean finger.

Urination

Infants urinate as often as every one to three hours or as infrequently as every four to six hours. In case of sickness or if the weather is very hot, urine output might drop by half and still be normal.

Urination should never be painful. If you notice any signs of distress while your infant is urinating, notify your child's healthcare provider because this could be a sign of infection or some other problem in the urinary tract. In a healthy child, urine is light to dark yellow in color. (The darker the color, the more concentrated the urine; the urine is more concentrated when the child is not drinking much liquid.) The presence of blood in the urine or a bloody spot on the diaper is not normal and should prompt a call to the healthcare provider. If this bleeding occurs with other symptoms, such as abdominal pain or bleeding in other areas, immediate medical attention is needed.

Jaundice

Jaundice can cause an infant's skin, eyes, and mouth to turn a yellowish color. The yellow color is caused by a buildup of bilirubin, a substance that is produced in the body during the normal process of breaking down old red blood cells and forming new ones.

Normally the liver removes bilirubin from the body. But, for many infants, in the first few days after birth, the liver is not yet working at its full power. As a result, the level of bilirubin in the blood gets too high, causing the infant's color to become slightly yellow—this is jaundice.

Although jaundice is common and usually not serious, in some cases, high levels of bilirubin could cause brain injury. All infants with jaundice need to be seen by a healthcare provider.

Many infants need no treatment. Their livers start to catch up quickly and begin to remove bilirubin normally, usually within a few days after birth. For some infants, healthcare providers prescribe phototherapy—a treatment using a special lamp—to help break down the bilirubin in their bodies.

If your infant has jaundice, ask your healthcare provider how long the child's jaundice should last after leaving the hospital, and schedule a follow-up appointment as directed. If jaundice lasts longer than expected, or an infant who did not have jaundice starts to turn yellowish after going home, a healthcare provider should be consulted right away. If you intend to get discharged early, particularly within 48 hours of birth, your infant's jaundice may peak later in the first week.

It is almost impossible to say how severe the jaundice level is by just looking at the baby's skin. Therefore, make every effort to keep follow-up appointments so the healthcare provider can check the level of jaundice with a simple blood test.

Sudden Infant Death Syndrome[1]

Since 1992, the American Academy of Pediatrics (AAP) has recommended that infants be placed to sleep on their backs to reduce the risk of sudden infant death syndrome (SIDS), also called "crib death." SIDS is the sudden and unexplained death of a baby under one year of age. Even though there is no way to know which babies might die of SIDS, there are some things that you can do to make your baby safer:

- Always place your baby on his or her back to sleep, even for naps. This is the safest sleep position for a healthy baby to reduce the risk of SIDS.

- Place your baby on a firm mattress, such as in a safety-approved crib. Research has shown that placing a baby to sleep on soft mattresses, sofas, sofa cushions, waterbeds, sheepskins, or other soft surfaces raises the risk of SIDS.

• Remove soft, fluffy, and loose bedding and stuffed toys from your baby's sleep area. Make sure you keep all pillows, quilts, stuffed toys, and other soft items away from your baby's sleep area.

• Do not use infant sleep positioners. Using a positioner to hold an infant on his or her back or side for sleep is dangerous and not needed.

• Make sure everyone who cares for your baby knows to place your baby on his or her back to sleep and about the dangers of soft bedding. Talk to child care providers, grandparents, babysitters, and all caregivers about SIDS risk. Remember, every sleep time counts.

• Make sure your baby's face and head stay uncovered during sleep. Keep blankets and other coverings away from your baby's mouth and nose. The best way to do this is to dress the baby in sleep clothing so you will not have to use any other covering over the baby. If you do use a blanket or another covering, make sure that the baby's feet are at the bottom of the crib, the blanket is no higher than the baby's chest, and the blanket is tucked in around the bottom of the crib mattress.

• Do not allow smoking around your baby. Do not smoke before or after the birth of your baby and make sure no one smokes around your baby.

• Do not let your baby get too warm during sleep. Keep your baby warm during sleep, but not too warm. Your baby's room should be at a temperature that is comfortable for an adult. Too many layers of clothing or blankets can overheat your baby.

Some mothers worry if the baby rolls over during the night. However, by the time your baby is able to roll over by herself, the risk for SIDS is much lower. During the time of greatest risk, two to four months of age, most babies are not able to turn over from their backs to their stomachs.

Chapter 68

Infant Feeding

Chapter Contents

Section 68.1

Breastfeeding

This section includes text excerpted from "Breastfeeding—
Making the Decision to Breastfeed," Office on Women's
Health (OWH), U.S. Department of Health and
Human Services (HHS), December 6, 2018.

When you breastfeed, you give your baby a healthy start that lasts a lifetime. Breastmilk is the perfect food for your baby. Breastfeeding saves lives, money, and time.

What Health Benefits Does Breastfeeding Give My Baby?

The cells, hormones, and antibodies in breastmilk help protect babies from illness. This protection is unique and changes every day to meet your baby's growing needs.

Research shows that breastfed babies have lower risks of:

- Asthma

- Leukemia (during childhood)

- Obesity (during childhood)

- Ear infections

- Eczema (atopic dermatitis)

- Diarrhea and vomiting

- Lower respiratory infections

- Necrotizing enterocolitis, a disease that affects the gastrointestinal tract in premature babies, or babies born before 37 weeks of pregnancy

- Sudden infant death syndrome (SIDS)

- Type 2 diabetes

What Is Colostrum and How Does It Help My Baby?

Your breastmilk helps your baby grow healthy and strong from day one.

Your first milk is liquid gold. Called liquid gold for its deep yellow color, colostrum is the thick first milk that you make during pregnancy and just after birth. This milk is very rich in nutrients and includes antibodies to protect your baby from infections.

Colostrum also helps your newborn's digestive system to grow and function. Your baby gets only a small amount of colostrum at each feeding, because the stomach of a newborn infant is tiny and can hold only a small amount.

Your milk changes as your baby grows. Colostrum changes into mature milk by the third to fifth day after birth. This mature milk has just the right amount of fat, sugar, water, and protein to help your baby continue to grow. It looks thinner than colostrum, but it has the nutrients and antibodies your baby needs for healthy growth.

What Are the Health Benefits of Breastfeeding for Mothers?

Breastfeeding helps a mother's health and healing following childbirth. Breastfeeding leads to a lower risk of these health problems in mothers:

- Type 2 diabetes

- Certain types of breast cancer

- Ovarian cancer

How Does Breastfeeding Compare to Formula Feeding?

- **Formula can be harder for your baby to digest.** For most babies, especially premature babies (babies born before 37 weeks of pregnancy), breastmilk substitutes like formula are harder to digest than breastmilk. Formula is made from cow's milk, and it often takes time for babies' stomachs to adjust to digesting it.

- **Your breastmilk changes to meet your baby's needs.** As your baby gets older, your breastmilk adjusts to meet your baby's changing needs. Researchers think that a baby's saliva transfers chemicals to a mother's body through breastfeeding. These chemicals help a mother's body create breastmilk that meets the baby's changing needs.

- **Life can be easier for you when you breastfeed.**
  Breastfeeding may seem like it takes a little more effort than
  formula feeding at first. But breastfeeding can make your life
  easier once you and your baby settle into a good routine. When
  you breastfeed, there are no bottles and nipples to sterilize. You
  do not have to buy, measure, and mix formula. And there are no
  bottles to warm in the middle of the night. When you breastfeed,
  you can satisfy your baby's hunger right away.

- **Not breastfeeding costs money.** Formula and feeding
  supplies can cost well over $1,500 each year. As your baby gets
  older she or he will eat more formula. But breastmilk changes
  with the baby's needs, and babies usually need the same amount
  of breastmilk as they get older. Breastfed babies may also be
  sick less often, which can help keep your baby's health costs
  lower.

- **Breastfeeding keeps mother and baby close.** Physical
  contact is important to newborns. It helps them feel more secure,
  warm, and comforted. Mothers also benefit from this closeness.
  The skin-to-skin contact boosts your oxytocin levels. Oxytocin is
  a hormone that helps breastmilk flow and can calm the mother.

Sometimes, formula feeding can save lives:

- Very rarely, babies are born unable to tolerate milk of any
  kind. These babies must have an infant formula that is
  hypoallergenic, dairy free, or lactose-free. A wide selection
  of specialist baby formulas now on the market includes
  soy formula, hydrolyzed formula, lactose-free formula, and
  hypoallergenic formula.

- Your baby may need formula if you have a health problem that
  won't allow you to breastfeed and you do not have access to
  donor breastmilk.

Talk to your doctor before feeding your baby anything besides your
breastmilk.

Can Breastfeeding Help Me Lose Weight?

Besides giving your baby nourishment and helping to keep your
baby from becoming sick, breastfeeding may help you lose weight.
Many women who breastfed their babies said it helped them get back

to their prepregnancy weight more quickly, but experts are still looking at the effects of breastfeeding on weight loss.

How Does Breastfeeding Benefit Society?

Society benefits overall when mothers breastfeed.

- **Breastfeeding saves lives.** Research shows that if 90 percent of families breastfed exclusively for six months, nearly 1,000 deaths among infants could be prevented each year.

- **Breastfeeding saves money.** Medical costs may be lower for fully-breastfed infants than never-breastfed infants. Breastfed infants usually need fewer sick care visits, prescriptions, and hospitalizations.

- **Breastfeeding also helps make a more productive workforce.** Mothers who breastfeed may miss less work to care for sick infants than mothers who feed their infants formula. Employer medical costs may also be lower.

- **Breastfeeding is better for the environment.** Formula cans and bottle supplies create more trash and plastic waste. Your milk is a renewable resource that comes packaged and warmed.

How Does Breastfeeding Help in an Emergency?

During an emergency, such as a natural disaster, breastfeeding can save your baby's life:

- Breastfeeding protects your baby from the risks of an unclean water supply.

- Breastfeeding can help protect your baby against respiratory illnesses and diarrhea.

- Your milk is always at the right temperature for your baby. It helps to keep your baby's body temperature from dropping too low.

- Your milk is always available without needing other supplies.

Section 68.2

Formula Feeding

This section includes text excerpted from "Infant Formula
Feeding," Centers for Disease Control and
Prevention (CDC), December 3, 2018.

If you are feeding your baby infant formula, there are some important things to know, such as how to choose an infant formula and how to prepare and store your infant's formula.

Choosing an Infant Formula

There is no particular brand of infant formula that is best for all babies. Choose an infant formula that is made especially for babies. The U.S. Food and Drug Administration (FDA) regulates commercial infant formulas which come in liquid and powder form. It is important to choose an iron-fortified infant formula. Most commercial infant formulas sold in the United States contain iron.

Other things to remember when choosing an infant formula:

- The FDA warns against using recipes to make homemade infant formula. Using homemade infant formula can lead to serious health concerns for your baby.

- Make sure the infant formula you have selected is not expired.

- The infant formula container should be in good condition. If there are any leaks, puffy ends, or rust spots, do not feed it to your infant.

You can ask your child's doctor or nurse if you have questions about choosing an infant formula for your baby. If you are thinking of switching infant formula brand or type, talk with your child's doctor or nurse.

Infant Formula Preparation and Storage

Carefully read and follow the instructions on the infant formula container. These steps will help you know how to prepare and store your infant's formula correctly. Preparing your infant's formula according to the instructions is important.

Here are additional pointers to keep in mind when preparing and storing your infant's formula.

Preparation

- Wash your hands well before preparing bottles or feeding your baby. Clean and sanitize the workspace where you will be preparing the infant formula.

- Bottles need to be clean and sanitized.

- Baby's milk or infant formula does not need to be warmed before feeding, but some people like to warm their baby's bottle. If you do decide to warm the bottle, never use a microwave. Microwaves heat milk and food unevenly, resulting in "hot spots" that can burn your baby's mouth and throat.

  - To warm a bottle: Place the bottle under running warm water, taking care to keep the water from getting into the bottle or on the nipple. Put a couple drops of infant formula on the back of your hand to see if it is too hot.

- If you use powdered infant formula:

  - Use water from a safe source to mix your infant formula. If you are not sure if your tap water is safe to use for preparing infant formula, contact your local health department.

  - Use the amount of water listed on the instructions of the infant formula container. Always measure the water first and then add the powder.

  - Too much water may not meet the nutritional needs of your baby

  - Too little water may cause your baby's kidneys and digestive system to work too hard and may cause your baby to become dehydrated

- If your baby is very young (younger than three months old), was born prematurely, or has a weakened immune system, you may want to take extra precautions in preparing your infant's formula to protect against Cronobacter.

Use Quickly or Store Safely

- Store unopened infant formula containers in a cool, dry, indoor place—not in vehicles, garages, or outdoors.

- Prepared infant formula can spoil if it is left out at room temperature.

- Use prepared infant formula within two hours of preparation and within one hour from when feeding begins.

- If you do not start to use the prepared infant formula within two hours, immediately store the bottle in the fridge and use it within 24 hours.

- Throw out any infant formula that is left in the bottle after feeding your baby. The combination of infant formula and your baby's saliva can cause bacteria to grow. Be sure to clean and sanitize the bottle before its next use.

How Much and How Often to Feed Infant Formula

Every baby is different. How much and how often your baby feeds will depend on your baby's needs. Here are a few things to know about infant formula feeding during the first days, weeks, and months of your baby's life.

First Days

- Your newborn baby's belly is tiny. She or he does not need a lot of infant formula with each feeding to be full.

- You can start by offering your baby 1 to 2 ounces of infant formula every 2 to 3 hours in the first days of life if your baby is only getting infant formula and no breast milk. Give your baby more if she or he is showing signs of hunger.

- Most infant formula-fed newborns will feed 8 to 12 times in 24 hours. Talk with your child's doctor or nurse about how much infant formula is right for your baby.

- As your baby grows, his or her belly grows too. Your baby will be able to drink more infant formula at each feeding, and the time between feedings will get longer.

First Weeks and Months

- Over the first few weeks and months, the time between feedings will get longer—about every 3 to 4 hours for most infant formula-fed babies. This means you may need to wake your baby to feed. You can try patting, stroking, undressing, or changing the diaper to help wake your baby to feed.

- Some feeding sessions may be long, and other feedings short. That is okay. Babies will generally take what they need at each feeding and stop eating when they are full.

6 to 12 Months Old

Continue feeding your baby when she or he shows signs of hunger. Most 6 to 12 month olds will need infant formula or solid foods about 5 to 6 times in 24 hours.

As your baby gradually starts eating more solid foods, the amount of infant formula she or he needs each day will likely start to decrease.

12 to 24 Months Old

When your toddler is 12 months old, you can switch from infant formula to fortified cow's milk. You can do this gradually. You may want to start by replacing one infant formula feeding with fortified cow's milk to help your child transition.

Chapter 69

Bonding with Your Baby

What's Happening?

Attachment is a deep, lasting bond that develops between a caregiver and child during the baby's first few years of life. This attachment is crucial to the growth of a baby's body and mind. Babies who have this bond and feel loved have a better chance to grow up to be adults who trust others and know how to return affection.

What You Might Be Seeing

Normal babies:

- Have brief periods of sleep, crying or fussing, and quiet alertness many times each day

- Often cry for long periods for no apparent reason

- Love to be held and cuddled

- Respond to and imitate facial expressions

- Love soothing voices and respond to them with smiles and small noises

- Grow and develop every day

This chapter includes text excerpted from "Bonding with Your Baby," Child Welfare Information Gateway, U.S. Department of Health and Human Services (HHS), February 18, 2007. Reviewed February 2019.

- Learn new skills quickly and can outgrow difficult behaviors in a matter of weeks

What You Can Do

No one knows your child like you do, so you are in the best position to recognize and fulfill your child's needs. Parents who give lots of loving care and attention to their babies help their babies develop a strong attachment. Affection stimulates your child to grow, learn, connect with others, and enjoy life. Here are some ways to promote bonding:

- Respond when your baby cries. Try to understand what she or he is saying to you. You can't "spoil" babies with too much attention—they need and benefit from a parent's loving care, even when they seem inconsolable.

- Hold and touch your baby as much as possible. You can keep her or him close with baby slings, pouches, or backpacks (for older babies).

- Use feeding and diapering times to look into your baby's eyes, smile, and talk to your baby.

- Read, sing, and play peek-a-boo. Babies love to hear human voices and will try to imitate your voice and the sounds you make.

- As your baby gets a little older, try simple games and toys. Once your baby can sit up, plan on spending lots of time on the floor with toys, puzzles, and books.

- If you feel you are having trouble bonding with your infant, don't wait to get help. Talk to your doctor or your baby's pediatrician as soon as you can.

Chapter 70

Working after Birth: Parental Leave Considerations

Chapter Contents

Section 70.1

Know Your Pregnancy Rights

This section contains text excerpted from the following sources:
Text under the heading "Pregnancy Rights" is excerpted from
"Know Your Pregnancy Rights," Office on Women's Health (OWH),
U.S. Department of Health and Human Services (HHS), January
30, 2019; Text under the heading "Pregnancy Discrimination" is
excerpted from "Pregnancy Discrimination," U.S. Equal
Employment Opportunity Commission (EEOC),
February 11, 2012. Reviewed February 2019.

Pregnancy Rights

When sharing your good news with coworkers, discrimination might
be the last thing on your mind. But the truth is that many women
are treated unfairly—or even fired—after revealing the news of their
pregnancy.

As long as a pregnant woman is able to perform the major functions
of her job, not hiring or firing her because she is pregnant is against
the law. It is against the law to dock her pay or demote her to a lesser
position because of pregnancy. It is also against the law to hold back
benefits for pregnancy because a woman is not married. All are forms
of pregnancy discrimination, and all are illegal.

Women are protected under the Pregnancy Discrimination Act
(PDA). It says that businesses with at least 15 employees must treat
women who are pregnant in the same manner as other job applicants
or employees with similar abilities or limitations.

The Family and Medical Leave Act (FMLA) also protects the jobs of
workers who are employed by companies with 50 employees or more
and who have worked for the company for at least 12 months. These
companies must allow employees to take 12 weeks of unpaid leave for
medical reasons, including pregnancy and childbirth. Your job cannot
be given away during this 12-week period.

Many state laws also protect pregnant women's rights.

These laws appear clear cut. But issues that arise on the job seldom
are.

Pregnancy Discrimination

Pregnancy discrimination involves treating a woman (an applicant
or employee) unfavorably because of pregnancy, childbirth, or a medical condition related to pregnancy or childbirth.

Pregnancy Discrimination and Work Situations

The PDA forbids discrimination based on pregnancy when it comes to any aspect of employment, including hiring, firing, pay, job assignments, promotions, layoff, training, fringe benefits, such as leave and health insurance, and any other term or condition of employment.

Pregnancy Discrimination and Temporary Disability

If a woman is temporarily unable to perform her job due to a medical condition related to pregnancy or childbirth, the employer or other covered entity must treat her in the same way as it treats any other temporarily disabled employee. For example, the employer may have to provide light duty, alternative assignments, disability leave, or unpaid leave to pregnant employees if it does so for other temporarily disabled employees.

Additionally, impairments resulting from pregnancy (for example, gestational diabetes or preeclampsia, a condition characterized by pregnancy-induced hypertension and protein in the urine) may be disabilities under the Americans with Disabilities Act (ADA). An employer may have to provide a reasonable accommodation (such as leave or modifications that enable an employee to perform her job) for a disability related to pregnancy, absent undue hardship (significant difficulty or expense). The ADA Amendments Act of 2008 makes it much easier to show that a medical condition is a covered disability.

Pregnancy Discrimination and Harassment

It is unlawful to harass a woman because of pregnancy, childbirth, or a medical condition related to pregnancy or childbirth. Harassment is illegal when it is so frequent or severe that it creates a hostile or offensive work environment or when it results in an adverse employment decision (such as the victim being fired or demoted). The harasser can be the victim's supervisor, a supervisor in another area, a coworker, or someone who is not an employee of the employer, such as a client or customer.

Pregnancy, Maternity, and Parental Leave

Under the PDA, an employer that allows temporarily disabled employees to take disability leave or leave without pay must allow an employee who is temporarily disabled due to pregnancy to do the same.

An employer may not single out pregnancy-related conditions for special procedures to determine an employee's ability to work. However, if an employer requires its employees to submit a doctor's statement concerning their ability to work before granting leave or paying sick benefits, the employer may require employees affected by pregnancy-related conditions to submit such statements.

Further, under the Family and Medical Leave Act (FMLA) of 1993, a new parent (including foster and adoptive parents) may be eligible for 12 weeks of leave (unpaid or paid if the employee has earned or accrued it) that may be used for the care of the new child. To be eligible, the employee must have worked for the employer for 12 months prior to taking the leave and the employer must have a specified number of employees.

Pregnancy and Workplace Laws

Pregnant employees may have additional rights under the FMLA, which is enforced by the U.S. Department of Labor (DOL). Nursing mothers may also have the right to express milk in the workplace under a provision of the Fair Labor Standards Act enforced by the U.S. Department of Labor's Wage and Hour Division (WHD).

Section 70.2

Family and Medical Leave Act

This section includes text excerpted from "Fact Sheet #28: The Family and Medical Leave Act," U.S. Department of Labor (DOL), February 5, 2013. Reviewed February 2019.

The Family and Medical Leave Act (FMLA) entitles eligible employees of covered employers to take unpaid, job-protected leave for specified family and medical reasons. This section provides general information about which employers are covered by the FMLA, when employees are eligible and entitled to take FMLA leave, and what rules apply when employees take FMLA leave.

Covered Employers

The FMLA only applies to employers that meet certain criteria. A covered employer is a:

- Private sector employer, with 50 or more employees in 20 or more workweeks in the current or preceding calendar year, including a joint employer or successor in interest to a covered employer

- Public agency, including a local, state, or federal government agency, regardless of the number of employees it employs

- Public or private elementary or secondary school, regardless of the number of employees it employs

Eligible Employees

Only eligible employees are entitled to take FMLA leave. An eligible employee is one who:

- Works for a covered employer

- Has worked for the employer for at least 12 months

- Has at least 1,250 hours of service for the employer during the 12 month period immediately preceding the leave*

- Works at a location where the employer has at least 50 employees within 75 miles

Special hours of service eligibility requirements apply to airline flight crew employees.

The 12 months of employment do not have to be consecutive. That means any time previously worked for the same employer (including seasonal work) could, in most cases, be used to meet the 12-month requirement. If the employee has a break in service that lasted seven years or more, the time worked prior to the break will not count unless the break is due to service covered by the Uniformed Services Employment and Reemployment Rights Act (USERRA), or there is a written agreement, including a collective bargaining agreement, outlining the employer's intention to rehire the employee after the break in service.

Leave Entitlement

Eligible employees may take up to 12 workweeks of leave in a 12-month period for one or more of the following reasons:

- The birth of a son or daughter or placement of a son or daughter with the employee for adoption or foster care

- To care for a spouse, son, daughter, or parent who has a serious health condition

- For a serious health condition that makes the employee unable to perform the essential functions of his or her job

- For any qualifying exigency arising out of the fact that a spouse, son, daughter, or parent is a military member on covered active duty or call to covered active duty status

An eligible employee may also take up to 26 workweeks of leave during a "single 12-month period" to care for a covered servicemember with a serious injury or illness, when the employee is the spouse, son, daughter, parent, or next of kin of the servicemember. The "single 12-month period" for military caregiver leave is different from the 12-month period used for other FMLA leave reasons.

Under some circumstances, employees may take FMLA leave on an intermittent or reduced schedule basis. That means an employee may take leave in separate blocks of time or by reducing the time she or he works each day or week for a single qualifying reason. When leave is needed for planned medical treatment, the employee must make a reasonable effort to schedule treatment so as not to unduly disrupt the employer's operations. If FMLA leave is for the birth, adoption, or foster placement of a child, use of intermittent or reduced schedule leave requires the employer's approval.

Under certain conditions, employees may choose, or employers may require employees, to "substitute" (run concurrently) accrued paid leave, such as sick or vacation leave, to cover some or all of the FMLA leave period. An employee's ability to substitute accrued paid leave is determined by the terms and conditions of the employer's normal leave policy.

Notice

Employees must comply with their employer's usual and customary requirements for requesting leave and provide enough information for their employer to reasonably determine whether the FMLA may apply to the leave request. Employees generally must request leave 30 days in advance when the need for leave is foreseeable. When the need for leave is foreseeable less than 30 days in advance or is unforeseeable, employees must provide notice as soon as possible and practicable under the circumstances.

When an employee seeks leave for a FMLA-qualifying reason for the first time, the employee need not expressly assert FMLA rights or even mention the FMLA. If an employee later requests additional leave for the same qualifying condition, the employee must specifically reference either the qualifying reason for leave or the need for FMLA leave.

Covered employers must:

1. Post a notice explaining rights and responsibilities under the FMLA. Covered employers may be subject to a civil money penalty for willful failure to post.

2. Include information about the FMLA in their employee handbooks or provide information to new employees upon hire

3. When an employee requests FMLA leave or the employer acquires knowledge that leave may be for a FMLA-qualifying reason, provide the employee with notice concerning his or her eligibility for FMLA leave and his or her rights and responsibilities under the FMLA

4. Notify employees whether leave is designated as FMLA leave and the amount of leave that will be deducted from the employee's FMLA entitlement

Certification

When an employee requests FMLA leave due to his or her own serious health condition or a covered family member's serious health condition, the employer may require certification in support of the leave from a healthcare provider. An employer may also require second or third medical opinions (at the employer's expense) and periodic recertification of a serious health condition.

Job Restoration and Health Benefits

Upon return from FMLA leave, an employee must be restored to his or her original job or to an equivalent job with equivalent pay, benefits, and other terms and conditions of employment. An employee's use of FMLA leave cannot be counted against the employee under a "no-fault" attendance policy. Employers are also required to continue group health insurance coverage for an employee on FMLA leave under the same terms and conditions as if the employee had not taken leave.

Other Provisions

Special rules apply to employees of local education agencies. Generally, these rules apply to intermittent or reduced schedule FMLA leave or the taking of FMLA leave near the end of a school term.

Salaried executive, administrative, and professional employees of covered employers who meet the Fair Labor Standards Act (FLSA) criteria for exemption from minimum wage and overtime under the FLSA regulations, 29 CFR Part 541, do not lose their FLSA-exempt status by using any unpaid FMLA leave. This special exception to the "salary basis" requirements for FLSA's exemption extends only to an eligible employee's use of FMLA leave.

Enforcement

It is unlawful for any employer to interfere with, restrain, or deny the exercise of or the attempt to exercise any right provided by the FMLA. It is also unlawful for an employer to discharge or discriminate against any individual for opposing any practice, or because of involvement in any proceeding, related to the FMLA. The Wage and Hour Division (WHD) is responsible for administering and enforcing the FMLA for most employees.

Most federal and certain congressional employees are also covered by the law but are subject to the jurisdiction of the U.S. Office of Personnel Management (OPM) or Congress. If you believe that your rights under the FMLA have been violated, you may file a complaint with the Wage and Hour Division or file a private lawsuit against your employer in court.

Section 70.3

Breastfeeding and Going Back to Work

This section contains text excerpted from the following sources: Text in this section begins with excerpts from "Breastfeeding and Going Back to Work," Office on Women's Health (OWH), U.S. Department of Health and Human Services (HHS), December 6, 2018; Text under the heading "Tips for Breastfeeding after Maternity Leave" is excerpted from "5 Tips: Breastfeeding after Maternity Leave," Office on Women's Health (OWH), U.S. Department of Health and Human Services (HHS), July 30, 2015. Reviewed February 2019.

Planning ahead for your return to work can help ease the transition. Learn as much as you can before the baby's birth, and talk with your employer about your options. Planning ahead can help you continue to enjoy breastfeeding your baby long after your maternity leave is over.

What Can I Do during My Pregnancy to Prepare for Breastfeeding after Returning to Work?

- Take a breastfeeding class, which may be offered at the hospital where you plan to deliver your baby. These classes offer tips on returning to work and continuing to breastfeed

- Join a breastfeeding support group to talk with other moms about breastfeeding while working.

- Watch videos of moms who successfully breastfed, including after returning to work.

- Talk with your boss about your plans to breastfeed before you go out on maternity leave.

- Encourage your boss to visit the Supporting Nursing Moms at Work: Employer Solutions (www.womenshealth.gov/supporting-nursing-moms-work?from=breastfeeding) site to get tips and solutions for supporting nursing mothers at work in all different types of workplaces.

- Discuss different types of schedules with your boss, such as starting back part-time at first or taking split shifts.

- Learn about your rights under the federal Break Time for Nursing Mothers law. The law requires some employers to

551

provide reasonable break time for employees to express milk for their nursing child for one year after their child's birth. These include a functional space and time for women to express milk each time they need to.

- Find out if your company offers a lactation support program for employees.

- Talk to other women at your company. Ask the lactation program director, your supervisor, the wellness program director, the employee human resources office, or other coworkers if they know of other women who breastfed after returning to work.

- Explore child care options. Find out whether a child care facility close to where you work is available, so that you can visit and breastfeed your baby during lunch or other breaks. Ask whether the facility has a place set aside for breastfeeding mothers. Make sure the facility will feed your baby with your pumped breastmilk.

What Can I Do While on Maternity Leave to Make Breastfeeding More Successful after I Return to Work?

- Take as many weeks off as you can. Taking at least six weeks of leave can help you recover from childbirth and settle into a good breastfeeding routine.

- Practice expressing your milk by hand or with a breast pump several days or weeks before you have to go back to work. It can feel very different to pump breastmilk compared to breastfeeding your baby. Some women find it helpful to get comfortable with their breast pump or hand expression while they are at home in a stress-free environment.

- A breast pump may be the best method for quickly removing milk during work. A hands-free breast pump may even allow you to work while pumping if you do office work.

- Pump breastmilk while your baby is napping or being looked after by others. Build up a supply of breastmilk for caregivers to give your baby while you are at work.

- Help your baby adjust to taking breastmilk from a bottle or cup. It may be helpful to have someone else give the bottle or cup to your baby at first. Wait at least a month after birth before introducing a bottle to your infant. Your baby may be able to drink from a cup at three or four months old.

• Talk with your family and your child care provider about your desire to breastfeed for as long as possible. Let them know you will need their support and how they can best help you. Follow these suggestions on how people in your network can support your breastfeeding goals.

What Can I Do When I Return to Work to Help Ease the Transition?

• Keep talking with your boss about your schedule and what is or isn't working for you. Under the Patient Protection and Affordable Care Act, most employers, with few exceptions, must offer a breastfeeding employee reasonable break times to pump for up to one year after her baby is born and a place other than a bathroom to comfortably, safely, and privately express breastmilk.

• When you arrive to pick up your baby from child care, see if you can take time to breastfeed your baby right away. This will give you and your baby time to reconnect before going home.

How Often Should I Pump at Work?

At work, you will need to pump during the times you would feed your baby if you were at home. As a general rule, in the first few months of life, babies need to breastfeed 8 to 12 times in 24 hours. As the baby gets older, the number of feedings may go down.

Pumping can take about 10 to 15 minutes once you are used to using your breast pump. Sometimes it may take longer. Many women use their regular breaks and lunch break to pump. Some women come to work early or stay late to make up the time needed to pump.

Where Should I Store My Breastmilk?

Breastmilk is food, so it is safe to keep it in an employee refrigerator or a cooler with ice packs. Talk to your boss about keeping your milk in an employee refrigerator if you think anyone will be concerned. If you work in a medical department, do not store milk in the same refrigerators where medical specimens are kept.

Label the milk container with your name and the date you expressed the milk. Try to keep the milk in the back of the refrigerator where the temperature is the most constant and coldest.

How Much Breastmilk Should I Send with My Baby during the Day?

You may need to pump two to three times each day at work to make enough milk for your baby while she or he is with a caregiver.

Research shows that breastfed babies between one and six months old take in an average of 2 to 3 ounces per feeding. As your baby gets older, your breastmilk changes to meet your baby's needs. So your baby will get the nutrition she or he needs from the same number of ounces at nine months as she or he did at three months.

Some babies eat less during the day when they are away from their mothers and then nurse more often at night. This is called "reverse-cycling." Or babies may eat during the day and still nurse more often at night. This may be more for the closeness with you that your baby craves. If your baby reverse-cycles, you may find that you do not need to pump as much milk for your baby during the day.

Tips for Breastfeeding after Maternity Leave

If you are pregnant or recently gave birth and you want to continue breastfeeding after you go back to work, here are five things that will make it easier.

1. **Know the law is on your side.** You may know that the Affordable Care Act (ACA) provides greater access to health coverage, but it also includes provisions around breastfeeding. The Break Time for Nursing Mothers law requires most employers of hourly workers to provide basic breastfeeding accommodations like time to pump and a functional, private space other than a bathroom. Many states also have laws that protect your right to pump, or "express milk," while at work.

2. **Plan ahead.** If you think you will need to pump at work, talk to your supervisor sooner rather than later. If possible, make a plan together before you go on maternity leave, so that things will be set up when you return. But if you are already back at work, talk with your employer.

3. **Think outside of the box.** Some workplaces may face more challenges than others when carving out adequate time and space for moms to pump. Supporting Nursing Moms at Work: Employer Solutions can help you and your employer navigate this sometimes complicated issue through their hundreds of creative, low-cost ideas to help nursing mothers continue breastfeeding after returning to work. And there's a good reason. Breastfeeding doesn't just benefit you and your baby— your employer benefits, too.

Breastfeeding helps keep babies healthy, which lowers healthcare costs and means you do not have to miss work for a doctor's appointment. Plus, research shows that working women whose breastfeeding goals are supported by their employers are more productive. Companies will also see lower turnover rates because women are more likely to go back to work if they know they'll have time and space to pump.

4. **Practice before you go back to work.** It is a good idea to practice pumping at home before you return to work. (You may be able to get a breast pump at no extra cost through your health insurance plan.) Once you are back at work, you'll probably need to pump two to three times during a typical eight-hour workday, or the number of times your baby needs to feed while you are away. Be sure to properly store your milk after each pumping session in a clean glass or bisphenol A (BPA) free plastic bottles or milk storage bags. Then keep it cool in a refrigerator or a cooler with ice packs—you can even freeze it.

5. **Support nursing moms.** You may not need to pump at work, but someone else in your life or workplace might. Your support can make a big difference to a nursing mom. One way you can help is by sending your friends, family, coworkers, and supervisors over to Supporting Nursing Moms at Work: Employer Solutions. If you've had to pump at work in the past, talk to new moms about what worked and did not work for you.

Part Eight

Additional Help and Information

Chapter 71

Glossary of Terms Related to Pregnancy and Birth

absorption: The process of taking in. For a person or an animal, absorption is the process of a substance getting into the body through the eyes, skin, stomach, intestines, or lungs.

acquired immunodeficiency syndrome (AIDS): A disease caused by the human immunodeficiency virus (HIV). People with AIDS are at an increased risk for developing certain cancers and for infections that usually occur only in individuals with a weak immune system.

adverse effect: An unexpected medical problem that happens during treatment with a drug or other therapy. Also called adverse event.

amino acid: One of several molecules that join together to form proteins. There are 20 common amino acids found in proteins.

anemia: A condition in which the number of red blood cells is below normal.

anesthetic: A drug that causes insensitivity to pain and is used for surgeries and other medical procedures.

antibiotic: A drug used to treat infections caused by bacteria and other microorganisms.

This glossary contains terms excerpted from documents produced by several sources deemed reliable.

antibody: A protein made by plasma cells (a type of white blood cell) in response to an antigen (a substance that causes the body to make a specific immune response). Each antibody can bind to only one specific antigen.

antigen: Any substance that causes the body to make an immune response against that substance. Antigens include toxins, chemicals, bacteria, viruses, or other substances that come from outside the body.

anxiety: Feelings of fear, dread, and uneasiness that may occur as a reaction to stress. A person with anxiety may sweat, feel restless and tense, and have a rapid heart beat.

assessment: The process of gathering evidence and documentation of a student's learning.

asthma: A chronic disease in which the bronchial airways in the lungs become narrowed and swollen, making it difficult to breathe.

autoimmune disease: A condition in which the body recognizes its own tissues as foreign and directs an immune response against them.

bacteria: A large group of single-cell microorganisms. Some cause infections and disease in animals and humans.

bacterial vaginosis (BV): The most common vaginal infection in women of childbearing age, which happens when the normal bacteria (germs) in the vagina get out of balance, such as from douching or from sexual contact.

birth control: The use of drugs, devices, or surgery to prevent pregnancy. There are many different types of birth control.

bladder: The organ in the human body that stores urine. It is found in the lower part of the abdomen.

blood: A tissue with red blood cells (RBCs), white blood cells (WBCs), platelets, and other substances suspended in fluid called plasma. Blood takes oxygen and nutrients to the tissues, and carries away wastes.

body mass index (BMI): A measure of body fat based on a person's height and weight.

breast cancer: Cancer that forms in tissues of the breast. The most common type of breast cancer is ductal carcinoma, which begins in the lining of the milk ducts (thin tubes that carry milk from the lobules of the breast to the nipple).

calcium: A mineral that is an essential nutrient for bone health. It is also needed for the heart, muscles, and nerves to function properly and for blood to clot.

calorie: A measurement of the energy content of food. The body needs calories as to perform its functions, such as breathing, circulating the blood, and physical activity.

cancer: A term for diseases in which abnormal cells in the body divide without control. Cancer cells can invade nearby tissues and can spread to other parts of the body through the blood and lymphatic system, which is a network of tissues that clears infections and keeps body fluids in balance.

carbohydrate: A sugar molecule. Carbohydrates can be small and simple (for example, glucose) or they can be large and complex (for example, polysaccharides such as starch, chitin, or cellulose).

cervix: The lower, narrow part of the uterus (womb). The cervix forms a canal that opens into the vagina, which leads to the outside of the body.

childbearing age: Range of ages during which a woman may become pregnant. For example: Can be defined as 16 to 49 years of age.

chromosome: A chromosome is an organized package of deoxyribonucleic acid (DNA) found in the nucleus of the cell. Different organisms have different numbers of chromosomes. Humans have 23 pairs of chromosomes—22 pairs of numbered chromosomes, called autosomes, and one pair of sex chromosomes, X and Y.

chronic disease: A disease that has one or more of the following characteristics: is permanent; leaves residual disability; is caused by nonreversible pathological alternation; requires special training of the patient for rehabilitation; or may be expected to require a long period of supervision, observation, or care.

chronic pain: Pain that can range from mild to severe, and persists or progresses over a long period of time.

computed tomography (CT): A procedure for taking X-ray images from many different angles and then assembling them into a cross-section of the body.

constipation: A decrease in frequency of stools or bowel movements with hardening of the stool.

diabetes: A disease in which blood glucose (blood sugar) levels are above normal. There are two main types of diabetes. Type 1 diabetes is caused by a problem with the body's defense system, called the immune system.

diet: What a person eats and drinks. Any type of eating plan.

ectopic pregnancy: A pregnancy that is not in the uterus. It happens when a fertilized egg settles and grows in a place other than the inner lining of the uterus. Most happen in the fallopian tube, but can happen in the ovary, cervix, or abdominal cavity.

endometriosis: A condition in which tissue that normally lines the uterus grows in other areas of the body, usually inside the abdominal cavity, but acts as if it were inside the uterus. Blood shed monthly from the misplaced tissue has no place to go, and tissues surrounding the area of endometriosis may become inflamed or swollen.

enzyme: A protein that speeds up chemical reactions in the body.

estrogen: A group of female hormones that are responsible for the development of breasts and other secondary sex characteristics in women. Estrogen is produced by the ovaries and other body tissues. Estrogen, along with progesterone, is important in preparing a woman's body for pregnancy.

exercise: A type of physical activity that involves planned, structured, and repetitive bodily movement done to maintain or improve one or more components of physical fitness.

fallopian tube(s): Part of the female reproductive system, one of a pair of tubes connecting the ovaries to the uterus.

gynecologist: A doctor who diagnoses and treats conditions of the female reproductive system and associated disorders.

hormone: Substance produced by one tissue and conveyed by the bloodstream to another to affect a function of the body, such as growth or metabolism.

human immunodeficiency virus (HIV): Human immunodeficiency virus (HIV) is the virus that infects and destroys the body's immune cells and causes a disease called AIDS, or acquired immunodeficiency syndrome.

hypertension: Also called high blood pressure, it is having blood pressure greater than 140 over 90 mmHg (millimeters of mercury). Long-term high blood pressure can damage blood vessels and organs, including the heart, kidneys, eyes, and brain.

immune system: A complex system of cellular and molecular components having the primary function of distinguishing self from not self and defense against foreign organisms or substances.

infertility: A condition in which a couple has problems conceiving, or getting pregnant, after 1 year of regular sexual intercourse without using any birth control methods. Infertility can be caused by a problem with the man or the woman, or both.

intestines: Also known as the bowels, or the long, tube-like organ in the human body that completes digestion or the breaking down of food. They consist of the small intestine and the large intestine.

lesion: An area of abnormal tissue. A lesion may be benign (not cancer) or malignant (cancer).

low birth weight: Having a weight at birth that is less than 2,500 grams, or 5 pounds, 8 ounces.

lupus: A chronic inflammatory disease that occurs when the body's immune system attacks its own tissues and organs. Also, called systemic lupus erythematosus (SLE).

magnetic resonance imaging (MRI): A noninvasive procedure that uses magnetic fields and radio waves to produce three-dimensional (3D) computerized images of areas inside the body.

menopause: The cessation of menstruation in women.

menstruating: The blood flow from the uterus that happens about every 4 weeks in a woman.

metabolism: The chemical changes that take place in a cell or an organism. These changes make energy and the materials cells and organisms need to grow, reproduce, and stay healthy. Metabolism also helps get rid of toxic substances.

miscarriage: An unplanned loss of a pregnancy. Also called a spontaneous abortion.

nipple: The protruding part of the breast that extends and becomes firmer upon stimulation. In breastfeeding, milk travels from the milk sinuses through the nipple to the baby.

nutrition: The taking in and use of food and other nourishing material by the body. Nutrition is a 3-part process. First, food or drink is consumed. Second, the body breaks down the food or drink into nutrients.

organ: A part of the body that performs a specific function. For example, the heart is an organ.

ovary (ovaries): Part of a woman's reproductive system, the ovaries produce her eggs. Each month, through the process called ovulation, the ovaries release eggs into the fallopian tubes, where they travel to the uterus, or womb. If an egg is fertilized by a man's sperm, a woman becomes pregnant and the egg grows and develops inside the uterus. If the egg is not fertilize, the egg and the lining of the uterus is shed during a woman's monthly menstrual period.

over-the-counter (OTC): Refers to a medicine that can be bought without a prescription (doctor's order). Also called nonprescription and OTC.

overweight: Overweight refers to an excessive amount of body weight that includes muscle, bone, fat, and water. A person who has a body mass index (BMI) of 25 to 29.9 is considered overweight.

ovulation: The release of a single egg from a follicle that developed in the ovary. It usually occurs regularly, around day 14 of a 28-day menstrual cycle.

penis: An external male reproductive organ. It contains a tube called the urethra, which carries semen and urine to the outside of the body.

perinatal: The time period immediately before and after birth.

physical activity: Any bodily movement that is produced by the contraction of skeletal muscle and that substantially increases energy expenditure.

physical fitness: A set of attributes that people possess or achieve that relates to the ability to perform physical activity and is comprised of skill-related, health-related, and physiological components.

pica: A craving to eat nonfood items, such as dirt, paint chips, and clay. Some children exhibit pica-related behavior.

placenta: During pregnancy, a temporary organ joining the mother and fetus. The placenta transfers oxygen and nutrients from the mother to the fetus, and permits the release of carbon dioxide and waste products from the fetus.

placental abruption: When the placenta separates from the uterine wall before delivery, which can mean the fetus doesn't get enough oxygen.

postpartum depression (PPD): A serious condition that requires treatment from a healthcare provider. With this condition, feelings of the baby blues (feeling sad, anxious, afraid, or confused after having a baby) do not go away or get worse.

preconception health: A woman's health before she becomes pregnant. It involves knowing how health conditions and risk factors could affect a woman or her unborn baby if she becomes pregnant.

pregnancy: The condition between conception (fertilization of an egg by a sperm) and birth, during which the fertilized egg develops in the uterus. In humans, pregnancy lasts about 288 days.

premature birth: The birth of a baby before 37 weeks of pregnancy. In humans, a normal pregnancy lasts about 40 weeks. The risk of premature birth may be increased by certain health problems in the mother, such as diabetes, heart disease, and kidney disease, or problems during pregnancy.

preterm birth: Also called premature birth, it is a birth that occurs before the 37th week of pregnancy.

prevention: Actions that reduce exposure or other risks, keep people from getting sick, or keep disease from getting worse.

progesterone: A female hormone produced by the ovaries. Progesterone, along with estrogen, prepares the uterus (womb) for a possible pregnancy each month and supports the fertilized egg if conception occurs. Progesterone also helps prepare the breasts for milk production and breastfeeding.

prognosis: The likely outcome or course of a disease; the chance of recovery or recurrence.

prostate: A gland in the male reproductive system. The prostate surrounds the part of the urethra (the tube that empties the bladder) just below the bladder, and produces a fluid that forms part of the semen.

protein: A molecule made up of amino acids. Proteins are needed for the body to function properly. They are the basis of body structures, such as skin and hair, and of other substances such as enzymes, cytokines, and antibodies.

puberty: Time when the body is changing from the body of a child to the body of an adult. This process begins earlier in girls than in boys, usually between ages 8 and 13, and lasts 2 to 4 years.

risk reduction: Actions that can decrease the likelihood that individuals, groups, or communities will experience disease or other health conditions.

saliva: The watery fluid in the mouth made by the salivary glands. Saliva moistens food to help digestion and it helps protect the mouth against infections.

semen: The fluid (which contains sperm) a male releases from his penis when he becomes sexually aroused or has an orgasm.

serum: The liquid part of blood that remains after clotting proteins and blood cells are removed.

sexually transmitted infections (STIs): Diseases that are spread by sexual activity. Also called sexually transmitted diseases (STDs).

sickle cell anemia: A blood disorder passed down from parents to children. It involves problems in the red blood cells. Normal red blood cells are round and smooth and move through blood vessels easily. Sickle cells are hard and have a curved edge.

stillbirth: When a fetus dies during birth, or when the fetus dies during the late stages of pregnancy when it would have been otherwise expected to survive.

sudden infant death syndrome (SIDS): The diagnosis given for the sudden death of an infant under one year of age that remains unexplained after a complete investigation. Because most cases of SIDS occur when a baby is sleeping in a crib, SIDS is also commonly known as crib death. Most SIDS deaths occur when a baby is between 1 and 4 months of age.

testicle (testis): The male sex gland. There are a pair of testes behind the penis in a pouch of skin called the scrotum. The testes make and store sperm, and make the male hormone testosterone.

toxic agent: Chemical or physical (for example, radiation, heat, cold, and microwaves) agents that, under certain circumstances of exposure, can cause harmful effects to living organisms.

umbilical cord: Connected to the placenta and provides the transfer of nutrients and waste between the woman and the fetus.

urinary tract infection: An infection anywhere in the urinary tract, or organs that collect and store urine and release it from your body (the kidneys, ureters, bladder, and urethra).

uterine contractions: During the birthing process, a woman's uterus tightens, or contracts. Contractions can be strong and regular (meaning that they can happen every 5 minutes, every 3 minutes, and so on) during labor until the baby is delivered. Women can have contractions before labor starts; these are not regular and do not progress, or increase in intensity or duration.

uterine fibroids: Common, benign (noncancerous) tumors that grow in the muscle of the uterus or womb. Fibroids often cause no symptoms and need no treatment, and they usually shrink after menopause.

uterus: A woman's womb, or the hollow, pear-shaped organ located in a woman's lower abdomen between the bladder and the rectum.

vagina: The muscular canal that extends from the cervix to the outside of the body. Its walls are lined with mucus membranes and tiny glands that make vaginal secretions.

vulva: The external female genital organ. It has five parts, including the urinary opening and the opening to the vagina.

weight-bearing exercise: Exercise that forces you to work against gravity, such as walking, hiking, jogging, climbing stairs, playing tennis, dancing, and lifting weights. This type of exercise is best for strengthening bone.

withdrawal: Symptoms that occur after chronic use of a drug is reduced abruptly or stopped.

X-ray: A type of high-energy radiation. In low doses, X-rays are used to diagnose diseases by making pictures of the inside of the body.

yoga: A mind and body practice with origins in ancient Indian philosophy. The various styles of yoga typically combine physical postures, breathing techniques, and meditation or relaxation.

Chapter 72

Directory of Organizations That Provide Help and Information about Pregnancy and Birth

Government Agencies That Provide Information about Pregnancy

Agency for Healthcare Research and Quality (AHRQ)
Office of Communications and Knowledge Transfer (OCKT)
5600 Fishers Ln.
Seventh Fl.
Rockville, MD 20857
Phone: 301-427-1364
Website: www.ahrq.gov

Centers for Disease Control and Prevention (CDC)
1600 Clifton Rd.
Atlanta, GA 30329-4027
Toll-Free: 800-CDC-INFO (800-232-4636)
Toll-Free TTY: 888-232-6348
Website: www.cdc.gov

Resources in this chapter were compiled from several sources deemed reliable; all contact information was verified and updated in February 2019.

Centers for Medicare & Medicaid Services (CMS)
7500 Security Blvd.
Baltimore, MD 21244
Toll-Free: 800-MEDICARE
(800-633-4227)
Toll-Free TTY: 877-486-2048
Website: www.cms.gov

Eunice Kennedy Shriver National Institute of Child Health and Human Development (NICHD)
NICHD Information Resource Center
P.O. Box 3006
Rockville, MD 20847
Toll-Free: 800-370-2943
Toll-Free TTY: 888-320-6942
Toll-Free Fax: 866-760-5947
Website: www.nichd.nih.gov
E-mail: NICHDInformation ResourceCenter@mail.nih.gov

Healthfinder®
1101 Wootton Pkwy
Rockville, MD 20852
Website: www.healthfinder.gov
E-mail: healthfinder@hhs.gov

National Cancer Institute (NCI)
9609 Medical Center Dr.
BG 9609, MSC 9760
Bethesda, MD 20892-9760
Toll-Free: 800-4-CANCER
(800-422-6237)
Phone: 301-435-3848
Website: www.cancer.gov
E-mail: cancergovstaff@mail.nih. gov

National Center for Complementary and Integrative Health (NCCIH)
9000 Rockville Pike
Bethesda, MD 20892
Toll-Free: 888-644-6226
Toll-Free TTY: 866-464-3615
Website: nccih.nih.gov
E-mail: info@nccih.nih.gov

National Heart, Lung, and Blood Institute (NHLBI)
Bldg. 31, 31 Center Dr.
Bethesda, MD 20892
Website: www.nhlbi.nih.gov
E-mail: nhlbiinfo@nhlbi.nih.gov

National Human Genome Research Institute (NHGRI)
Office of Communications and Public Liaison Branch (OCPL)
Bldg. 31, Rm. 4B09, 31 Center Dr., MSC 2152
9000 Rockville Pike
Bethesda, MD 20892-2152
Phone: 301-402-0911
Fax: 301-402-2218
Website: www.genome.gov
E-mail: nhgripressoffice@mail. nih.gov

National Institute of Arthritis and Musculoskeletal and Skin Diseases (NIAMS)
NIAMS Information Clearinghouse
1 AMS Cir.
Bethesda, MD 20892-3675
Toll-Free: 877-22-NIAMS (877-226-4267)
Phone: 301-495-4484
TTY: 301-565-2966
Fax: 301-718-6366
Website: www.niams.nih.gov
E-mail: NIAMSinfo@mail.nih.gov

National Institute of Diabetes, Digestive and Kidney Diseases (NIDDK)
Toll-Free: 800-860-8747
Toll-Free TTY: 866-569-1162
Website: www.niddk.nih.gov
E-mail: healthinfo@niddk.nih.gov

National Institute of Environmental Health Sciences (NIEHS)
P.O. Box 12233, MD K3-16
Research Triangle Park, NC 27709-2233
Phone: 919-541-3345
Fax: 919-541-4395
Website: www.niehs.nih.gov

National Institute of Mental Health (NIMH)
Office of Science Policy, Planning, and Communications (OSPPC)
6001 Executive Blvd.
Rm. 6200, MSC 9663
Bethesda, MD 20892-9663
Toll-Free: 866-615-NIMH (866-615-6464)
Phone: 301-443-4513
TTY: 301-443-8431
Toll-Free TTY: 866-415-8051
Fax: 301-443-4279
Website: www.nimh.nih.gov
E-mail: nimhinfo@nih.gov

National Institute of Neurological Disorders and Stroke (NINDS)
NIH Neurological Institute
P.O. Box 5801
Bethesda, MD 20824
Toll-Free: 800-352-9424
Website: www.ninds.nih.gov
E-mail: braininfo@ninds.nih.gov

National Institutes of Health (NIH)
9000 Rockville Pike
Bethesda, MD 20892
Phone: 301-496-4000
TTY: 301-402-9612
Website: www.nih.gov

Office of Minority Health (OMH)
Tower Oaks Bldg. 1101 Wootton Pkwy
Ste. 600
Rockville, MD 20852
Phone: 240-453-2882
Fax: 240-453-2883
Website: www.minorityhealth.hhs.gov

U.S. Department of Health and Human Services (HHS)
200 Independence Ave. S.W.
Washington, DC 20201
Toll-Free: 877-696-6775
Website: www.hhs.gov

U.S. Food and Drug Administration (FDA)
10903 New Hampshire Ave.
Silver Spring, MD 20993-0002
Toll-Free: 888-INFO-FDA (888-463-6332)
Website: www.fda.gov

U.S. National Library of Medicine (NLM)
8600 Rockville Pike
Bethesda, MD 20894
Toll-Free: 888-FIND-NLM (888-346-3656)
Phone: 301-594-5983
Website: www.nlm.nih.gov

Women, Infants, and Children (WIC)
Website: www.fns.usda.gov/wic

Private Agencies That Provide Information about Pregnancy

American Academy of Family Physicians (AAFP)
11400 Tomahawk Creek Pkwy
Leawood, KS 66211-2680
Toll-Free: 800-274-2237
Phone: 913-906-6000
Fax: 913-906-6075
Website: www.aafp.org

American Academy of Pediatrics (AAP)
345 Park Blvd.
Itasca, IL 60143
Toll-Free: 800-433-9016
Fax: 847-434-8000
Website: www.aap.org
E-mail: csc@aap.org

American Association of Birth Centers (AABC)
3123 Gottschall Rd.
Perkiomenville, PA 18074
Toll-Free: 866-54-BIRTH (866-54-24784)
Phone: 215-234-8068
Fax: 215-234-8829
Website: www.birthcenters.org
E-mail: aabc@birthcenters.org

American College of Allergy, Asthma and Immunology (ACAAI)
85 W. Algonquin Rd.
Ste. 550
Arlington Heights, IL 60005
Phone: 847-427-1200
Fax: 847-427-9656
Website: www.acaai.org
E-mail: mail@acaai.org

American College of Nurse-Midwives (ACNM)
8403 Colesville Rd.
Ste. 1550
Silver Spring, MD 20910
Phone: 240-485-1800
Fax: 240-485-1818
Website: www.midwife.org

The American College of Obstetricians and Gynecologists (ACOG)
409 12th St. S.W.
P.O. Box 70620
Washington, DC 20024-2188
Toll-Free: 800-673-8444
Phone: 202-638-5577
Website: www.acog.org

American College of Surgeons (ACS)
633 N. Saint Clair St.
Chicago, IL 60611-3295
Toll-Free: 800-621-4111
Phone: 312-202-5000
Fax: 312-202-5001
Website: www.facs.org
E-mail: postmaster@facs.org

American Diabetes Association (ADA)
2451 Crystal Dr.
Ste. 900
Arlington, VA 22202
Toll-Free: 800-DIABETES
(800-342-2383)
Website: www.diabetes.org
E-mail: askada@diabetes.org

American Institute of Ultrasound in Medicine (AIUM)
14750 Sweitzer Ln.
Ste. 100
Laurel, MD 20707-5906
Toll-Free: 800-638-5352
Phone: 301-498-4100
Fax: 301-498-4450
Website: www.aium.org

American Medical Association (AMA)
AMA Plaza, 330 N. Wabash Ave.
Ste. 39300
Chicago, IL 60611-5885
Website: www.ama-assn.org

American Pregnancy Association (APA)
3007 Skyway Cir. N.
Ste. 800
Irving, TX 75038
Toll-Free: 800-672-2296
Phone: 972-550-0140
Website: www. americanpregnancy.org
E-mail: info@ americanpregnancy.org

American Public Human Services Association (APHSA)
1101 Wilson Blvd.
Sixth Fl.
Arlington, VA 22209
Phone: 202-682-0100
Fax: 202-289-6555
Website: www.aphsa.org
E-mail: memberservice@aphsa.org

American Society for Reproductive Medicine (ASRM)
1209 Montgomery Hwy
Birmingham, AL 35216-2809
Phone: 205-978-5000
Fax: 205-978-5005
Website: www.asrm.org
E-mail: asrm@asrm.org

American Society of Anesthesiologists (ASA)
1061 American Ln.
Schaumburg, IL 60173-4973
Phone: 847-825-5586
Fax: 847-825-1692
Website: www.asahq.org
E-mail: info@asahq.org

Association of Maternal and Child Health Programs (AMCHP)
1825 K St. N.W.
Ste. 250
Washington, DC 20006
Phone: 202-775-0436
Fax: 202-478-5120
Website: www.amchp.org

Association of Women's Health, Obstetric and Neonatal Nurses (AWHONN)
1800 M St. N.W.
Ste. 740S
Washington, DC 20036
Toll-Free: 800-673-8499
Phone: 202-261-2400
Fax: 202-728-0575
Website: www.awhonn.org
E-mail: customerservice@awhonn.org

Center for Health Care Strategies, Inc. (CHCS)
200 American Metro Blvd.
Ste. 119
Hamilton, NJ 08619
Phone: 609-528-8400
Fax: 609-586-3679
Website: www.chcs.org

Center for Research on Reproduction and Women's Health (CRRWH)
University of Pennsylvania Health System (UPHS)
1355 Biomedical Research Bldg.
II/III 421 Curie Blvd.
Philadelphia, PA 19104-6160
Phone: 215-898-0147
Fax: 215-573-5408
Website: www.med.upenn.edu/crrwh

Childbirth and Postpartum Professional Association (CAPPA)
P.O. Box 547
Flowery Branch, GA 30542
Phone: 770-965-9777
Toll-Free Fax: 888-688-5241
Website: www.cappa.net
E-mail: info@cappa.net

Childbirth Connection
1875 Connecticut Ave. N.W.
Ste. 650
Washington, DC 20009
Phone: 202-986-2600
Fax: 202-986-2539
Website: www.
childbirthconnection.org
E-mail: info@
nationalpartnership.org

Cleveland Clinic
9500 Euclid Ave.
Cleveland, OH 44195
Toll-Free: 800-223-2273
Website: www.clevelandclinic.
org

DONA International
35 E. Wacker Dr.
Ste. 850
Chicago, IL 60601-2106
Toll-Free: 888-788-DONA
(888-788-3662)
Website: www.dona.org
E-mail: DONA@dona.org

Guttmacher Institute
1301 Connecticut Ave. N.W.
Ste. 700
Washington, DC 20036
Toll Free: 877-823-0262
Phone: 202-296-4012
Fax: 202-223-5756
Website: www.guttmacher.org

Hyperemesis Education and Research Foundation (HER)
9600 S.E. 257th Dr.
Damascus, OR 97089
Website: www.hyperemesis.org
E-mail: info@helpHER.org

Institute for Women's Policy Research (IWPR)
1200 18th St. N.W.
Ste. 301
Washington, DC 20036
Phone: 202-785-5100
Fax: 202-833-4362
Website: www.iwpr.org
E-mail: iwpr@iwpr.org

The International Childbirth Education Association (ICEA)
110 Horizon Dr.
Ste. 210
Raleigh, NC 27615
Toll-Free: 800-624-4934
Phone: 919-674-4183
Fax: 919-459-2075
Website: www.icea.org
E-mail: info@icea.org

International Council on Infertility Information Dissemination (INCIID)
5765 F Burke Centre Pkwy
P.O. Box 330
Burke, Virginia 22015
Website: www.inciid.org
E-mail: INCIIDinfo@inciid.org

La Leche League International (LLLI)
110 Horizon Dr.
Ste. 210
Raleigh, NC 27615
Toll-Free: 800-LALECHE
(800-525-3243)
Phone: 919-459-2167
Fax: 919-459-2075
Website: www.llli.org
E-mail: info@llli.org

Lamaze International
2025 M St. N.W.
Ste. 800
Washington, DC 20036-3309
Toll-Free: 800-368-4404
Phone: 202-367-1128
Fax: 202-367-2128
Website: www.lamaze.org
E-mail: info@lamaze.org

March of Dimes (MOD)
1550 Crystal Dr.
Ste. 1300
Arlington, VA 22202
Toll-Free: 888-MODIMES
(888-663-4637)
Website: www.marchofdimes.org

Midwives Alliance of North America (MANA)
P.O. Box 373
Montvale, NJ 07645
Toll-Free: 844-626-2674
Website: www.mana.org

Motherisk Program
Toll-Free: 877-439-2744
Phone: 416-813-6780
Website: www.motherisk.org

National Advocates for Pregnant Women (NAPW)
875 Sixth Ave.
Ste. 1807
New York, NY 10001
Phone: 212-255-9252
Fax: 212-255-9253
Website: www.
advocatesforpregnantwomen.org

National Coalition on Health Care (NCHC)
1111 14th St. N.W.
Ste. 900
Washington, DC 20005
Phone: 202-638-7151
Website: www.nchc.org

National Rural Health Association (NRHA)
4501 College Blvd.
Ste. 225
Leawood, KS 66211-1921
Phone: 816-756-3140
Fax: 816-756-3144
Website: www.ruralhealthweb.
org
E-mail: mail@NRHArural.org

Organization of Teratology
Information Specialist
(OTIS)
5034A Thoroughbred Ln.
P.O. Box 210202
Brentwood, TN 37027
Toll-Free: 866-626-OTIS
(866-626-6847)
Phone: 615-649-3082
Website: www.mothertobaby.org
E-mail: ContactUs@
mothertobaby.org

Planned Parenthood
Federation of America
(PPFA)
123 William St.
10th Fl.
New York, NY 10038
Toll-Free: 800-230-PLAN
(800-230-7526)
Phone: 212-541-7800
Website: www.
plannedparenthood.org

Power To Decide the
Campaign to prevent
unplanned pregnancy
1776 Massachusetts Ave. N.W.
Ste. 200
Washington, DC 20036
Phone: 202-478-8500
Fax: 202-478-8588
Website: www.
thenationalcampaign.org
E-mail: info@powertodecide.org

Preeclampsia Foundation
3840 W. Eau Gallie Blvd.
Ste. 104
Melbourne, FL 32934
Toll-Free: 800-665-9341
Phone: 321-421-6957
Website: www.preeclampsia.org
E-mail: info@preeclampsia.org

RESOLVE: The National
Infertility Association
7918 Jones Branch Dr.
Ste. 300
McLean, VA 22102
Phone: 703-556-7172
Fax: 703-506-3266
Website: www.resolve.org
E-mail: info@resolve.org

Robert Wood Johnson
Foundation (RWJF)
50 College Rd. E.
Princeton, NJ 08540-6614
Toll-Free: 877-843-7953
Phone: 609-627-6000
Website: www.rwjf.org

Sidelines National Support
Network
3167 Bern Dr.
Laguna Beach, CA 92651
Phone: 612-492-1353
Website: www.sidelines.org
E-mail: sidelines@sidelines.org

Urban Institute
2100 M St. N.W.
Washington, DC 20037
Phone: 202-833-7200
Website: www.urban.org

Index

Index

Page numbers followed by 'n' indicate a footnote. Page numbers in *italics* indicate a table or illustration.

A

A1C test, blood-glucose levels 294
abdominal cramps
  pregnancy loss symptoms 354, 432
  preterm labor symptoms 443
abnormal fetal position, fetal
  problems 502
abortion
  placental complications 381
  unintended pregnancy 48
"About Pregnancy Loss (before 20
  Weeks of Pregnancy)"
  (NICHD) 429n
absorption, defined 559
abstinence (sexual activity)
  sexually transmitted disease (STD)
    prevention 404
  unwanted pregnancy prevention 49
acquired immunodeficiency syndrome
  (AIDS)
  defined 559
  high-risk pregnancy 257
  STDs in pregnant women 402
ADA *see* Americans with Disabilities
  Act

adolescents
  cigarette smoke exposure 226
  epilepsy 297
  hepatitis B vaccination 411
  human immunodeficiency virus
    (HIV) 402
  injectable birth control 54
  sickle cell disease 307
adoption, leave entitlement 548
adverse effect
  defined 559
  teen pregnancy 262
"Adverse Effects" (Youth.gov) 262n
Advil (ibuprofen), drug facts
  label 158
AFP *see* alpha-fetoprotein
afterbirth
  HIV medicines 414
  see also placenta
age
  carpal tunnel syndrome (CTS) 85
  contraception 51
  genetic counseling 17
  infertility 30
  pelvic-floor disorders 93
  puberty 28
  unintended pregnancies 48
  urinary incontinence 95
Agency for Healthcare Research and
  Quality (AHRQ), contact 569